Minimally Invasive Foot and Ankle Surgery

A Percutaneous Approach

Minimally Invasive Foot and Ankle Surgery

A Percutaneous Approach

EDITORS

Ettore Vulcano, MD

Chief of Orthopedic Surgery
Director of Foot and Ankle Surgery
Associate Professor of Orthopedic Surgery
Columbia University at Mount Sinai
Medical Center
Miami Beach, Florida

A. Holly Johnson, MD

Orthopedic Foot and Ankle Surgeon
Hospital for Special Surgery
Associate Professor
Weill Cornell Medical School
New York, New York

Oliver N. Schipper, MD

Orthopaedic Foot and Ankle Surgeon
Anderson Orthopaedic Clinic
Annandale, Virginia

Wolters Kluwer

Philadelphia • Baltimore • New York • London
Buenos Aires • Hong Kong • Sydney • Tokyo

Acquisitions Editor: Tulie McKay
Senior Development Editor: Stacey Sebring
Editorial Coordinator: Sunmerrilika Baskar
Marketing Manager: Kirsten Watrud
Senior Production Project Manager: Alicia Jackson
Manager: Graphic Arts & Design: Steve Druding
Manufacturing Coordinator: Lisa Bowling
Prepress Vendor: Straive

1st edition

9 8 7 6 5 4 3 2 1

Printed in United States of America

Cataloging-in-Publication Data available on request from the Publisher

ISBN: 978-1-9751-9870-1

shop.lww.com

MPP1223

To our families

Contributors

Assil-Ramin Alimy
MD/PhD Candidate
Department of Trauma and Orthopaedic Surgery
University Medical Center Hamburg-Eppendorf
Hamburg, Germany

Paulo Carvalho, MD, PhD(c)
Orthopedic Foot and Ankle Surgeon
Barcelona University PhD Student
Barcelona, Spain
Orthopedic Foot and Ankle Surgeon
Hospital da Ordem Terceira Chiado
Lisbon, Portugal

Manuel Cuervas-Mons, MD, PhD, FEBOT
Orthopedic Foot and Ankle Surgeon
University Hospital Gregorio Marañon
Madrid, Spain

Véronique Darcel, MD
Orthopaedic Foot and Ankle Surgeon
Maison de Santé Protestante de Bordeaux Bagatelle
Bordeaux, France

Serrano Mariano De Prado, MD
Director of Foot and Ankle Surgery
Honorary Professor
University of Murcia, Spain
Hospital Quirónsalud Murcia
Hospital Ruber Internacional
Madrid, Spain

Alirio J. deMeireles, MD, MBA
Orthopedic Surgery Resident
Columbia University Irving Medical Center
New York, New York

Tyler Gonzalez, MD, MBA
Assistant Professor of Orthopedic Surgery
University of South Carolina School of Medicine/Prisma Health
Columbia, South Carolina

Akshay Jain, MD
Orthopedic Foot and Ankle Fellow
Hospital for Special Surgery
New York, New York

A. Holly Johnson, MD
Orthopedic Foot and Ankle Surgeon
Hospital for Special Surgery
Associate Professor
Weill Cornell Medical School
New York, New York

Philip B. Kaiser, MD
Orthopaedic Foot and Ankle Surgeon
California Pacific Orthopaedics
San Francisco, California

Jonathan R. M. Kaplan, MD
Associate Chief of Foot and Ankle Division
Director of Minimally Invasive Foot and Ankle Surgery
Associate Professor of Orthopaedic Surgery
Department of Orthopaedic Surgery
Duke University
Durham, North Carolina

Olivier Laffenêtre, MD
Exclusive Foot and Ankle Surgeon
Foot and Ankle Institute
Clinique Blomet
Paris, France
Chief of Foot and Ankle Department
Pellegrin University Hospital
Bordeaux, France

Peter Lam, MBBS(Hons), FRACS, FAOA
Orthopaedic Foot and Ankle Surgeon
Orthopaedic and Arthritis Specialist Centre
Sydney, Australia

Thomas L. Lewis, BSc(Hons), MBChB(Hons), MFSTEd, FRCS(Tr & Orth)
Trauma and Orthopaedic Surgery Registrar
King's Foot and Ankle Unit
King's College Hospital National Health Service Foundation Trust
London, United Kingdom

Adam Lukasiewicz, MD
Orthopedic Foot and Ankle Surgeon
Hughston Clinic
Birmingham, Alabama

Patrick J. Maloney, MD
Orthopaedic Foot and Ankle Surgeon
Institute for Foot and Ankle Reconstruction at Mercy
Mercy Medical Center
Baltimore, Maryland

Gerard F. Marciano, MD
Resident in Orthopedic Surgery
Department of Orthopedics
Columbia University Irving Medical Center
New York, New York

Christopher P. Miller, MD, MHS
Chief
Division of Foot and Ankle Surgery
Department of Orthopaedic Surgery
Assistant Professor
Harvard Medical School
Beth Israel Deaconess Medical Center
New England Baptist Hospital
Boston, Massachusetts

Roslyn J. Miller, FRCS(Tr & Orth(Ed))
Orthopaedic Foot and Ankle Surgeon
University Hospital Hairmyres
Honorary Professor
Glasgow Caledonian University
Glasgow, United Kingdom

Conor I. Murphy, MD
Orthopedic Foot & Ankle Surgeon
TMI Sports Medicine and Orthopedic Surgery
Arlington, Texas

Gustavo A. Nunes, MD, PhD(c)
Orthopedic Foot and Ankle Surgeon
Cote Brasília Clinic
Brasília, Brazil

Taylor L. Paskey, MD
Orthopedic Surgery Resident
New York–Presbyterian Hospital
Columbia University Medical Center
New York, New York

Barbara Piclet-Legré, MD
Orthopedic Foot and Ankle Surgeon
Centre du Pied
Marseilles, France

Eduard Rabat, MD
Orthopedic and Trauma Surgeon
Orthopedic Foot and Ankle Surgeon
Chief, Foot and Ankle Unit at Institut Rabat–Hospital Quirónsalud Barcelona
Barcelona, Spain

Robbie Ray, MBChB, ChM(T&O), FRCS(T&O), FEBOT
Consultant, Orthopedic Foot and Ankle Surgeon
King's Foot and Ankle Unit
King's College Hospital National Health Service Foundation Trust
London, United Kingdom

David J. Redfern, FRCS
Consultant Orthopaedic Foot and Ankle Surgeon
Cleveland Clinic
London, United Kingdom

Oliver N. Schipper, MD
Orthopaedic Foot and Ankle Surgeon
Anderson Orthopaedic Clinic
Annandale, Virginia

Josep Torrent, MD
Orthopedic Foot and Ankle Surgeon
Institut Rabat–Hospital Quirónsalud Barcelona
Barcelona, Spain

Andrea Veljkovic, MD
Orthopedic Foot and Ankle Surgeon
St. Paul's Hospital
Research Director for Foot and Ankle Reconstruction
University of British Columbia
Vancouver, British Columbia, Canada

Joel Vernois, MD, MBA
Orthopaedic Foot and Ankle Surgeon
NHS Brighton and Sussex University Hospital
Brighton and Hove, United Kingdom

Ettore Vulcano, MD
Chief of Orthopedic Surgery
Director of Foot and Ankle Surgery
Associate Professor of Orthopedic Surgery
Columbia University at Mount Sinai Medical Center
Miami Beach, Florida

Hazibullah Waizy, MD
Orthopedic Foot and Ankle Surgeon
Orthoprofis
Hannover Medical School
Hanover, Germany

Alastair Younger, MB, ChB, MSc, ChM, FRCSC
Orthopaedic Foot & Ankle Surgeon
Professor
Head of Distal Extremities
Department of Orthopaedics
University of British Columbia
Director of Foot and Ankle Research
St. Paul's Hospital
CHEOS Surgeon Scientist
Providence Health Care
Past President
British Columbia Orthopaedic Association
Vancouver, British Columbia, Canada

Preface

It is a new era for foot and ankle surgery. In the last few years, there has been a dramatic spread of percutaneous approaches in the United States, fueled by the work spanning almost two decades of our European and Australian friends. These colleagues from "across the pond" have studied, evolved, and perfected keyhole surgery to optimize outcomes and minimize those complications observed with the earlier techniques.

Today, percutaneous surgery has not only changed the way we perform surgery, but it has revolutionized how we approach and visualize deformity correction. Until a few years ago, the idea of translating the first metatarsal head 100% in a hallux valgus correction or osteotomizing the lesser metatarsals without fixating them would have been heresy. For a growing number of us, it is now the gold standard for management of forefoot pathology. As we have become more comfortable with the burr and its tactile feedback, we have expanded its use to address ankle, hindfoot, midfoot, and forefoot conditions as well. No matter what surgery I'm performing, I almost always set up the burr in the room to address at least one part of the procedure.

The goal of this internationally written book is to present an array of percutaneous surgical techniques that go beyond the bunion correction. My coeditors and I hope that the content of this volume will inspire you to adopt percutaneous surgery in your practice, adding one more weapon to your surgical armamentarium, whether you are using it alone or in conjunction with more traditional techniques.

Lastly, I want to acknowledge the perseverance of those surgeons who, in the last 20 years, continued to popularize percutaneous surgery despite the criticism of many. Without them, we absolutely would not be able to publish this volume today.

Ettore Vulcano, MD

Contents

PART 1 Forefoot

SECTION 1
Hallux Valgus

1 Chevron-Akin

David J. Redfern

INTRODUCTION

Hallux valgus surgery remains one of the core skills expected of the foot and ankle specialist surgeon. Reliably good to excellent outcomes are rightly expected by patients but perhaps often without full understanding of the complexities of such surgery and the long learning curves involved. Experience is required not only in the surgical craft itself but also in decision-making, patient education, management of patient expectations, and postoperative compliance. It is only by attention to all these details that the surgeon can fully optimize outcomes in these patients.

Minimally invasive chevron-Akin (MICA) for the treatment of hallux valgus was first described in 2011 by Redfern and Vernois, and their subsequent publications have described evolution and refinement of this technique.[1-7] Despite initial skepticism from those wary of the concept of percutaneous minimal incision surgery with fluoroscopic guidance rather than large incisions and soft-tissue dissection to allow direct vision, the literature has grown in support of MICA both in terms of reliability of outcomes, very low infection rates, fewer soft-tissue complications, and less postoperative pain.[8-19]

The MICA technique has been shown to be versatile in terms applicability to the treatment of severe hallux valgus as well as mild to moderate deformities and revision surgery scenarios.[20-23]

MICA incorporates the strengths of modern open hallux valgus surgical principles, with osteotomies held in position by rigid internal fixation, but with the additional benefits of preservation of the biological soft-tissue envelope. MICA is performed with the use of percutaneous instrumentation under fluoroscopic guidance.

The key elements of MICA are as follows:

1. Extracapsular distal diaphyseal-metaphyseal first metatarsal osteotomy
2. Rigid internal fixation of the first metatarsal osteotomy achieved with two fully threaded oblique screws of exacting configuration
3. Combined with distal soft-tissue release (division of the lateral head of the flexor hallucis brevis only) if dictated by persisting first metatarsophalangeal incongruence or lateral sesamoid uncovering
4. Combined with the hallux proximal phalanx Akin osteotomy to complete correction if required
5. Percutaneous recontouring of the medial border of the first metatarsal and bunionectomy
6. Immediate postoperative full weight bearing

CLINICAL ASSESSMENT

A thorough history and examination should be undertaken. Assessment should include the nature of the presenting symptoms, their location (ie, bunion pain, joint pain, sesamoid complex pain, metatarsalgia), hallux valgus reducibility, hallux range of motion, lesser toe deformity, midfoot or hindfoot symptoms, gastrocnemius tension, and underlying health.

RADIOGRAPHS

Standing anteroposterior and lateral radiographs should be obtained. From these, the hallux valgus angle (HVA) and intermetatarsal angle (IMA) can be assessed as well as the length and width of the first metatarsal. These parameters will facilitate the surgeon assessing the severity of deformity and planning the required first metatarsal displacement. It is important to remember that mild to moderate deformities are likely to become worse with time and hence require larger displacements than indicated by current measurements if the risk of recurrence is to be minimized. The presence of radiological degenerative change should be noted and considered in conjunction with the clinical findings.

PATIENT SELECTION

In principle, the MICA technique is indicated in patients of all ages, but caution is advised in patients with advanced age or those with a history of osteoporosis and osteopenia. If contemplating surgery in such individuals, then they ought to be capable of partial weight bearing if required. This author assesses the feedback from the Shannon cutting burr during the osteotomy in such cases, and if subjectively "soft bone," then patients are advised to 50% weight bear for the first 4 weeks postoperatively in order to protect the first metatarsal osteotomy. Bilateral MICA corrections in patients with compromised bone density is not recommended as they may not be able to adequately off-load one side or the other should there be concern.

Bilateral Surgery

This author has not observed any increased rate of complications from undertaking bilateral simultaneous MICA hallux valgus corrections in patients with normal bone density. In younger patients with bilateral symptomatic deformities, it is preferable to undertake correction of both feet at the single sitting.

◆ OPERATIVE TECHNIQUE

Theatre Setup

General anesthetic and/or regional (ankle) anesthetic block is administered. The patient should be positioned supine with their feet overhanging the end of the operating table. Use of a tourniquet is not required but may be used based on surgeon preference. If a tourniquet is used, then it is vital that adequate cooling irrigation of the burr is employed during use, so as to avoid thermal injury. The burr driver system should be able to deliver saline irrigation and capable of delivering high torque at low speeds. Fluoroscopy is required and preferably mini C-arm for its lower dose of radiation to both patient and surgeon and better maneuverability for switching easily from anteroposterior to lateral and oblique views during the surgery (Table 1.1). For a right-handed surgeon, the C-arm is positioned to the right of the patient and the surgeon to the left (independent of which foot is to be operated on). The scrub nurse should be to the left or tangential to the surgeon and the trolley positioned to allow the surgeon to access the instruments easily. The surgeon requires a working arc of 90° (Figure 1.1A). The patient's preoperative weight-bearing radiographs should be displayed in theatre for reference during surgery (Figure 1.1B).

Table 1.1

Equipment Required for MICA

Equipment	
Burrs	2 mm × 20 mm Shannon burr 2 mm × 12 mm Shannon burr 3.1 wedge burr
Burr driver	System with control of speed and torque and saline irrigation for cooling
Required instruments	Beaver blade and percutaneous elevators (straight and curved)
Optional instruments	MICA jig
Fluoroscopy	Mini C-arm (large C-arm if unavailable)

MICA, minimally invasive chevron-Akin.

Osteotomy Creation

After preparation of the skin and sterile draping, the surgeon will begin by making a portal through which the distal chevron osteotomy is created. The incision is dorsolateral at the level of the distal metaphyseal-diaphyseal junction of the first metatarsal (Figures 1.1C and 1.2A). A small working space is created using a straight elevator ensuring that the dorsomedial cutaneous nerve is not damaged. A 2 mm × 20 mm Shannon burr is then "shown" to the bone through this portal at the base of the flare of the distal first metatarsal metaphysis, and fluoroscopy is used to ensure that the plane of entry of the burr is correct (Figure 1.2A). In order to maintain the length and sagittal plane profile of the first metatarsal, the burr should be directed approximately 10° to 20° (distal) beyond perpendicular and 10° to 20° (plantar) beyond parallel to the first metatarsal. If the burr is directed perpendicular to the first metatarsal, it will result in slight shortening of the metatarsal due to the 2-mm kerf of the burr. Similarly, without plantar direction of the burr, slight elevation of the distal metatarsal will occur due to the 2-mm kerf.

The initial insertion site of the burr through both near and far cortices becomes the apex of the chevron osteotomy, and it is therefore vital that the plane is correct (Figure 1.2B).

The chevron is then cut in two stages. First, the dorsal limb is cut in a plane perpendicular to the axis of the metatarsal. The plantar limb cut is parallel to the floor (as if foot on floor), and should be shorter than the dorsal limb cut (Figure 1.2C). It is also important to avoid inadvertent "reverse" cuts (creating an "X" cut rather than "V"/chevron) due to the center of burr rotation lying within the bone—the center of rotation should lie medial to the first metatarsal. The burr hand movements when creating the osteotomies are a combination of translation with modest rotation. It is essential that the surgeon has experience with using the burr and such technique concepts before attempting to learn the MICA hallux valgus correction.

Initial Guidewire Insertion

Once the osteotomy has been created, then the proximal screw guidewire is inserted via the proximal metaphyseal flare via an additional skin portal and advanced so as to pick up the lateral metatarsal cortex approximately 12 mm proximal to the osteotomy site (Figure 1.2D). Once the wire has penetrated the lateral cortex, it is not advanced any further until the osteotomy has been displaced.

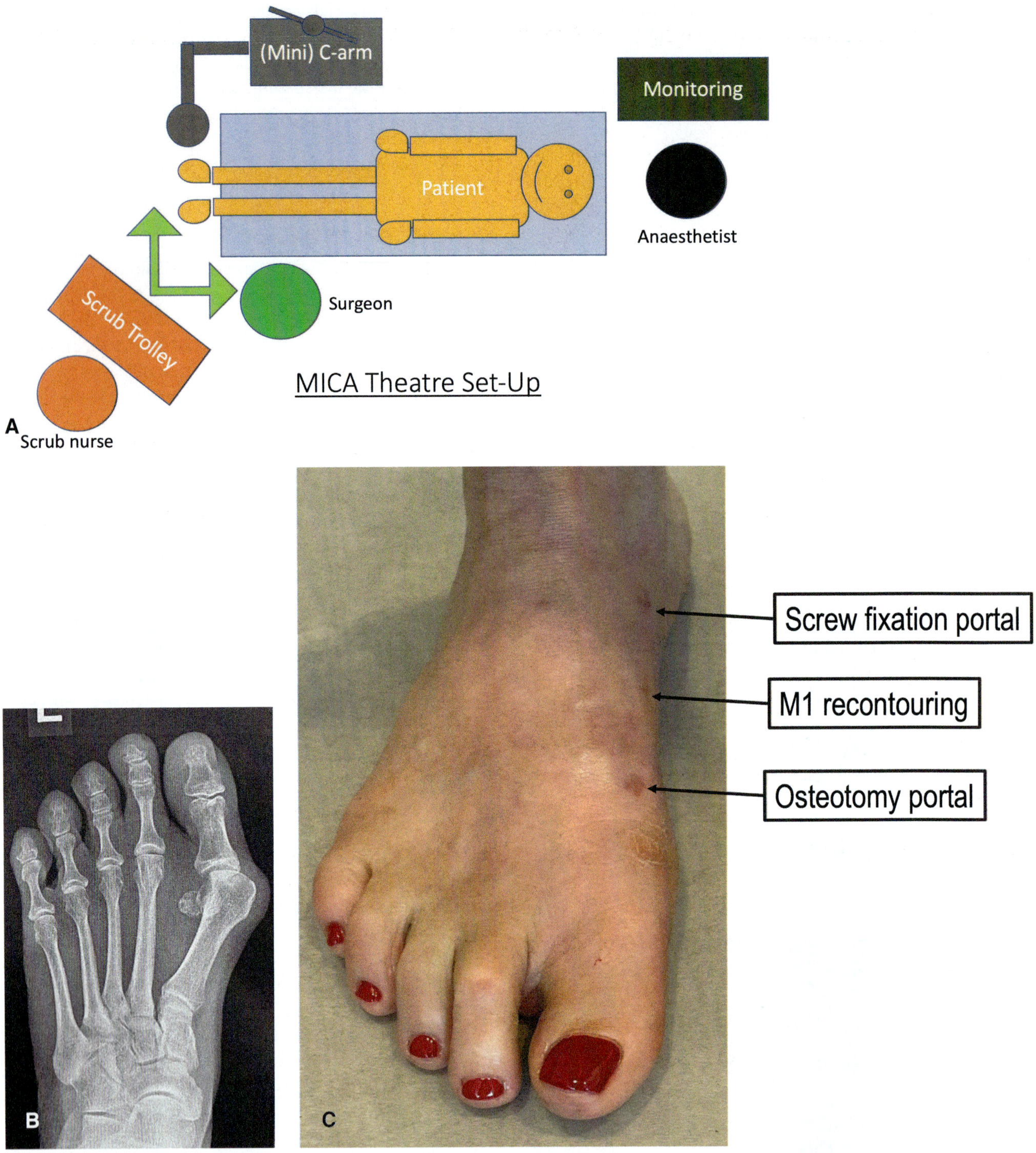

Figure 1.1 **A.** Minimally invasive chevron-Akin (MICA) theatre setup. **B.** Preoperative weight-bearing anteroposterior radiograph of moderate to severe hallux valgus deformity. **C.** Portals for MICA first metatarsal osteotomy.

Osteotomy Displacement and Screw Insertion

The osteotomy is then displaced using a combination of levers and elevators (Figure 1.3A and B). The displacement maneuver internally rotates the proximal metatarsal fragment and laterally translates the head fragment. It is important to avoid external rotation of the head fragment by adding varus force to the hallux during the displacement maneuver. At this point, the coronal plane rotation of the first metatarsal can also be corrected. Both anteroposterior and lateral view fluoroscopy should be used to ensure correct plane of displacement.

The obtuse chevron osteotomy shape with short plantar tail serves to protect against inadvertent elevation of the head fragment and improve stability of the osteotomy without

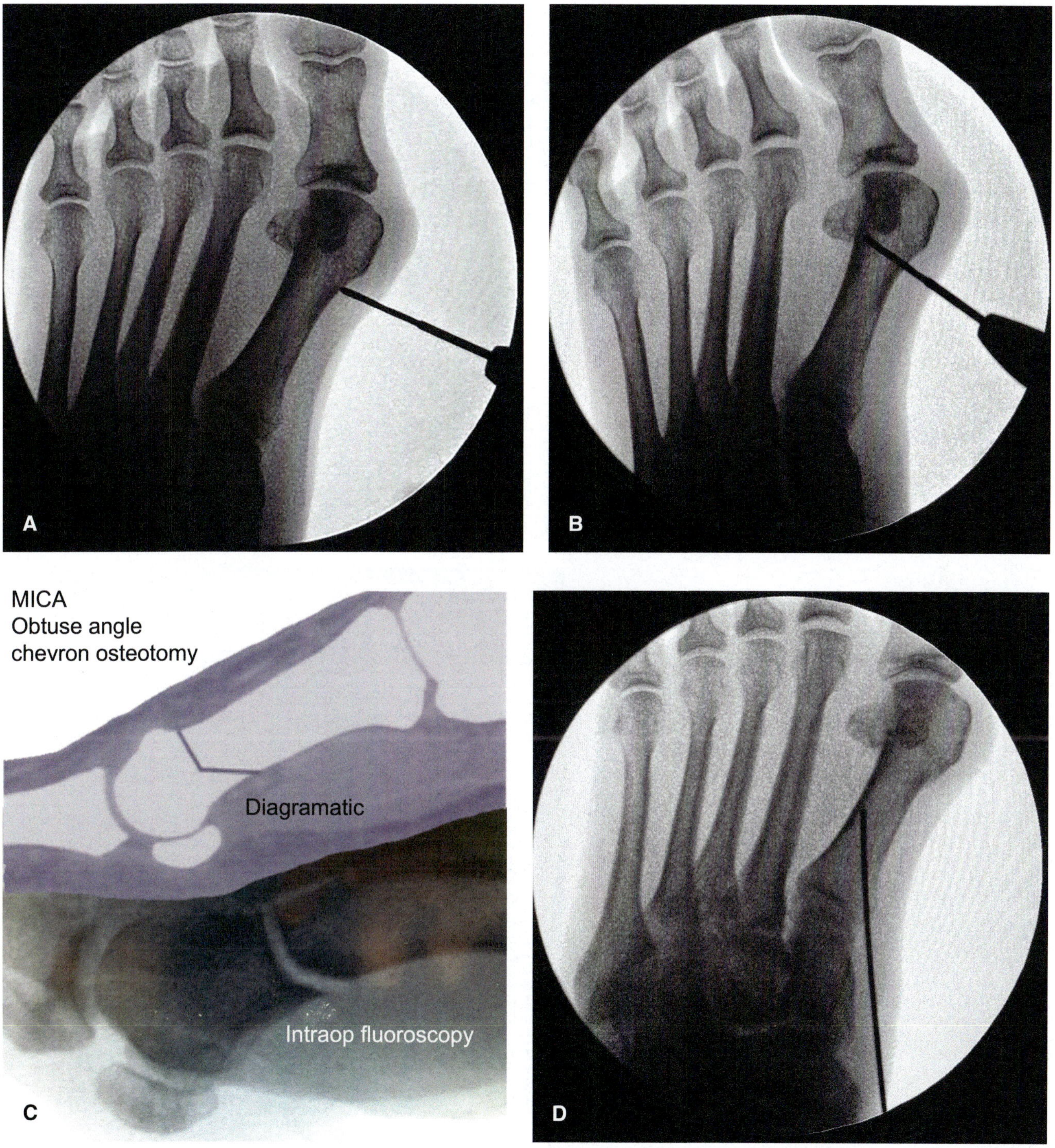

Figure 1.2 **A.** Initial 2-mm Shannon burr placement at distal diaphyseal-metaphyseal junction. **B.** Advancement of 20-mm Shannon burr under fluoroscopic guidance, setting plane of apex of chevron osteotomy. **C.** Diagrammatic and corresponding fluoroscopic appearance of obtuse, short-tailed chevron osteotomy. **D.** Insertion of 1.4-mm guidewire under fluoroscopic guidance in anteroposterior and lateral planes.

compromising the ability to correct rotation and without compromising the bicortical fix of the proximal screw (as long as the point of traversing the lateral wall is greater than 12 mm from the osteotomy). The guidewire is then advanced into the head fragment and the appropriate screw length measured. A 4-mm chamfered head screw is preferred. The wire is then driven through the foot and clipped with a hemostat. This gives the surgeon control of both ends of the wire should this break during drilling and also avoids inadvertent removal of the wire during drilling. Drilling and screw insertion then follow.

Once the proximal screw has been inserted, then the distal antirotation screw guidewire and screw insertion follows. The second distal screw is important to avoid rotational

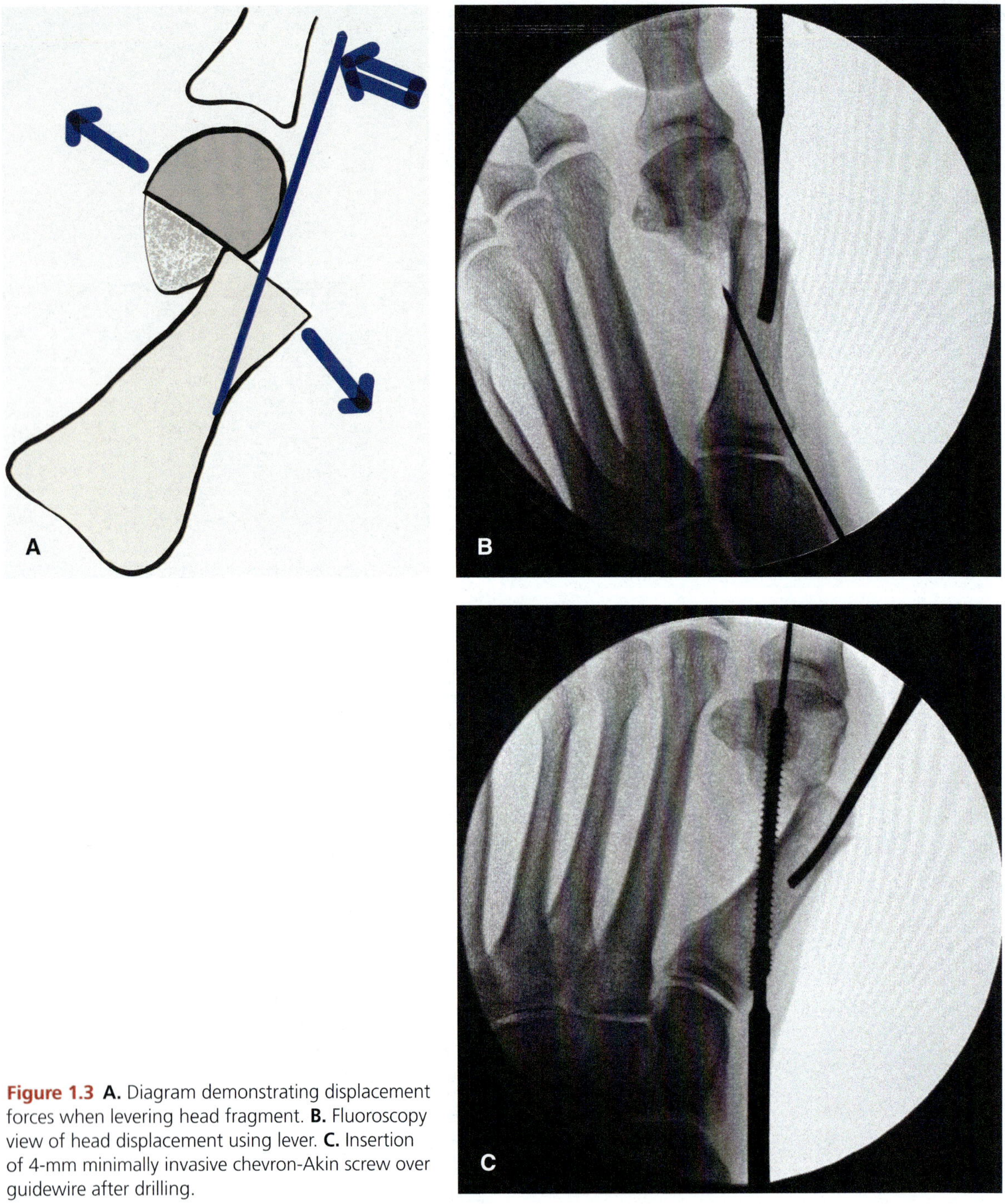

Figure 1.3 **A.** Diagram demonstrating displacement forces when levering head fragment. **B.** Fluoroscopy view of head displacement using lever. **C.** Insertion of 4-mm minimally invasive chevron-Akin screw over guidewire after drilling.

instability in larger displacements (>50% of the metatarsal width). A narrower (3-mm) MICA screw is preferred for this role—unless a larger bone patient. It is often easier to use a larger guidewire (2 mm diameter) initially, which is stiffer and less able to skive, to obtain the desired plane and then exchange this for the fine 0.9-mm guidewire required for the 3-mm MICA screw insertion (Figures 1.3C and 1.4). In male or larger feet with large displacements, a 4-mm MICA screw may be more appropriate for the distal screw.

Recontouring of Medial Border of Metatarsal

The residual proximal metatarsal fragment "spike" is then recontoured via an additional portal (Figure 1.1C). The 20 mm × 2 mm burr is again used for this, cutting from plantar lateral to dorsomedial direction (Figure 1.5A). If there is residual prominence of the medial eminence (bunion), then this can also be removed at this stage with a 3.1-mm wedge

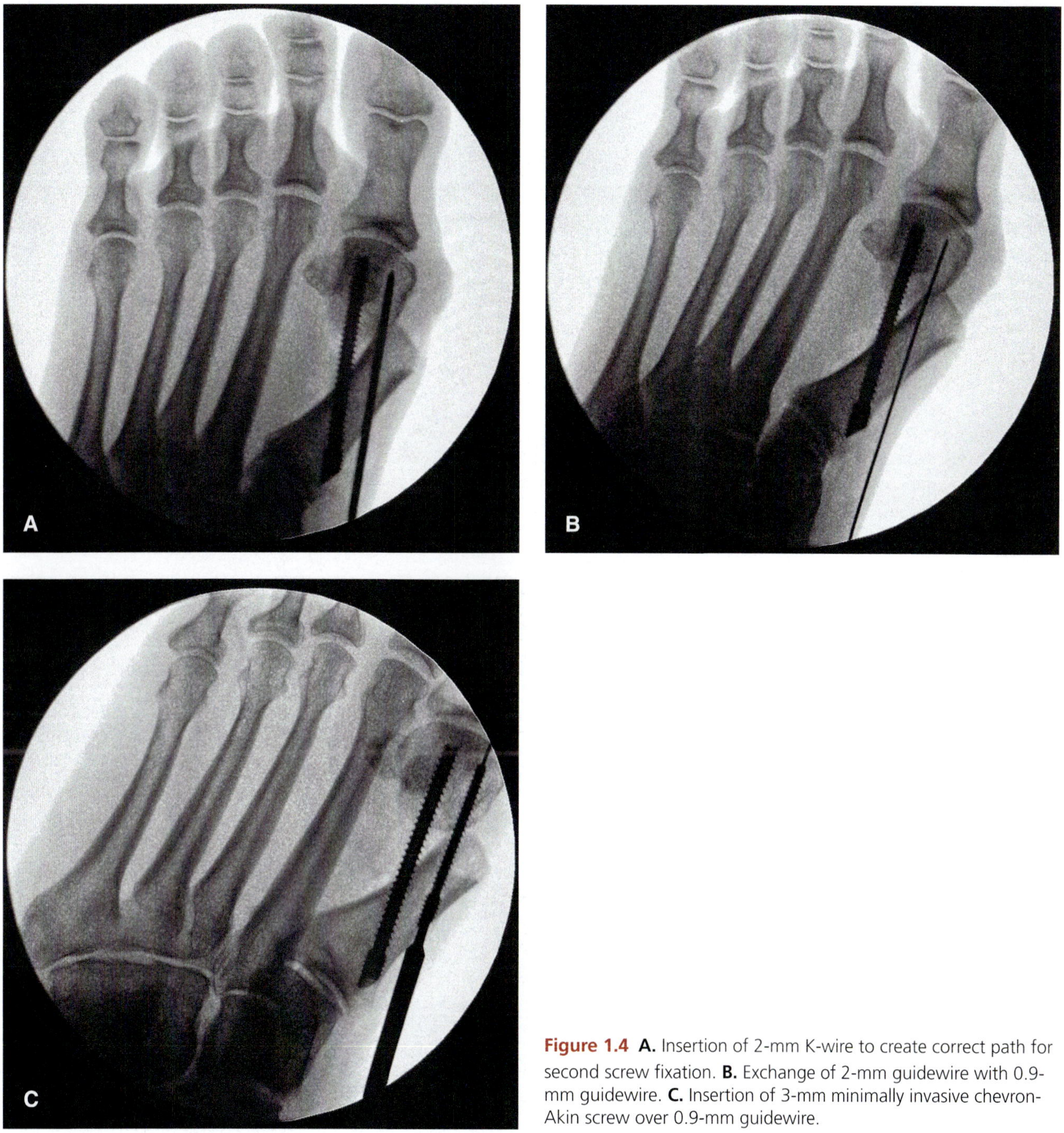

Figure 1.4 **A.** Insertion of 2-mm K-wire to create correct path for second screw fixation. **B.** Exchange of 2-mm guidewire with 0.9-mm guidewire. **C.** Insertion of 3-mm minimally invasive chevron-Akin screw over 0.9-mm guidewire.

burr. This is termed recontouring of the medial and dorsomedial first metatarsal border.

Commercial Jigs to Assist With Displacement and Screw Fixation

Various jigs are available from different orthopedic companies to assist the surgeon with steps 2 to 4 above, which otherwise require cadaver lab training and surgeon learning curve to become familiar with and achieve reproducible displacement and stable fixation. Key to stable fixation is the initial proximal screw, which is acting as a positional screw (rather than a lag screw) with three points of fixation.

Distal Soft-Tissue Release

The surgeon then needs to assess whether a distal soft-tissue release is required. The surgeon should never undertake this prior to performing the chevron osteotomy and fixation. Otherwise, control of the head fragment via ligamentotaxis will be lost and the surgeon will be unable to counteract the tendency of the head fragment to drift into valgus during the

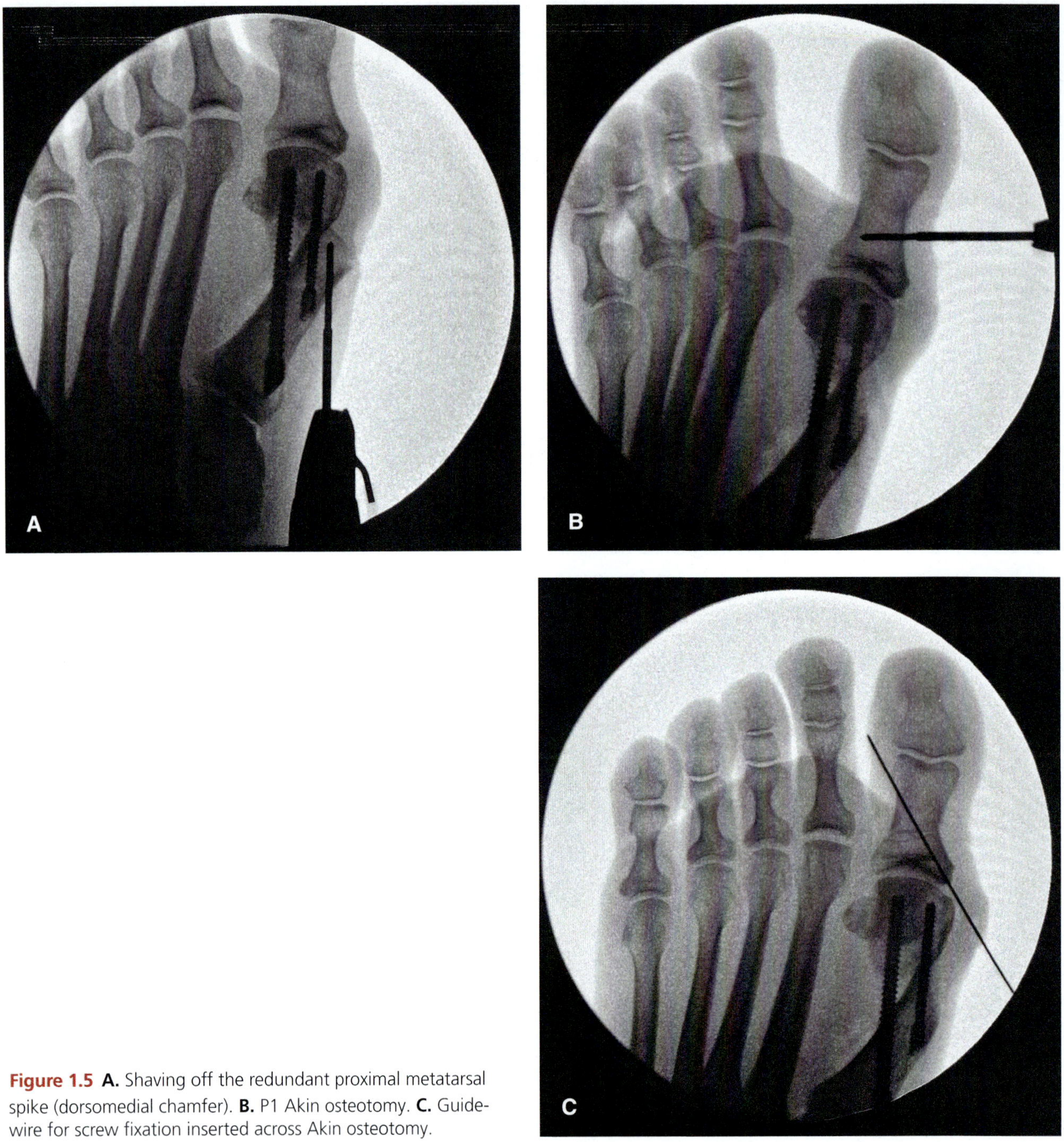

Figure 1.5 **A.** Shaving off the redundant proximal metatarsal spike (dorsomedial chamfer). **B.** P1 Akin osteotomy. **C.** Guidewire for screw fixation inserted across Akin osteotomy.

levering maneuver. There are two indications for a modified distal soft-tissue release:

i. If there is incongruity of the first metatarsophalangeal joint (MTPJ) after performing the chevron osteotomy with displacement and fixation (ie, residual hallux valgus). This may indicate that the surgeon has not managed to achieve sufficient translational ± rotational correction in the chevron first metatarsal osteotomy. The lateral sesamoid in this situation will remain uncovered and a persisting deforming force—hence the need for a distal soft-tissue release.

ii. If there is residual adherence of the fibular sesamoid to the lateral metatarsal head despite adequate chevron displacement and first MTPJ congruence. This situation may arise in chronic, more severe deformities and is less frequently encountered than situation (i).

The distal soft-tissue release involves isolated division of the lateral head of flexor hallucis brevis distal to the lateral (fibular) sesamoid. The lateral collateral ligament of the first MTPJ should be preserved. A Beaver blade is used to undertake the release. This is introduced into the dorsal lateral corner of the first MTPJ and carefully advanced plantar ward into the plantar plate (sesamoid-phalangeal ligament) in this position. The sesamoid-phalangeal ligament is then divided by cautiously rotating the Beaver blade tip in the direction of the first web space while simultaneously drawing the hallux into varus—drawing the ligament over the blade while turning the blade through the ligament at the same time. The tissue is robust, and the surgeon should feel it give (and often hear it too) as the cut is completed. There is very little excursion of the blade. The flexor hallucis longus is not at risk as long as the position of the cut is as detailed above, but injury to this structure has been reported.[13]

Akin Osteotomy

An Akin osteotomy is added if there is significant hallux valgus interphalangeus (valgus deviation within the proximal phalanx of the hallux). The osteotomy is performed via a midaxial portal on the medial border of the hallux, and the surface position for this portal is assessed as the midpoint between the hallux MTPJ and the hallux interphalangeal joint.

The osteotomy is performed with a 12-mm Shannon burr under fluoroscopy. An incomplete osteotomy is performed, leaving the lateral cortex intact. The entry point in the proximal phalanx is at the proximal diaphyseal-metaphyseal junction, and the burr is preferably directed slightly obliquely in a proximal direction as the osteotomy is created, which makes subsequent screw fixation easier (Figure 1.5B).

The cut is completed in dorsal and plantar directions using rotational movements of the burr but leaving the lateral cortex intact. It is helpful to push the burr through the dorsolateral and plantar lateral corners otherwise the osteotomy will likely not close. Additional sweeps of the burr in the same path will remove more bone and create greater corrections, but generally, one pass of the burr is sufficient. Applying varus force to the hallux then closes the osteotomy.

Fixation of the Akin osteotomy is preferable otherwise there is a risk the hallux will angulate in the sagittal plane and develop a dorsiflexion deformity. Fixation is achieved with a 3-mm screw via a midmedial portal. A stab incision is made proximal to the base of the hallux P1 in the intended plane of insertion of the guidewire for the cannulated screw. The blade is inserted up to the base of the P1 medially and then the guidewire passed. The desired screw length is then estimated, and the guidewire is driven through the other side of the hallux and clipped with a hemostat. Due to the curvature of the plantar surface of the P1, the guidewire should be directed in a dorsal direction as advanced laterally to avoid inadvertent exit from the proximal phalanx and loss of fixation. Drilling with the appropriate cannulated drill is then followed by screw insertion (Figures 1.5 and 1.6).

Closure

All portals should be irrigated with saline using a syringe with a venous catheter attached. This removes any bony debris that could either cause stiffness or a symptomatic lumpy portal once the skin has healed. The osteotomy and screw insertion portals are then sutured and adhesive strips are applied to all the portals. Chlorhexidine- or saline-soaked dressing gauze (surgeon preference) is then applied such that the correction is splinted. This will dry and become firm postoperatively and provides a comfortable splint for the patient. A covering of wool and crepe bandaging is then applied. Intraoperative fluoroscopy images should be saved.

◆ POSTOPERATIVE MANAGEMENT

The operative and postoperative period is formed of phases. The first phase is that of the surgery itself. The second is the wound healing phase, third is the bone healing phase, and thereafter, the fourth phase is the rehabilitation.

Phase 1, the wound healing phase, requires strict elevation of the foot. Patients are allowed to weight bear as tolerated in a stiff postoperative shoe; immediately postoperatively, they must be carefully instructed to take short steps to ensure that body weight remains in the hindfoot during gait. They should be instructed to keep the foot strictly elevated apart from getting up once an hour for toileting and sustenance. Appropriate venous thromboembolism prophylaxis must be considered. The percutaneous incisions heal rapidly with appropriate elevation. While 1 week of elevation is often sufficient, this author generally recommends 2 weeks of strict elevation, at which point they are reviewed in the outpatient department. At 2 weeks, there is more certainty of sufficient healing for suture removal.

Phase 2 involves protecting the foot until adequate bone healing has occurred. Strict use of the stiff-soled postoperative shoe must continue whenever weight bearing until 6 weeks after surgery.

Phase 3 involves a switch in emphasis from protection of the healing bones to rehabilitation and returned to function. Patients are seen at 5 to 6 weeks in the outpatient department for both clinical and radiological review (weight-bearing anteroposterior and lateral views). Patients should be allowed to return to their own footwear from 6 weeks onward and gradually increase their activity but should be instructed to avoid impact work such as running and racquet sports until at least 3 months after surgery.

Physical therapy is recommended from 6 weeks after surgery to optimize return to normal gait and restoration of joint motion etc. Patients should be made aware that the foot will remain swollen until approximately 5 to 6 months after surgery and that this reflects the underlying bone healing and remodeling. This understanding of the biology is helpful with compliance.

Outpatient review takes place at 2 weeks, 6 weeks, 6 months, and as needed thereafter if there are any patient concerns.

◆ OUTCOMES

There have been numerous recent publications on the topic of MICA hallux valgus correction, and to this author's

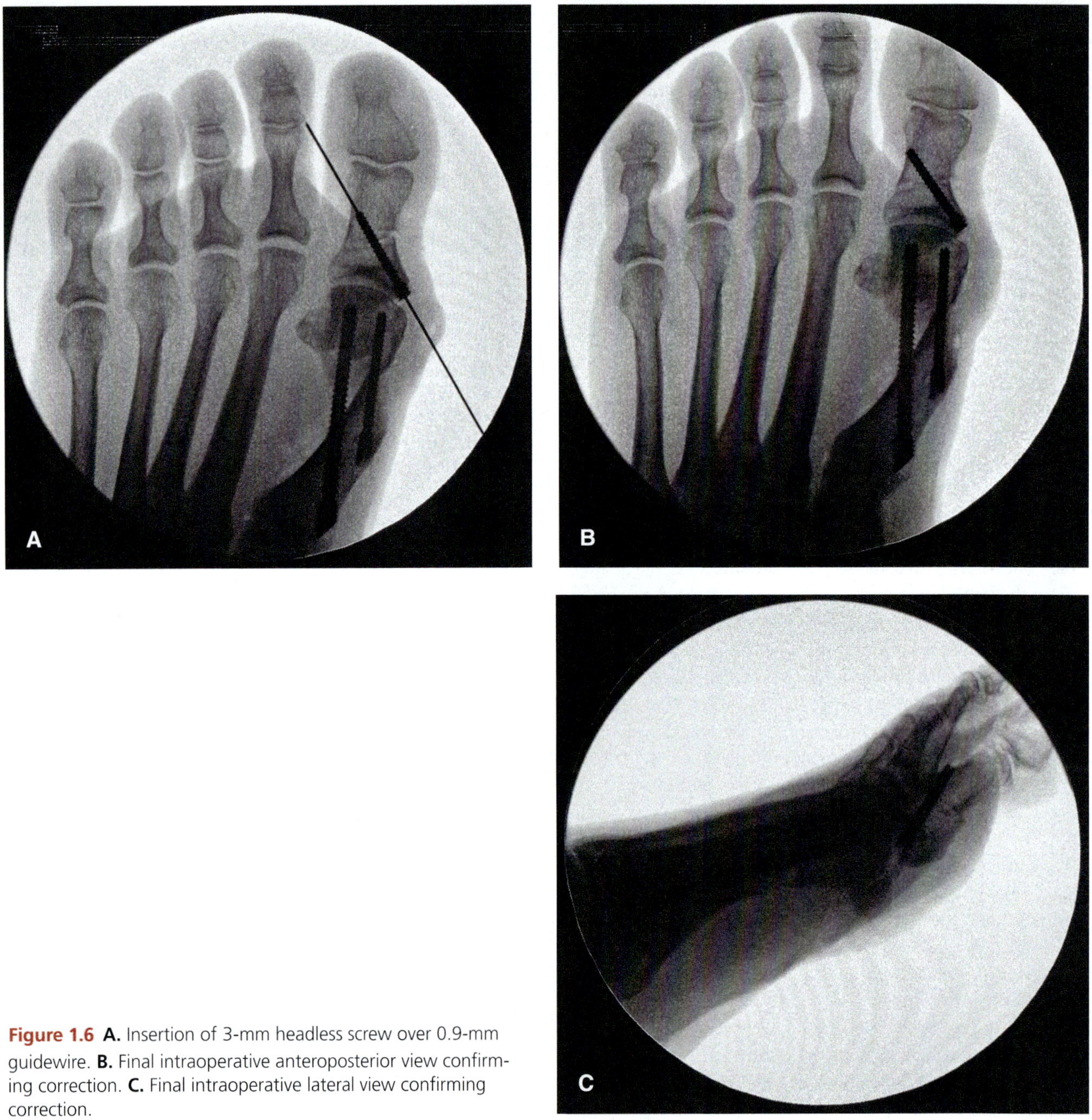

Figure 1.6 **A.** Insertion of 3-mm headless screw over 0.9-mm guidewire. **B.** Final intraoperative anteroposterior view confirming correction. **C.** Final intraoperative lateral view confirming correction.

knowledge, no published studies to date have shown inferiority of outcome when compared with open scarf-Akin correction (even where this includes a learning curve). There is prospective comparative study evidence that the MICA technique is associated with less pain than the open scarf-Akin technique.[8,9] This has been a consistent observation in this author's practice.

In 2017, Lee et al. published a prospective, randomized study (level II evidence) of 50 patients undergoing either percutaneous chevron-Akin (PECA) or open scarf-Akin.[8] Data was collected preoperatively and at day 1, 2 weeks, 6 weeks, and 6 months postoperatively. Outcome measures included the American Orthopedic Foot and Ankle Society Hallux-Metatarsophalangeal-Interphalangeal (AOFAS-HMI) score, visual analogue pain score, HVA, and 1 to 2 IMA. Twenty-five patients underwent PECA procedure, and 25 patients received scarf-Akin procedure. Both groups showed significantly improved AOFAS-HMI scores after surgery. Final outcome scores, HVA, and IMA were similar at final follow-up. However, the PECA group showed significantly lower pain level (visual analog scale) in the early postoperative phase (postoperative day 1 to postoperative week 6, $P < .001$ and $P = .004$, respectively). No serious complications were observed in either group. The authors concluded that both groups showed comparable good to excellent clinical and radiologic outcomes at final follow-up, but the PECA group had significantly less pain in the first 6 weeks following surgery.

Subsequent studies from United Kingdom, United States, Asia, and Europe have re-affirmed excellent results with the MICA technique.[8-18]

Lewis et al. have published results of a 2-year prospective study of 292 patients (333 feet) who underwent MICA hallux valgus correction.[13] They observed an improvement in all domains of MOXFQ scores, quality of life, and pain scores as well as good radiological correction and a very low rate of symptomatic recurrence (0.9%). Hardware removal was required in 6.3% of patients. Other UK studies have reported similarly good results, including correction of severe hallux valgus deformities. The majority of recovery and improvement occurs in the first 6 months after surgery, but improvement continues for up to 2 years.[24]

Tay et al. from Singapore reported similar results for both MICA and open scarf-Akin at 2 years after surgery but significantly less pain in the MICA group postoperatively.[16]

Mikhail et al. from United States published their results with 248 MICA and observed 91.6% patient satisfaction with the outcome of surgery.[14] Neufeld et al. also from United States published the results of 94 MICA corrections and observed 94% good or excellent patient satisfaction. They observed 5% reoperation rate including three hardware removals.[17] Summaries of recent published results appear in Table 1.2.

Table 1.2

Summary of Recent Published Studies Regarding MICA Hallux Valgus Correction

Group (Geographical Origin)	Number of Patients (Duration of Follow-up)	Results/Conclusion
Lewis et al. (United Kingdom)[13]	292 (2 y)	The third-generation MICA provided significant improvement in clinical outcome measures at the 2-y follow-up and can be successfully used for correction of a range of hallux valgus deformities with a low rate of symptomatic recurrence (0.9%). Hardware removal reported in 6.3% cases
Lewis et al. (United Kingdom)[22]	106 (2 y)	MICA for the treatment of severe hallux valgus deformity enables substantial deformity correction and is associated with significant improvements in clinical PROMs 2 y following surgery
Mikhail et al. (United States)[14]	248	91.6% patient satisfaction and low postoperative narcotic requirements
Neufeld et al. (United States)[17]	94	94% of patients reported good or excellent satisfaction with the procedure. The reoperation rate was 5%, including 3 hardware removals, 1 irrigation and débridement, and 1 neurolysis
Chan et al. (Singapore)[11]	13 (2 y)	All patients 0/10 visual analogue score pain postoperatively and SF-36 improved in all patients
Tay et al. (Singapore)[16]	60 (2 y)	A matched cohort study comparing MICA and scarf-Akin techniques. Similar outcomes at 2 y but significantly less pain MICA group in postoperative period
Kurashige et al. (Japan)[21]	40	MICA improved moderate to severe hallux valgus both radiologically and clinically
Hromádka et al. (Czech Republic)[15]	76	They reported their first experience with MICA and concluded that the technique offers the possibility to correct mild, moderate, and partially severe deformities
Lewis et al. (United Kingdom)[24]	61	Over a 17-mo period, 61 consecutive cases were performed with outcome data available for 58 of these (95%). Technical proficiency was reached after 38 cases. Operation time and radiation exposure significantly decreased after this transition point ($P < .05$). There was no difference in complication rate or radiographic deformity correction regardless of position along the learning curve ($P > .05$)

MICA, minimally invasive chevron-Akin; PROM, patient-reported outcome measure.

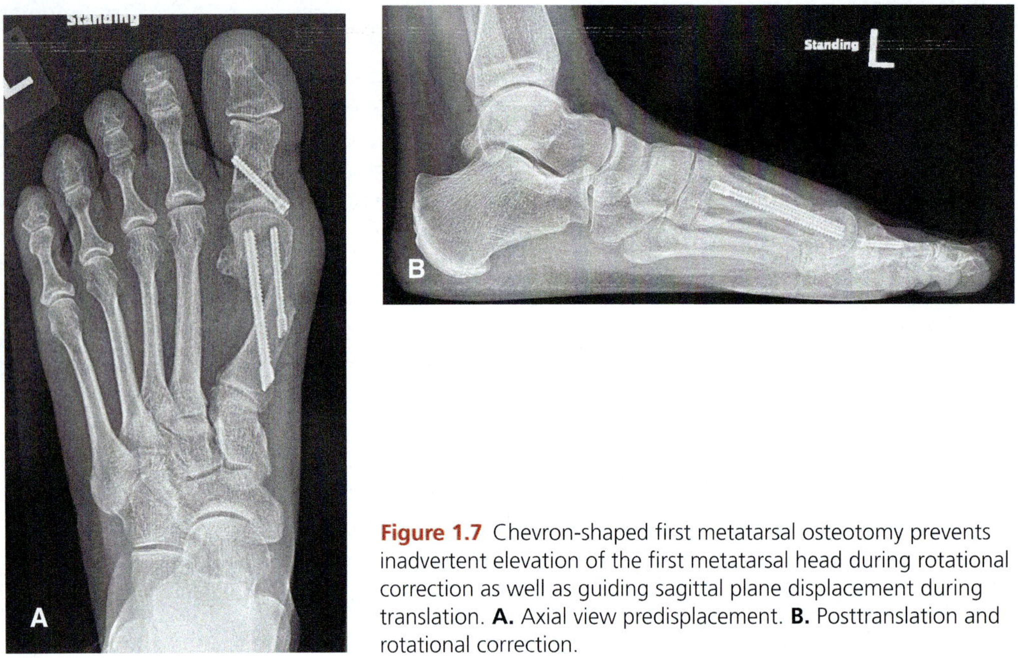

Figure 1.7 Chevron-shaped first metatarsal osteotomy prevents inadvertent elevation of the first metatarsal head during rotational correction as well as guiding sagittal plane displacement during translation. **A.** Axial view predisplacement. **B.** Posttranslation and rotational correction.

Postoperative stiffness is a concern with traditional procedures that seems to be lessened with a minimally invasive technique. While this has yet to be adequately independently confirmed by other authors in the literature, a study by Frigg et al. tried to explore this.[18] In their MICA group, extension increased by 10°, while it remained unchanged in the scarf group. This is not adequately explained by the authors who suggested that it may be secondary to first metatarsal shortening they created in their MICA group.

◆ COMPLICATIONS

The list of potential complications is the same as for all hallux valgus surgery. However, the risk of infection is lower, wound and scar problems far fewer, and level of pain postoperatively substantially lower than with open techniques. The risk of stiffness in the hallux MTPJ is also appears to be lower.[18]

The risk of hardware removal is probably slightly higher (~5%) than with the scarf-Akin procedure. It is important to pay attention to achieve a smooth dorsomedial first metatarsal border during the initial corrective surgery to minimize the incidence of such problems. If symptomatic, it is usually the metalwork in the first metatarsal rather than hallux Akin that is problematic and more likely the distal screw than proximal. Sometimes, it is a combination of the distal screw and the surrounding bone that causes symptoms. Presentation is usually beyond 5 to 6 months when the majority of swelling has resolved, and the patient is returning to a wider variety of footwear including narrower and more fashionable shoes.

Removal of the distal M1 screw and "recontouring" of the surrounding bone to remove any prominence involves a day-case admission and brief general or regional anesthetic. The additional surgery can usually be undertaken via the original portals rather than new incisions, and once the screw has been located with the guidewire, then the screwdriver is inserted over this and the screw removed. A 3.1 mm wedge bur can then usually be inserted into this hole, and working medially, the unwanted residual bone prominence is easily removed.

Patients can usually return to normal footwear within 7 days after surgery with instructions to avoid impact activity such as running or racket sports for 4 weeks but without further restriction.

◆ TECHNIQUE TIPS

Overall, the initial learning curve for MICA has been shown to be relatively short and safe.[24] However, as with any technique, it is a longer-term commitment to master the craft. The following are important principles to adhere to:

1. *Attention to the correct plane of the chevron osteotomy*
   The plane should be tailored to the specific patient circumstances and ensuring compensating for the characteristics of the cutting instrument. In most cases, trying to preserve a neutral first metatarsal length is optimal. The burr has a kerf of 2 to 2.5 mm, which will tend to elevate and shorten the first metatarsal unless the surgeon compensates for this in the plane of the osteotomy. However, it is also possible to overcompensate and lengthen with the plane of the osteotomy, which can increase pressures across the MTPJ and create symptoms of stiffness and pain. Lengthening in most circumstances should therefore be avoided as much as substantial shortening. Similarly, it is also relatively easy to over elevate or plantaris the first metatarsal head if the lateral view is not checked on the fluoroscopy regularly during the chevron displacement and fixation. Sagittal plane malpositioning (angulation or translation) is poorly tolerated as with overshortening or overlengthening and should be avoided. The chevron-shaped osteotomy rather than straight helps to avoid inadvertent elevation mal positioning by blocking dorsal head translation, especially at

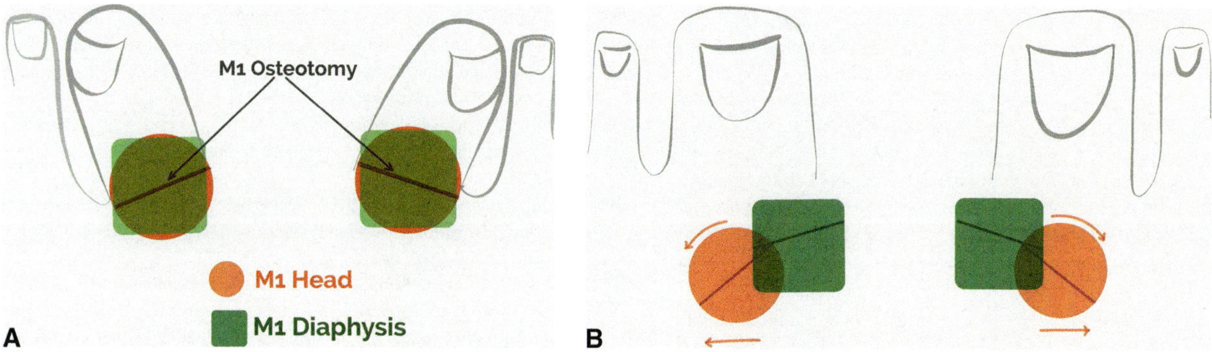

Figure 1.8 Postoperative anteroposterior **(A)** and lateral views **(B)** obtained at 6 weeks after surgery.

the point when the surgeon is correcting the first metatarsal rotation (Figure 1.7).

2. *Attention to stable fixation*
   Achieving stable fixation is vital in maintaining the osteotomy position during the postoperative period. It is therefore essential that the surgeon ensures that the proximal screw fixation passes through the lateral cortex of the metatarsal, proximal to the osteotomy, to provide secure angular stability (Figures 1.8 and 1.9). A short plantar limb and large first metatarsal head displacement are both helpful to achieve optimal screw configuration.
3. *"Lock-out" the first tarsometatarsal joint medial excursion*
   It is notable that even in relatively mild deformities, the first metatarsal displacement achieved can easily approach 90+%. Because the osteotomy is extracapsular, it is not confined by the capsule, and the mechanism of displacement (Figure 1.3A) brings about internal rotation of the proximal first metatarsal (as well as lateral translation of the head fragment) and "locks out" maximal medial excursion of the first tarsometatarsal joint. This will reduce the capacity for recurrence, explaining the reported recurrence rate of less than 1%.[13]
4. *Err on the side of lengthening rather than shortening with initial chevron plane*
   It is easy to remove a little more bone if the plane of the osteotomy is a little too distally angulated, but the die is cast if the surgeon shortens too much with the initial plane of the osteotomy.
5. *Adjust technique if taking on severe deformities*
   With experience, severe deformities can be tackled and greater than 100% displacement performed if necessary. If considering displacements of greater than 100%, then the plane of osteotomy will need to be adjusted to accommodate for the shortening that will occur once the head fragment moves off the end of the proximal fragment. The osteotomy needs to be directed slightly more distally to accommodate for this.[23]

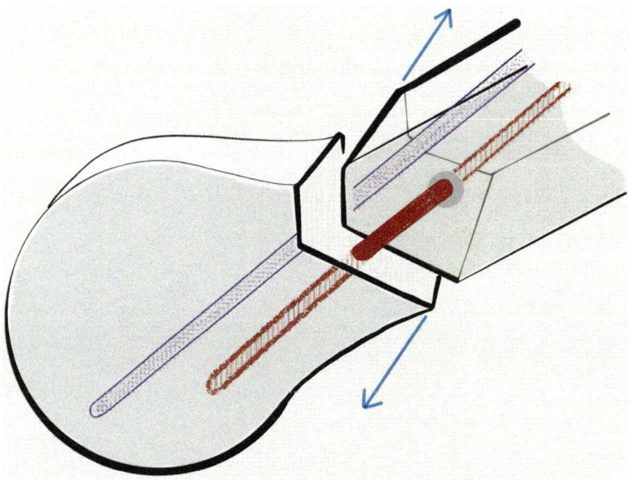

Figure 1.9 Lateral view of distal first metatarsal diaphysis, chevron osteotomy, and metatarsal head, demonstrating the plane of displacement and configuration of fixation screws. The proximal screw (*red* in the figure) can be seen to exit the lateral wall of the distal metatarsal, proximal to the osteotomy and then continuing into the head fragment.

There is a strong base of peer-reviewed literature confirming MICA correction of hallux valgus as a powerful and reproducible tool associated with little postoperative pain and excellent outcomes. It has been shown effective in mild to severe hallux valgus deformities and is associated with a relatively short and safe learning curve after initial cadaveric training. The majority of recovery and improvement occurs within 6 months of MICA surgery, but further improvement can be seen for up to 2 years.

References

1. Redfern D, Gill I, Harris M. Early experience with a minimally invasive modified chevron and Akin osteotomy for correction of hallux valgus. *J Bone Joint Surg Br.* 2011;93-B(SUPP IV):482.
2. Vernois J. The treatment of the hallux valgus with a percutaneous chevron osteotomy. *J Bone Joint Surg Br.* 2011;93-B(SUPP IV):482.
3. Vernois J, Redfern DJ. Percutaneous chevron; the union of classic stable fixed approach and percutaneous technique. *Fuß Sprunggelenk.* 2013;11(2):70-75.
4. Redfern D, Perera AM. Minimally invasive osteotomies. *Foot Ankle Clin.* 2014;19(2):181-189.
5. Redfern D, Vernois J, Legré BP. Percutaneous surgery of the forefoot [review]. *Clin Podiatr Med Surg.* 2015;32(3):291-332.
6. Redfern D, Vernois J. Minimally invasive chevron Akin (MICA) for correction of hallux valgus. *Tech Foot Ankle Surg.* 2016;15(1):3-11.
7. Redfern D. Minimally invasive chevron Akin (MICA) for correction of hallux valgus. *Tech Foot Ankle Surg.* 2020;19(3):132-141.

8. Lee M, Walsh J, Smith MM, Ling J, Wines A, Lam P. Hallux valgus correction comparing percutaneous chevron/Akin (PECA) and open scarf/Akin osteotomies. *Foot Ankle Int.* 2017;38(8):838-846.
9. Lai MC, Rikhraj IS, Woo YL, Yeo W, Ng YCS, Koo K. Clinical and radiological outcomes comparing percutaneous chevron-Akin osteotomies vs open scarf-Akin osteotomies for hallux valgus. *Foot Ankle Int.* 2018;39(3):311-317.
10. Altenberger S, Kriegelstein S, Gottschalk O, et al. The minimally invasive chevron and Akin osteotomy (MICA) [in German; review]. *Oper Orthop Traumatol.* 2018;30(3):148-160.
11. Chan CX, Gan JZ, Chong HC, et al. Two year outcomes of minimally invasive hallux valgus surgery. *Foot Ankle Surg.* 2019;25(2):119-126.
12. Holme TJ, Sivaloganathan SS, Patel B, Kunasingam K. Third-generation minimally invasive chevron Akin osteotomy for hallux valgus. *Foot Ankle Int.* 2020;41(1):50-56.
13. Lewis TL, Ray R, Miller G, Gordon DJ. Third-generation minimally invasive chevron and Akin osteotomies (MICA) in hallux valgus surgery: two-year follow-up of 292 cases. *J Bone Joint Surg Am.* 2021;103(13):1203-1211.
14. Mikhail CM, Markowitz J, Lenarda LD, Guzman J, Vulcano E. Clinical and radiographic outcomes of percutaneous chevron-Akin osteotomies for the correction of hallux valgus deformity. *Foot Ankle Int.* 2022;43(1):32-41.
15. Hromádka R, Klouda J, Popelka S, Bek J, Kodat L, Barták V. Miniinvazivní operace hallux valgus: první zkušenost [Minimally invasive hallux valgus surgery: first experience]. *Acta Chir Orthop Traumatol Cech.* 2021;88(2):137-143. Czech.
16. Tay AYW, Goh GS, Koo K, Yeo NEM. Third-generation minimally invasive chevron-Akin osteotomy for hallux valgus produces similar clinical and radiological outcomes as scarf-Akin osteotomy at 2 years: a matched Cohort study. *Foot Ankle Int.* 2022;43(3):321-330.
17. Neufeld SK, Dean D, Hussaini S. Outcomes and surgical strategies of minimally invasive chevron/Akin procedures. *Foot Ankle Int.* 2021;42(6):676-688.
18. Frigg A, Zaugg S, Maquieira G, Pellegrino A. Stiffness and range of motion after minimally invasive chevron-Akin and open scarf-Akin procedures. *Foot Ankle Int.* 2019;40(5):515-525.
19. Dearden PMC, Whitehouse MR, Lam P, Dracopoulos G. The learning curve of third-generation percutaneous chevron and Akin osteotomy (PECA) for hallux valgus. *J Foot Ankle Surg.* 2023;62(1):162-167.
20. Vernois J, Redfern DJ. Percutaneous surgery for severe hallux valgus. *Foot Ankle Clin.* 2016;21(3):479-493.
21. Kurashige T. Radiographic and clinical results of minimally invasive chevron Akin osteotomy for moderate to severe hallux valgus deformities. *Foot Ankle Spec.* 2021;19386400211045911.
22. Lewis TL, Ray R, Gordon DJ. Minimally invasive surgery for severe hallux valgus in 106 feet. *Foot Ankle Surg.* 2022;28(4):503-509.
23. Redfern D, Vernois J. Minimally invasive revision forefoot surgery. *Tech Foot Ankle Surg.* 2020;19(2):62-68.
24. Lewis TL, Ray R, Gordon DJ. Time to maximum clinical improvement following minimally invasive chevron and Akin osteotomies (MICA) in hallux valgus surgery. *Foot Ankle Surg.* 2022;28(7):928-934.

2 Surgical Technique for Percutaneous Transverse Distal First Metatarsal Osteotomy and Akin Bunionectomy

Oliver N. Schipper

◆ INTRODUCTION

The percutaneous extra-articular transverse distal first metatarsal osteotomy and Akin osteotomy technique (PETA) offers several potential benefits over the percutaneous distal first metatarsal chevron osteotomy and Akin osteotomy technique. First, a transverse osteotomy allows for easier rotational correction of the pronation component of a hallux valgus deformity. Second, more bone is preserved at the first metatarsal head, allowing for increased bony screw purchase, as opposed to a chevron osteotomy where the screws may be placed within the central apex of the chevron with less bony purchase at the first metatarsal head. Third, the transverse osteotomy is quicker to perform. Finally, the transverse osteotomy allows for a medial midaxial incision rather than a dorsomedial incision for the chevron osteotomy, which reduces the risk of iatrogenic dorsomedial sensory nerve branch injury. A prior biomechanical study attempted to compare the biomechanical strength of the percutaneous chevron osteotomy versus the percutaneous transverse osteotomy but found no significant difference in ultimate load, yield load, and ultimate stiffness between the two osteotomies.[1] The study was limited by poor screw placement, and therefore, further studies are needed to determine if the transverse osteotomy is biomechanically and clinically superior to the chevron osteotomy.

◆ PREOPERATIVE PLANNING

- Consider patient bone quality
  - Younger patients may have better bone quality, which increases the risk of bone and skin thermal injury with use of the Shannon and wedge burrs. The surgeon should pause every 10 seconds to clean the burr flutes and allow the burr to cool.
- Patients should be counseled that foot swelling is normal for 6 months postoperatively.
- If clear first tarsometatarsal joint radiographic instability or symptomatic first tarsometatarsal joint arthritis is present, lapidus bunionectomy is the preferred procedure over PETA.

◆ INDICATIONS

- Mild to severe flexible hallux valgus deformities (including patients with planovalgus foot deformity) in which the 1 to 2 intermetatarsal angle is not greater than the width of the first metatarsal head
- Revision of recurrent hallux valgus deformities, including after lapidus bunionectomy

◆ PREPARATION AND PATIENT POSITIONING

- The surgical technician should have all equipment on the Mayo stand prior to starting the case (Figure 2.1). The Mayo stand is placed to the right of the surgeon, and the surgeon typically stands to the left of the patient's foot if right handed (opposite if left handed).
- The patient is positioned supine with the operative foot off of the bed distally and externally rotated slightly away from the

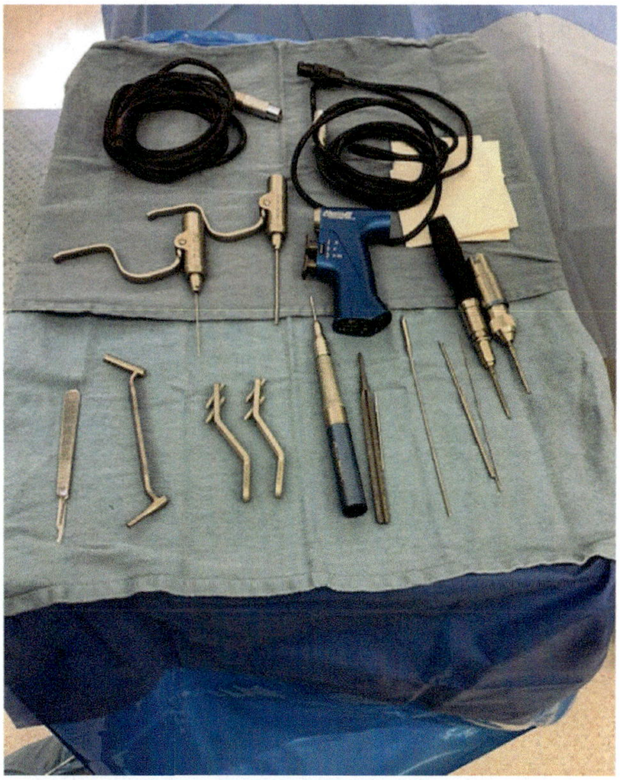

Figure 2.1 Equipment setup on Mayo stand for percutaneous extra-articular transverse distal first metatarsal osteotomy and Akin osteotomy (PETA) technique prior to starting procedure.

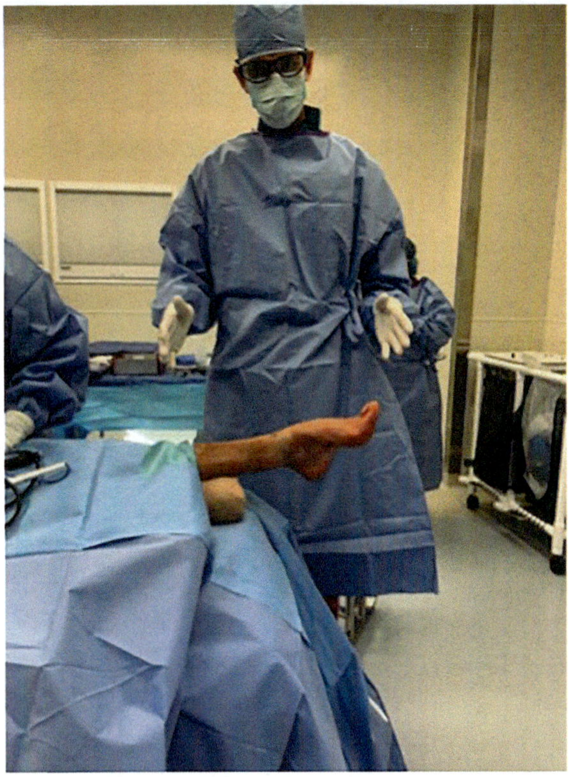

Figure 2.2 The operative leg is elevated on a bump and the entire foot is off the end of the operative table.

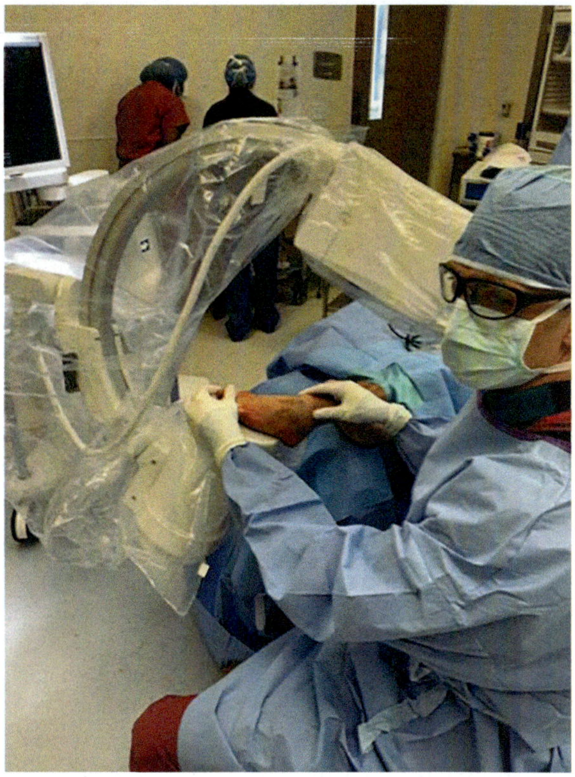

Figure 2.3 The mini C-arm is positioned to the right of the patient and the surgeon typically sits or stands to the left of the foot if right handed. The opposite is true for left-handed surgeons.

body to facilitate AP and lateral fluoroscopy views of the forefoot with minimal adjustment of the mini C-arm (Figure 2.2).

- The operative leg is elevated on a bump or blankets. The nonoperative leg may be frog-legged proximally away from the field and taped in order to avoid interfering with the C-arm.
- The mini C-arm is typically positioned to the right of the patient for right-handed surgeons and to the left of the patient for left-handed surgeons, although this may be altered based on surgeon preference (Figure 2.3).

SURGICAL TECHNIQUE

Distal First Metatarsal Osteotomy

1. Tips
   - Copious refrigerated (37 °F) bulb syringe irrigation is used at all times with the burr, during guidewire insertion, and when overdrilling the guidewire to prevent skin and bone thermal injury.
   - Burring is paused every 5 to 10 seconds in order to reduce heat generation, especially in younger patients with good bone quality.
2. The 4:1 reducer is attached to the handpiece, and the core console is set to 4:1 reducer attachment at 5,000 rpm once the handpiece has been attached to the power cord.
3. The procedure is performed without a tourniquet.
   - Use of tourniquet may increase the chance of thermal bone necrosis and therefore nonunion/delayed union.
   - The patient may be placed in 10° to 20° of Trendelenburg to reduce bony bleeding during the procedure.
4. A medial ankle peripheral nerve block or first ray field block is performed using a combination of lidocaine 1% and ropivacaine 0.5%.
5. The central longitudinal axis of the first metatarsal shaft (midaxial) is marked out on a lateral fluoroscopy view of the foot (Figure 2.4).
6. Using fluoroscopic guidance, a 3- to 4-mm medial, midaxial, percutaneous, longitudinal incision is made at the distal metaphyseal-diaphyseal junction of the first metatarsal at the base of the first metatarsal head flare (Figure 2.5).
   - No periosteal stripping is necessary.
   - The incision is midaxial in order to avoid the dorsomedial sensory nerve.
7. (Optional) The first metatarsal head medial eminence may be resected prior to the osteotomy or after fixation of the osteotomy and removal of the residual distal medial shaft bone spike. Preservation of the medial eminence allows for greater shift of the first metatarsal head during hallux valgus correction, and therefore, the author recommends waiting to perform the medial eminence resection until after fixation of the osteotomy and removal of the residual distal medial shaft bone spike (Figure 2.6).

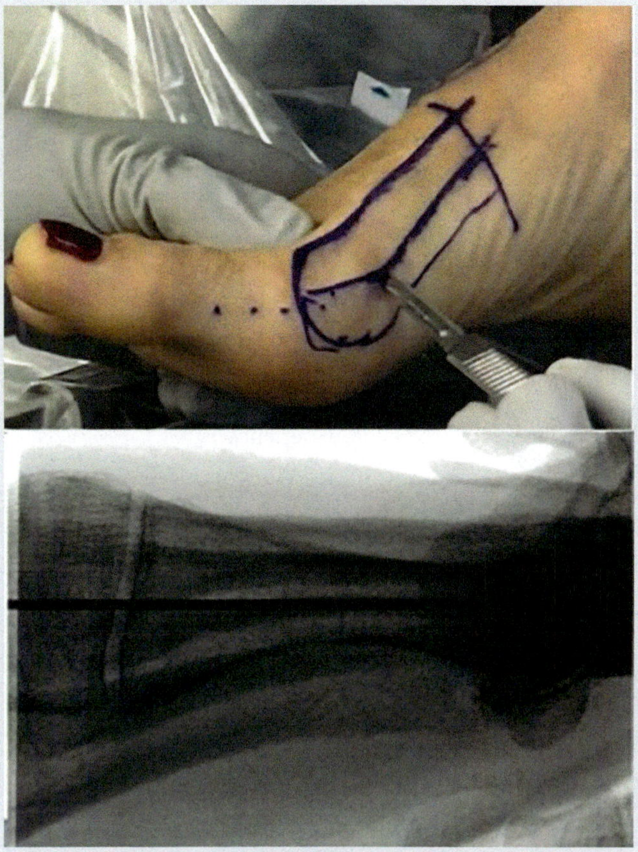

Figure 2.4 The central longitudinal axis of the first metatarsal shaft (midaxial) is marked out using a lateral fluoroscopy view of the foot.

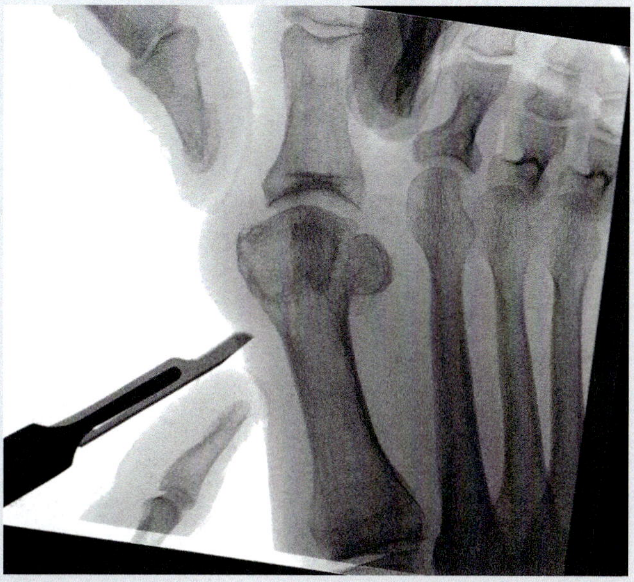

Figure 2.5 A 3- to 4-mm medial, midaxial, percutaneous, longitudinal incision is made at the distal metaphyseal-diaphyseal junction of the distal first metatarsal at the base of the first metatarsal head flare.

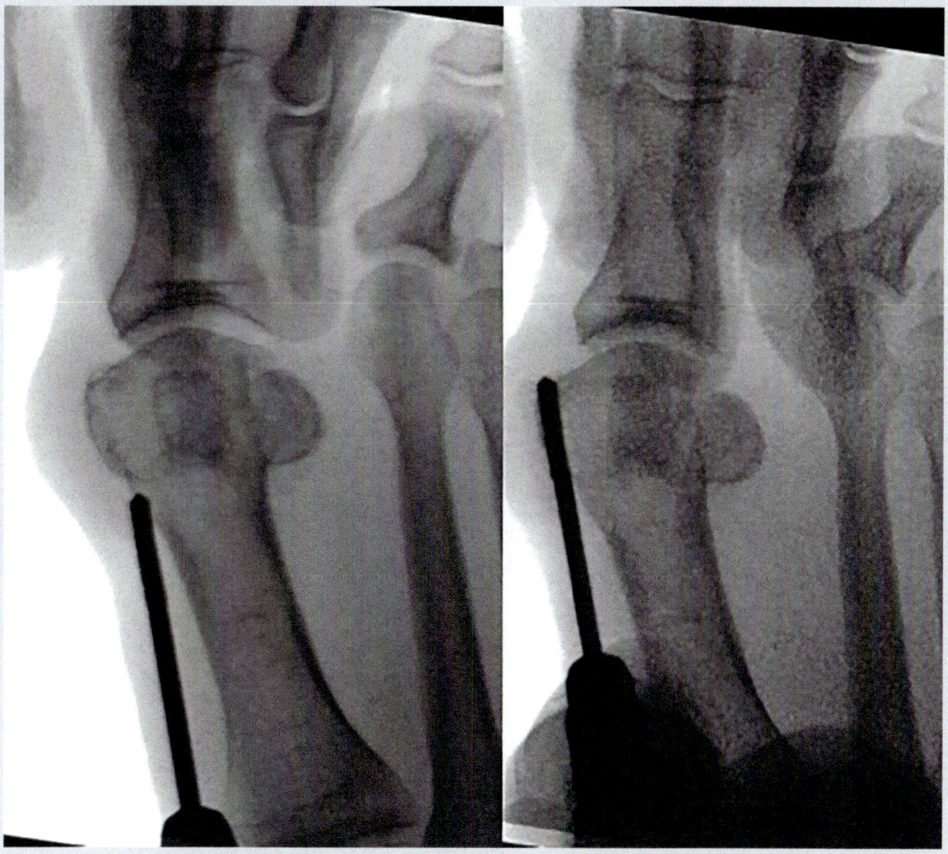

Figure 2.6 AP fluoroscopy view of the foot showing first metatarsal head medial eminence resection.

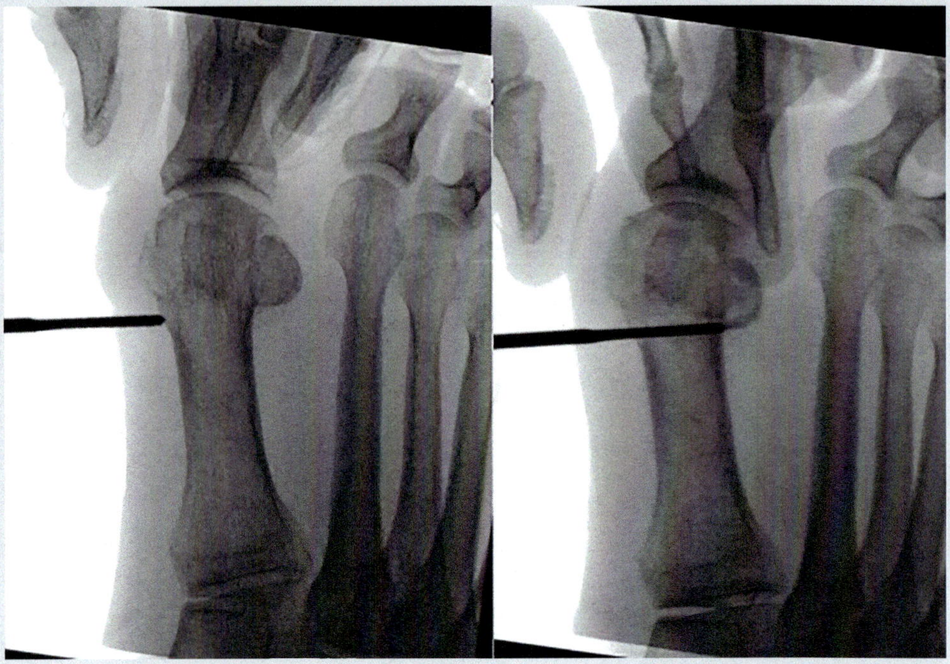

Figure 2.7 The 2.2 × 22 mm Shannon burr is inserted through the same incision used for medial eminence resection under AP fluoroscopic guidance into the base of the medial first metatarsal head flare and angled 10° distally relative to the second metatarsal shaft.

- Using an overhand grip, the 3.1-mm wedge burr is inserted directly into the medial eminence using AP fluoroscopic guidance with the burr handpiece over top of the first metatarsal shaft angling dorsal to plantar.
- The medial eminence is then resected (2 mm) with rotation of the burr plantar. Then, using a sawlike oscillating motion, resect the remaining central and dorsal medial eminence bone.
  - The surgeon may need to drop the handpiece below the first metatarsal to resect the very dorsomedial portion of the medial eminence.
  - Bone debris is expressed through the skin incision.

8. The 2.2 × 22 mm Shannon burr is then inserted through the same incision used for medial eminence resection under AP fluoroscopic guidance into the base of the medial first metatarsal head flare midaxially to avoid the dorsomedial sensory nerve.
   - The burr is angled 10° distal to the second metatarsal shaft to reduce the risk of transfer metatarsalgia and prevent shortening of the first ray due to the 2.2-mm kerf from the burr (Figure 2.7).
   - Do not angle too distal with the burr, as this can overtension the first ray and possibly lead to instability at the first tarsometatarsal joint.
9. Once the burr tip has reached the lateral cortex, an AP fluoroscopy view is obtained to confirm the trajectory of the burr. The burr is then passed through the lateral cortex (Figure 2.7).
10. For each limb of the transverse distal first metatarsal osteotomy, the surgeon should envision the end point of their hand position prior to each cut. First, in order to complete the dorsal vertical limb, the hand is rotated plantarly and the burr is rotated dorsally, using the medial skin incision as the center of rotation (fulcrum). The cut is finished with dorsomedial translation for the dorsomedial cortex. As the osteotomy is performed, the surgeon should gently oscillate the burr to ensure that they have cut the far cortex.
11. Next, the burr is returned to the center of the osteotomy. In order to complete the plantar limb of the transverse osteotomy, the hand is rotated dorsally and the burr is rotated plantarly, using the medial skin incision as the center of rotation for the osteotomy. The cut is finished with plantarmedial translation for the plantarmedial cortex.
12. Ensure that the osteotomy is complete prior to attempting to shift head in order to prevent a small cortical bridge from limiting head translation.
    - The surgeon will typically feel a slight pop or give in the osteotomy once complete.
    - Traction is pulled on the hallux to distract the osteotomy and ensure it is complete prior to shifting.
13. An elevator is inserted across the osteotomy site to distract the osteotomy and free any remaining periosteum attachments, allowing for easier lateral shift of the first metatarsal head (Figure 2.8).
14. If using a jig, the paddle of the jig is inserted into the medial first metatarsal incision and placed midaxially over the medial first metatarsal head. The first metatarsal shaft metal pin is inserted through the jig at the osteotomy site into the first metatarsal shaft and locked into the jig (Figure 2.9).
    - Pull traction and valgus on the hallux to facilitate pin entry into the osteotomy site.
    - Ensure that the jig is all the way down to bone at the osteotomy site.

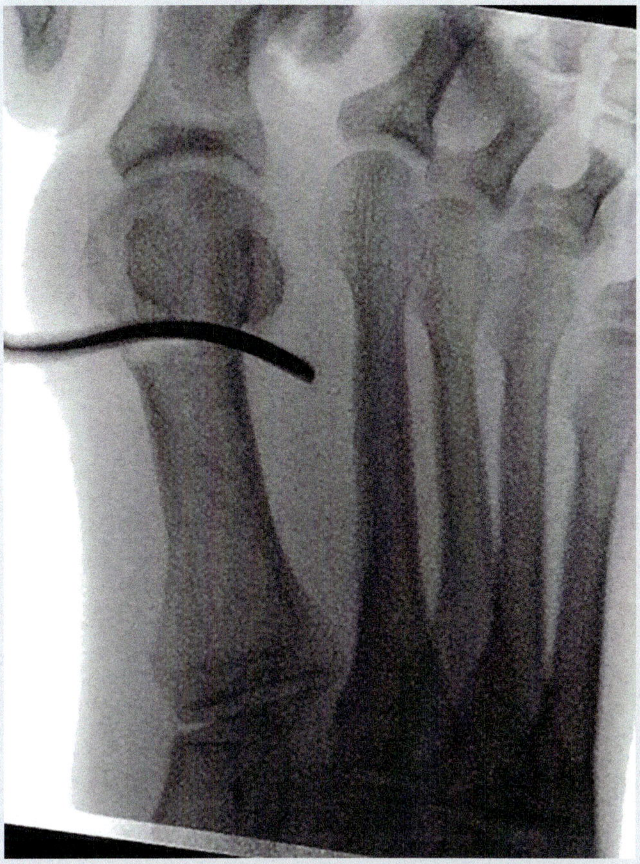

Figure 2.8 An elevator is inserted across the osteotomy site in order to distract the osteotomy site and free up any remaining periosteum.

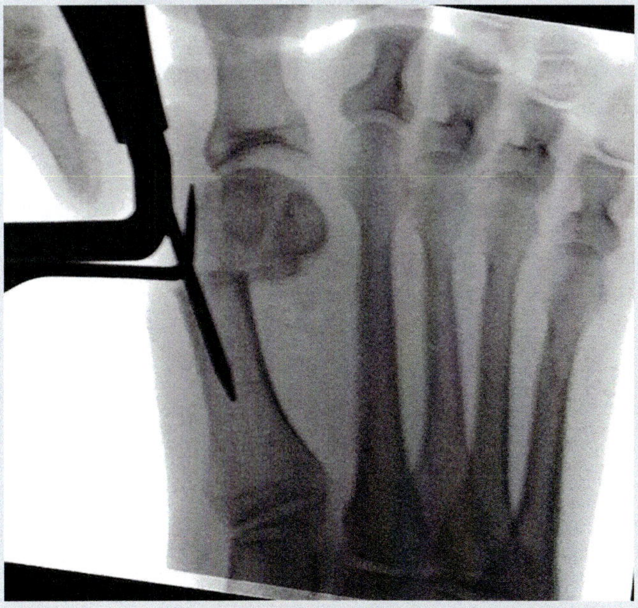

Figure 2.9 The paddle of the jig is inserted into the medial first metatarsal incision and placed midaxially over the medial first metatarsal head. The metal pin is then placed through the jig at the osteotomy site into the first metatarsal shaft and locked into the jig.

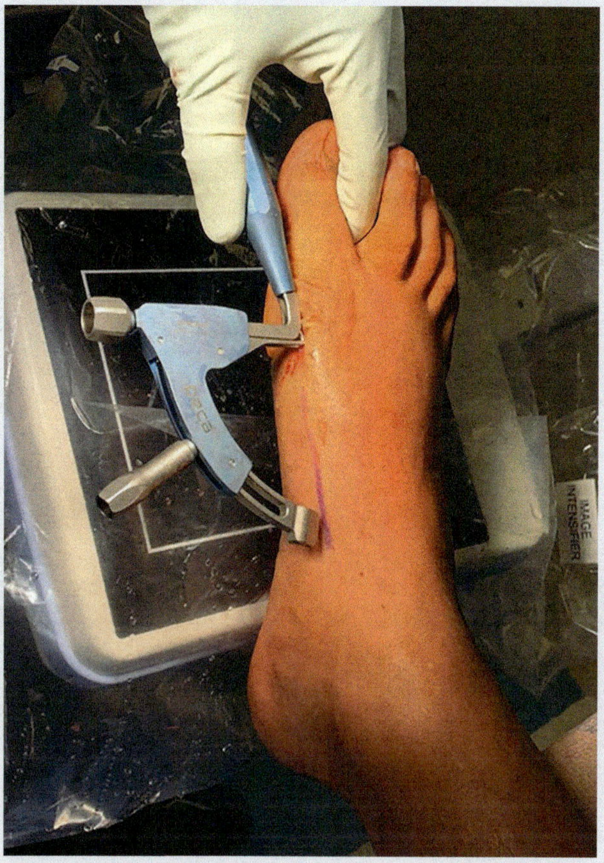

Figure 2.10 The jig is placed all the way down to bone at the osteotomy site. The hallux is supinated and pulled into varus with the handpiece compressed against the hallux in order to correct the hallux valgus deformity.

15. The arm for wire guides is extended and locked into place.
16. The hallux is supinated and pulled into varus with the handpiece compressed against the hallux in order to correct the hallux valgus deformity (Figure 2.10).
    - The dial on the jig is turned in order to obtain further correction of the hallux valgus deformity (Figure 2.11).
17. Using the jig, the first threaded tip guidewire for a 4.0-mm fully threaded, cannulated headless screw is inserted proximally at the base of the medial first metatarsal.
    - The guidewire should exit the lateral distal first metatarsal shaft cortex approximately 8 to 10 mm from the osteotomy site for stability of the construct (Figure 2.12).
18. Again, using the jig, the second threaded tip guidewire for a 4.0-mm fully threaded, cannulated headless screw is inserted distal to the proximal guidewire (Figure 2.13).
19. Wire position is checked on AP and lateral fluoroscopy views of the foot (Figure 2.14).
    - The jig is removed if adequate wire position has been obtained.
    - Wire may be repositioned with the jig removed if necessary.
20. (If not using a jig) Once the capital fragment is mobile, traction is pulled on the hallux and the thick end of the

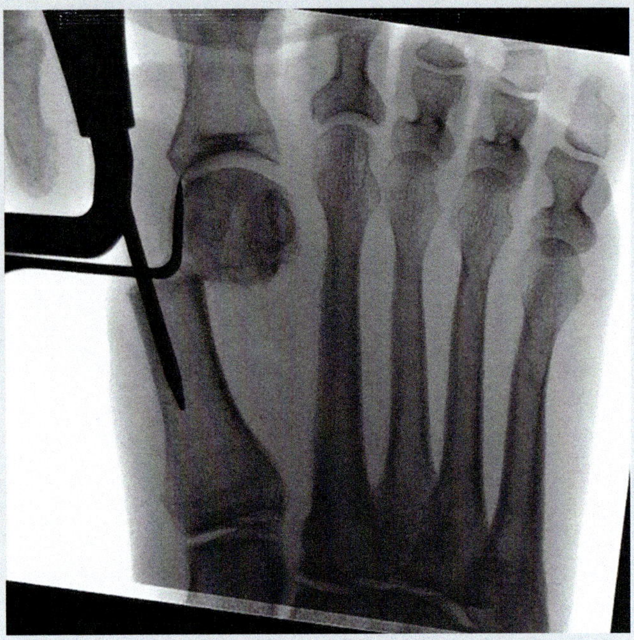

Figure 2.11 The dial on the jig is turned in order to obtain correction of the hallux valgus deformity.

head-shifting tool is inserted through the distal first metatarsal incision into the first metatarsal shaft. Again, traction is pulled on the hallux, and the hallux is supinated with varus stress to shift the first metatarsal head laterally relative to the shaft and lock out the first tarsometatarsal joint into varus. Proper sagittal alignment and rotation of the head relative to the shaft are checked on AP and lateral fluoroscopy views of the foot (Figure 2.15).
- Guidewire position is confirmed on AP and lateral fluoroscopy views of the foot.

21. A small longitudinal 4-mm incision is made over each of the guidewire insertion sites.
22. Each guidewire is then measured and overdrilled.
    - For an odd reading, 5 mm is taken off of the measurement, and for an even reading, 4 mm is taken off of the measurement in order to avoid prominent screw hardware.
    - The surgeon should always drill into the first metatarsal head, and if good bone quality, drill up to 2 to 4 mm from the tip of the guidewire.
23. The proximal first metatarsal 4.0-mm percutaneous chevron Akin (PECA) screw is inserted on power through the chamfered screw insertion sleeve to prevent skin injury. Screw insertion is finished by hand.
24. The distal first metatarsal 4.0-mm PECA screw is inserted on power through the chamfered screw insertion sleeve to prevent skin injury. Screw insertion is finished by hand.
25. AP and lateral fluoroscopy views are checked to confirm that the screw heads are not prominent and that the screw tips are not within the first metatarsophalangeal joint (Figure 2.16).
    - Typically, the screw tips are 2 to 4 mm from the articular surface.

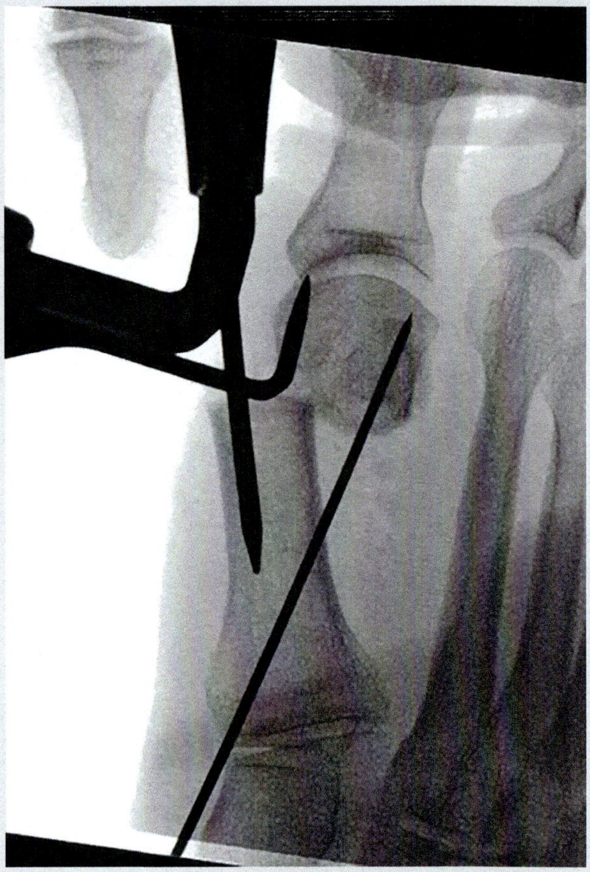

Figure 2.12 Using the jig, the first threaded tip guidewire is inserted for a 4.0-mm fully threaded, cannulated headless screw proximally at the base of the medial first metatarsal. The wire should exit the lateral distal first metatarsal shaft cortex at least approximately 8 to 10 mm from osteotomy site.

26. The medial spike of first metatarsal shaft bone is excised using a 3-mm wedge burr or 2.2 × 22 mm Shannon burr typically through the distal screw insertion incision, although this can also be performed through the osteotomy incision if preferred. The medial spike is cut using a sawlike oscillating motion from plantar to dorsal (to avoid damaging dorsomedial sensory nerve) and then completed with rotation of the burr tip dorsally to cut the dorsomedial portion of the distal first metatarsal shaft (Figure 2.17).
    - Maintain a lateral pressure on the burr to prevent it from skiving medially over the shaft.
    - The surgeon only needs to leave 1 to 2 mm of bone between the area of medial distal first metatarsal spike excision and the distal screw.
    - The free bone fragment may then either be removed with a hemostat through the osteotomy incision using a mosquito clamp or synovial rongeur, or pushed into the osteotomy site as bone graft.
    - A synovial rongeur may be used to remove any remaining sharp bony prominence through the osteotomy incision.
27. A percutaneous lateral release is rarely necessary but may be performed with fluoroscopic guidance.[2] The order of lateral release is sequential and includes the lateral

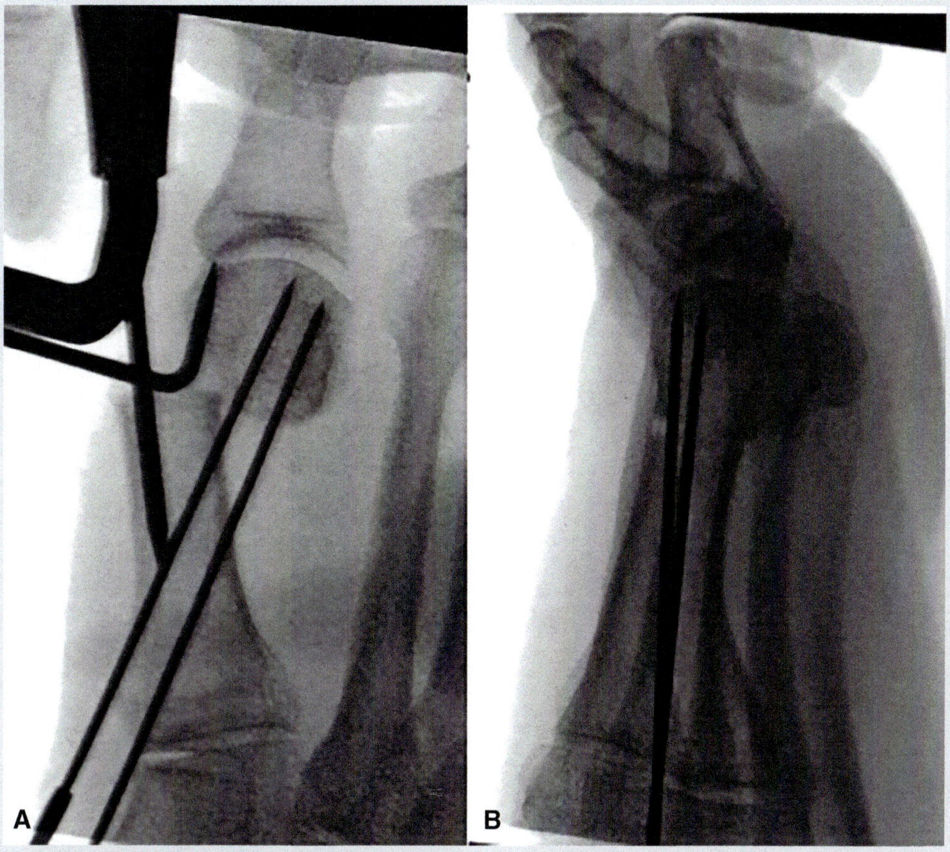

Figure 2.13 The second threaded tip guidewire for a 4.0-mm fully threaded, cannulated headless screw is inserted distal to the proximal guidewire, and wire position is checked on AP **(A)** and **(B)** lateral fluoroscopy views of the foot after removing the jig.

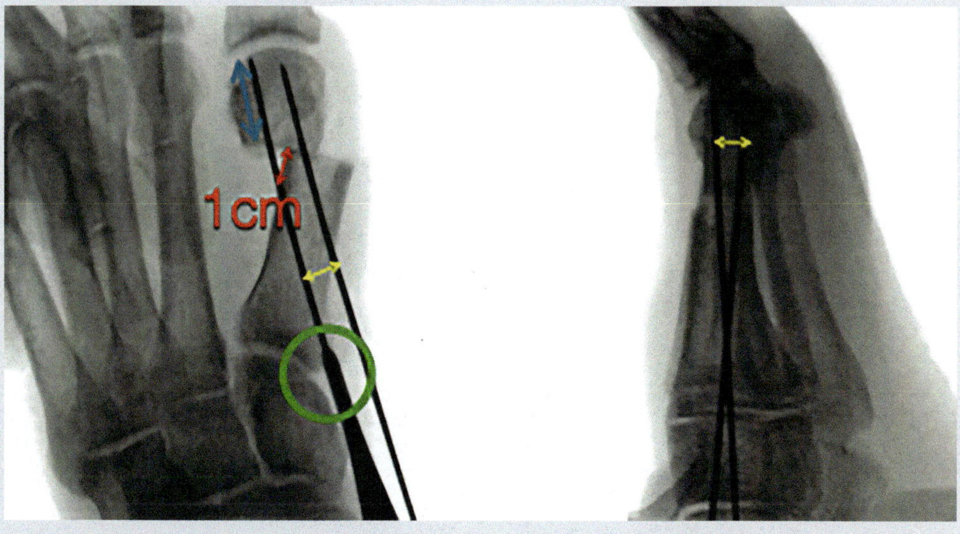

Figure 2.14 The proximal guidewire is inserted at the base of the first metatarsal (*green circle*), exits the lateral first metatarsal cortex at least 8 to 10 mm from the osteotomy site (*red arrow*), and runs parallel to the lateral first metatarsal head cortex (*blue arrow*). There is spacing between the two guidewires on the AP and lateral views (*yellow arrows*).

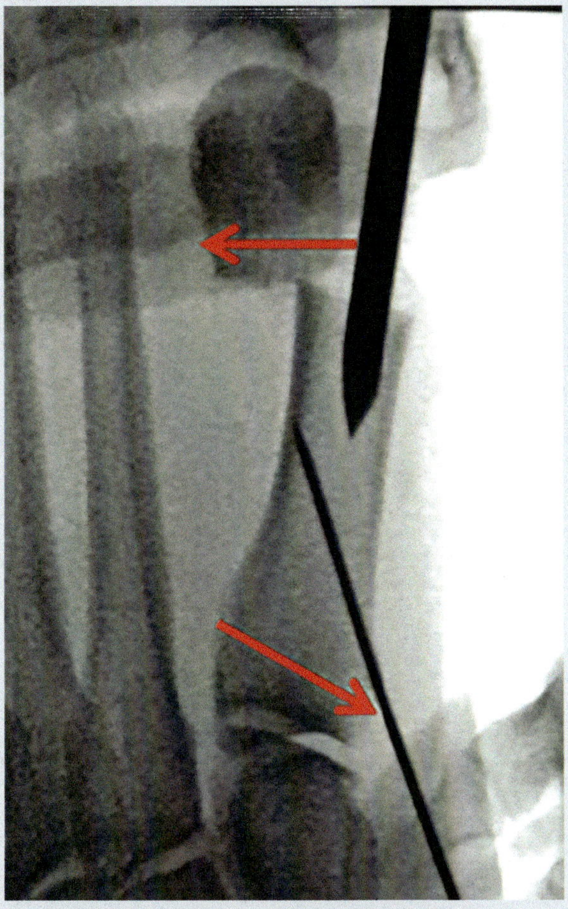

Figure 2.15 The thick end of the head-shifting tool is inserted through the distal first metatarsal incision into the first metatarsal shaft. The first metatarsal head is shifted laterally relative to the shaft while the first tarsometatarsal joint is locked out in varus (*arrows*).

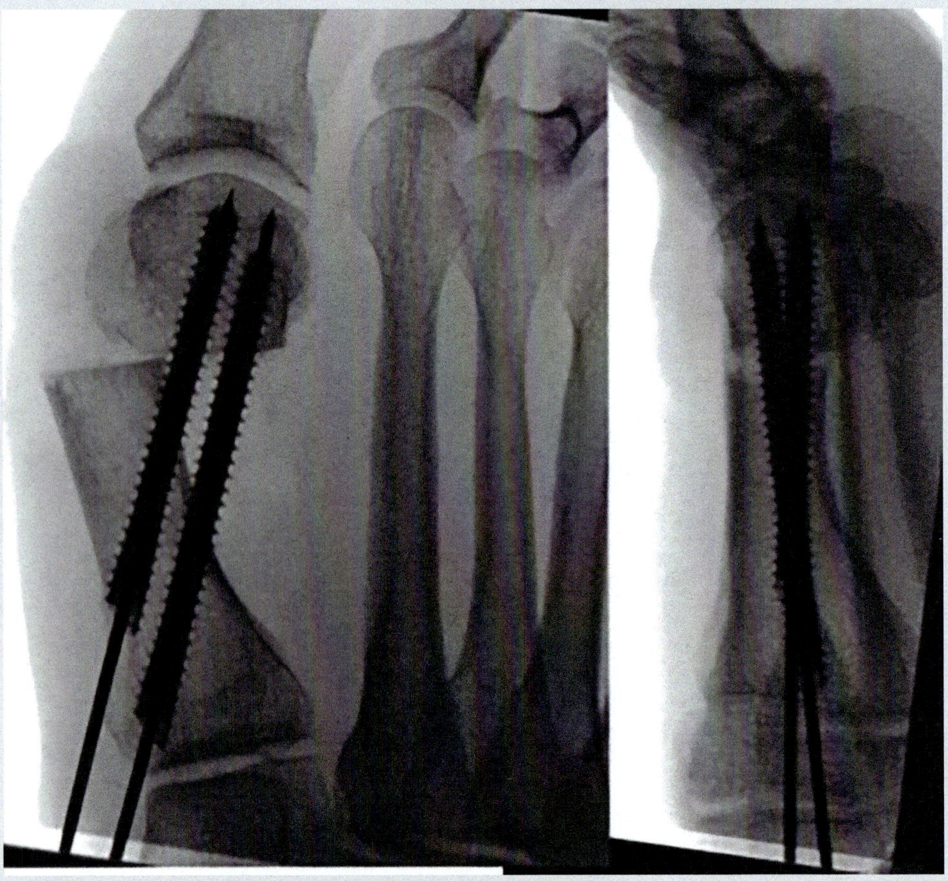

Figure 2.16 An AP fluoroscopy view of the foot is checked to confirm that the screw heads are not prominent and that the screw tips are not within the first metatarsophalangeal joint.

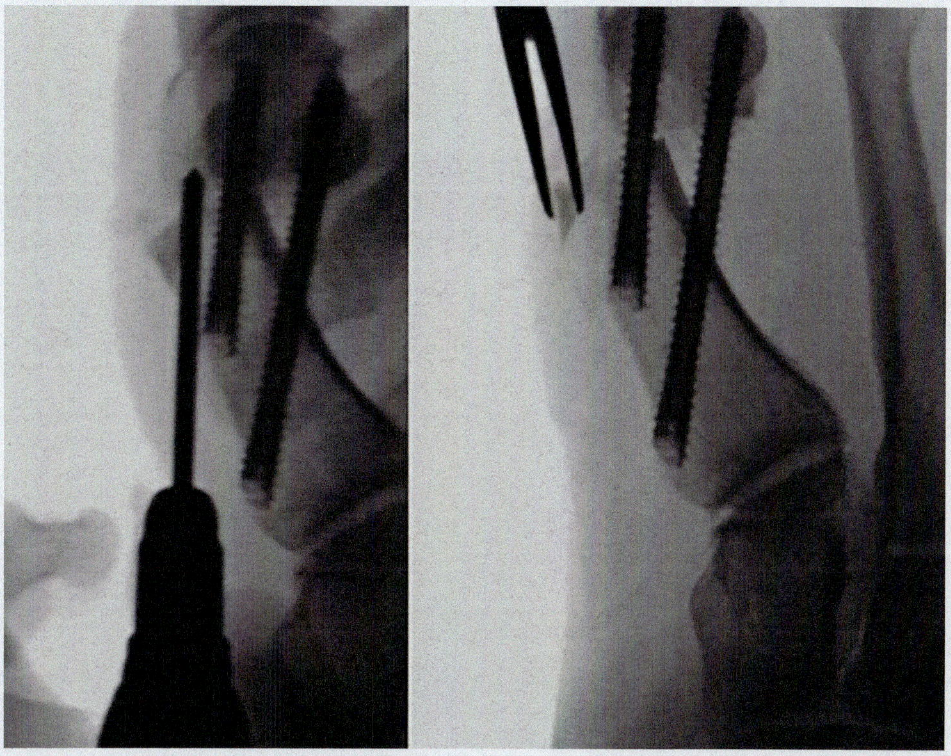

Figure 2.17 The medial distal first metatarsal shaft spike is cut using a sawlike oscillating motion from plantar to dorsal through the distal screw insertion incision.The free bone fragment is then removed through the osteotomy incision.

metatarsosesamoid ligament, followed by the adductor hallucis tendon, and finally, the lateral phalangeosesamoid ligament. Release of the adductor hallucis tendon or lateral phalangeosesamoid ligament may increase the risk of developing hallux varus.

Akin Osteotomy

1. An Akin osteotomy is commonly performed for further correction of hallux valgus deformity or hallux interphalangeus deformity. Using an AP fluoroscopy view of the foot, a medial longitudinal midaxial incision is made at the proximal diaphysis of the hallux proximal phalanx.
2. The 2 × 12 mm Shannon burr is inserted midaxially and angled retrograde toward the lateral proximal metaphysis of the hallux proximal phalanx while preserving the lateral cortex (Figure 2.18).
3. The dorsal limb of the Akin osteotomy is completed while holding the hallux interphalangeal joint dorsiflexed to prevent damage to the extensor hallucis longus tendon.
   - The goal is to maintain central lateral cortex, but the dorsolateral cortex must be cut in order to close down Akin osteotomy.
4. The plantar limb is completed with the hallux interphalangeal joint plantarflexed to prevent damage to the flexor hallucis longus tendon.
   - The goal is to maintain central lateral cortex, but the plantarlateral cortex must be cut in order to close down Akin osteotomy.
5. With varus stress, the medial hallux proximal phalanx Akin osteotomy is closed down in order to correct the residual hallux valgus deformity.
6. A 1.0-mm guidewire for the 3.0-mm PECA screw is then placed percutaneously from the medial base of the hallux proximal phalanx across the Akin osteotomy site and just through the distal lateral cortex.

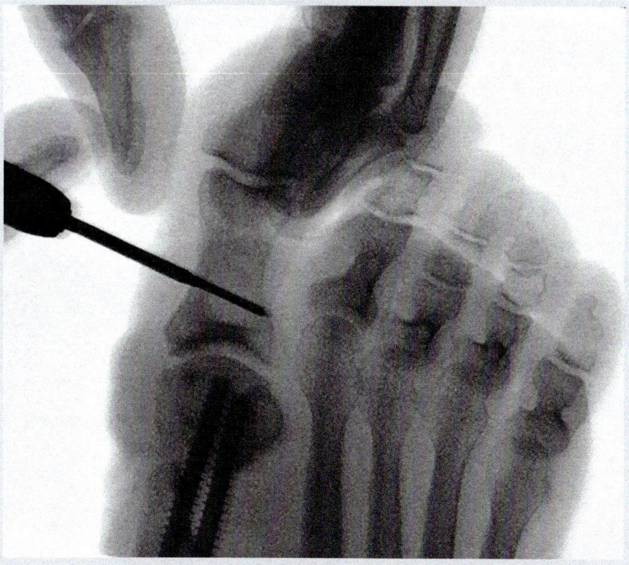

Figure 2.18 The 2 × 12 mm Shannon burr is inserted midaxially and angled retrograde toward the lateral proximal metaphysis of the hallux proximal phalanx while preserving the lateral cortex.

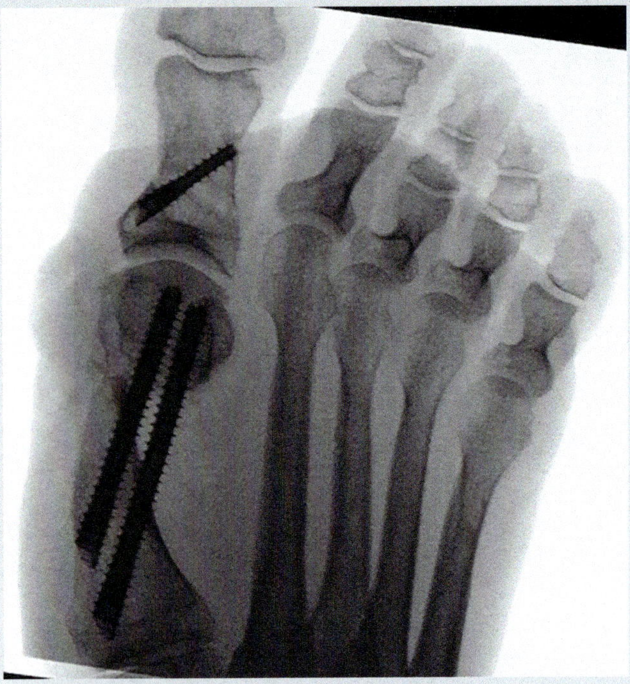

Figure 2.19 The 3.0-mm headless chamfered screw is inserted across the Akin osteotomy after closing down the medial cortex.

7. Guidewire position is checked on AP and lateral fluoroscopy views of the foot and then measured.
   - Always take 2 mm off of Akin screw guidewire measurement to ensure that the screw is not prominent and reduce risk of hardware irritation.
8. The guidewire is advanced through lateral hallux and out of the skin. It is then clamped with a hemostat in order to prevent wire removal with overdrilling.
9. The wire is overdrilled through both cortices, and a 3.0-mm PECA screw is inserted (Figure 2.19).
10. The incisions are closed with a single 3.0-mm monofilament suture or adhesive strips.
11. The incisions are dressed with a nonadherent layer, 4 × 4 in gauze, cotton wrap, and ace wrap.

◆ POSTOPERATIVE CARE

- The bunion dressing is left in place for 1 to 2 weeks and kept dry.
- The dressing and sutures are removed at 1 to 2 weeks.
- Immediate weight bearing as tolerated is allowed once the nerve block has worn off **in a heel-bearing postoperative** shoe for 4 weeks followed by supportive sneakers for 2 months.
- A soft forefoot compression sleeve may be applied at 4 weeks postoperatively to assist with edema reduction.
- Physical therapy is offered at the 2-week postoperative visit to begin at 5 weeks postoperatively.
- Patient may start stationary bike at 2 weeks, walking for exercise at 4 weeks, elliptical at 6 weeks, and running/heels/sports at 3 months postoperatively.

◆ COMPLICATIONS

- Infection
- Wound problems
- Hardware irritation
- Osteotomy nonunion
- Dorsomedial sensory nerve injury

References

1. Aiyer A, Massel DH, Siddiqui N, Acevedo JI. Biomechanical comparison of 2 common techniques of minimally invasive hallux valgus correction. *Foot Ankle Int.* 2021;42(3):373-380.
2. Dalmau-Pastor M, Malagelada F, Cordier G, et al. Anatomical study of minimally invasive lateral release techniques for hallux valgus treatment. *Foot Ankle Int.* 2020;41(8):984-992.

3 Basal Closing Wedge Osteotomy

Gustavo A. Nunes and Joel Vernois

◆ INTRODUCTION

Hallux valgus consists of a complex pathology with a multifactorial etiology involving anatomical, hereditary, and biomechanics factors.[1,2] There are numerous surgical techniques described, including distal, diaphyseal, or proximal osteotomies. Regardless of the technique chosen, the multiple intrinsic factors involved in the pathophysiology of this disease must be corrected.[3,4]

The basal closing wedge osteotomy (BCWO) of the first metatarsal is a popular procedure used for years to treat hallux valgus associated with metatarsus primus varus.[5,6] As a proximal metatarsal procedure, this osteotomy provides a great potential for correction and is traditionally recommended for moderate to severe hallux valgus with large intermetatarsal angle (IMA).[5,6] This technique was first described in 1901 by Loison as a lateral basal closing wedge of the first metatarsal fixed with Kirschner wires (K-wires).[7] Over time, this procedure underwent some modifications and was consolidated as an oblique wedge osteotomy with a medial hinge at the base of the first metatarsal fixed with screws.[8-10] With the more recent introduction of minimally invasive surgery, this technique has once again evolved.[11] BCWO can be performed percutaneously, thus combining the benefits of a stable osteotomy fixed by screws with minimal soft-tissue manipulation.[12,13] The purpose of this chapter is to present the general technical considerations for percutaneous BCWO.

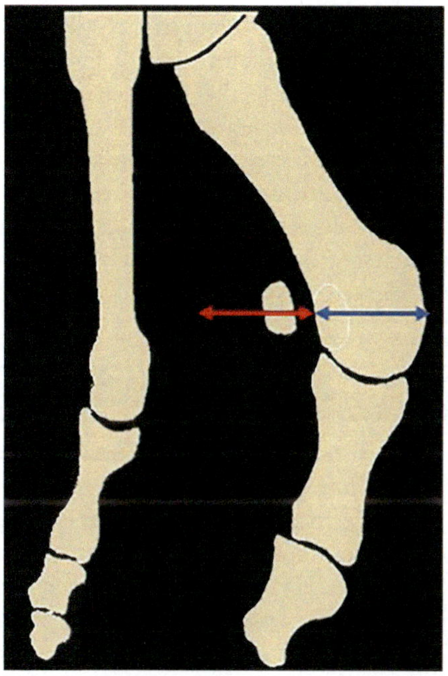

Figure 3.1 Schematic view of a severe hallux valgus with a large intermetatarsal angle in which the size of the first metatarsal head is not wide enough to cover the intermetatarsal space after a 100% lateral translation.

◆ INDICATIONS AND CONTRAINDICATIONS

The indication for the percutaneous BCWO is moderate to severe hallux valgus cases with an incongruent first metatarsal phalangeal joint (1MTPJ) in patients with good bone quality. This technique is preferred over the distal osteotomies in those cases with a severe deformity due to a large IMA, in which the size of the first metatarsal head would not be wide enough to appropriately close the intermetatarsal space following a 100% lateral translation[12,13] (Figure 3.1).

BCWO can also be performed in other circumstances. In patients with moderate to severe hallux valgus with congruent 1MTPJ due to a pathological distal metatarsal articular angle (DMMA), the percutaneous BCWO can be used as long as it is associated with a distal procedure.[3,14] Hypermobility of the first tarsometatarsal joint (1TMTJ) is not necessarily a contraindication as with the percutaneous BCWO the proximal fragment is fixed in the most medialized position, as is done with the percutaneous chevron osteotomy.[12,13,15] Because the BCWO resects a basal wedge, thus shortening the first metatarsal, in patients with associated transfer metatarsalgia with plantar callosities, the authors recommend adding a minimally invasive distal metatarsal osteotomy of the second, third, and fourth metatarsals.[16] One of the limitations of the BCWO is the lack of rotational correction of the first ray in light of the integrity of the dorsomedial hinge. Given the attention that the three-dimensional correction of bunions is attracting the readers need to understand the implications of the BCWO and therefore the need to possibly having to add a distal metatarsal osteotomy to correct the sesamoid position.[17,18]

◆ PATIENT HISTORY AND PHYSICAL EXAMINATION

Patient history includes duration of symptoms, impact of the bunion on activity levels, footwear restrictions, and associated clinical comorbidities such as diabetes, vasculopathy, and rheumatologic conditions.

A comprehensive physical examination of a patient with hallux valgus should be carried out with the patient weight bearing as well as non–weight bearing and must include assessment of the gait, the hindfoot, midfoot, and forefoot alignment. Special attention should be directed toward the 1MTPJ evaluating its position, range of motion, deformity reducibility, and areas of tenderness. Any limitation in either dorsiflexion or plantarflexion of the 1MTPJ should be noted and compared to the contralateral foot as it can suggest intra-articular degeneration.[19] The first ray hypermobility is clinically assessed through the first ray splay test (Figure 3.2A) and the range of motion analysis of the 1TMTJ.[15] The associated lesser toe deformities, plantar callosities, metatarsalgia, and gastrocnemius contracture must also be documented.[19]

◆ IMAGING STUDIES

Weight-bearing three-view radiographs are crucial for the evaluation of hallux valgus and play an important role in classifying the severity of the deformity and its surgical treatment. The most commonly used measurements include the hallux valgus angle (HVA), the IMA between the first and second rays (IMA), the DMMA, and the sesamoids position according to the Hardy and Clapham classification.[20] The true IMA can be assessed with a radiographic splay test[15] (Figure 3.2B).

The congruence and presence of degenerative signs of the 1MTPJ and 1TMTJ should also be noted. The 1TMTJ asymmetry may be an indirect sign of a first ray hypermobility.[17] Lastly, the frontal plane view allows for evaluation of the rotational deformity.

The latter can be calculated on the AP radiographs using the lateral shape of the metatarsal head as described by Okuda et al. or on weight-bearing computed tomography (WBCT) through the alpha angle described by Mahmoud et al.[18]

Magnetic resonance imaging has a secondary role in the evaluation of hallux valgus. Its main indication is to evaluate degenerative signs of the 1MTPJ, including lesions of the cartilage or the hallux-sesamoid complex. It may also be useful to evaluate abnormalities of the muscles, tendons, collateral ligaments, and plantar plate.[20]

◆ PREOPERATIVE PLANNING AND PREPARATION

The equipment used includes Beaver blade, periosteal elevator, rasp, 2 × 20 mm Shannon and 3.1-mm wedge burrs, power tool (dedicated low-speed, high torque handpiece), and C-arm fluoroscopy. Intravenous antibiotics are given during induction as per physician preference. The procedure is performed under general anesthesia and always without tourniquet. The patient is positioned supine with the feet hanging off the end of the table, supported by the C-arm. For the right-handed surgeon, the authors' preference is for the C-arm to be positioned on the patient's right side, whereas the surgeon stands on the patient's left side. For left-handed surgeon, the position is reversed.

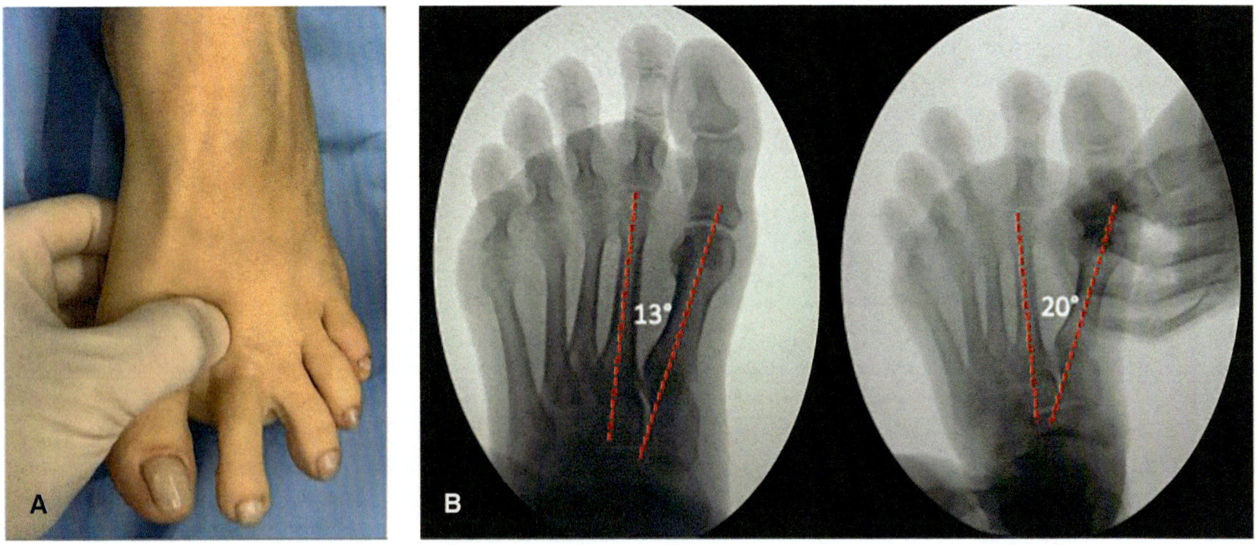

Figure 3.2 **A.** Clinical splay test. **B.** Fluoroscopic image showing the increase of the intermetatarsal angle with the splay test.

SURGICAL TECHNIQUE

1. The first step is to manually increase the IMA and the first ray dorsiflexion. While the first metatarsal is maintained in the most medial (squeezing the first space) and dorsiflexed position, a 2-mm K-wire is inserted from the base of the first metatarsal, parallel to the TMTJ, to the base of the second metatarsal, thus stabilizing the deformity (Figure 3.3).
2. With a Beaver blade, a dorsal portal is created at the proximal third of the first metatarsal, just lateral to the extensor hallucis longus (Figure 3.4).
3. Through this portal, a 2 × 20 mm Shannon burr is introduced in the middle of the first metatarsal in a perpendicular way, cutting the dorsal and plantar cortex.
4. With the burr inside the bone, the surgeon performs an oblique osteotomy going from medial proximal to lateral and distal, preserving the dorsomedial cortex (Figure 3.5).
5. Sequentially, a large diameter burr is introduced into the osteotomy site to increase the osteotomy wedge and the power of correction of this procedure. Using a 3.1-mm wedge burr, the gesture described above is cautiously performed again in order to maintain the dorsomedial cortex intact (Figure 3.6).
6. The osteotomy is then closed manually correcting the deformity. To close the osteotomy wedge, the surgeon has to perform a reduction maneuver with lateralization and plantarization of the distal fragment (Figure 3.7A).

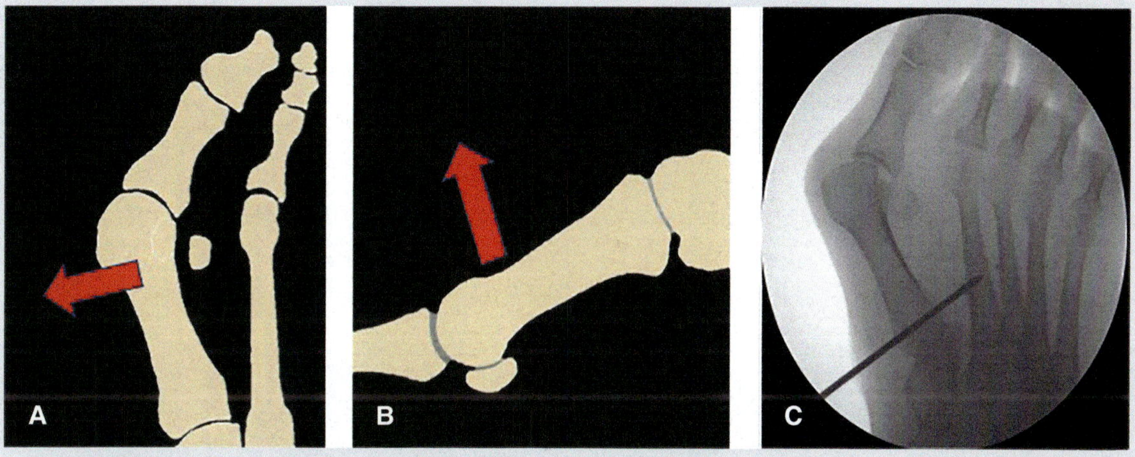

Figure 3.3 **A.** The first intermetatarsal space is squeezed, medializing the first metatarsal. **B.** At the same time, a dorsiflexion force is applied under the first ray. **C.** A 2-mm Kirschner wire is inserted from the base of the first metatarsal to the second metatarsal, stabilizing this position.

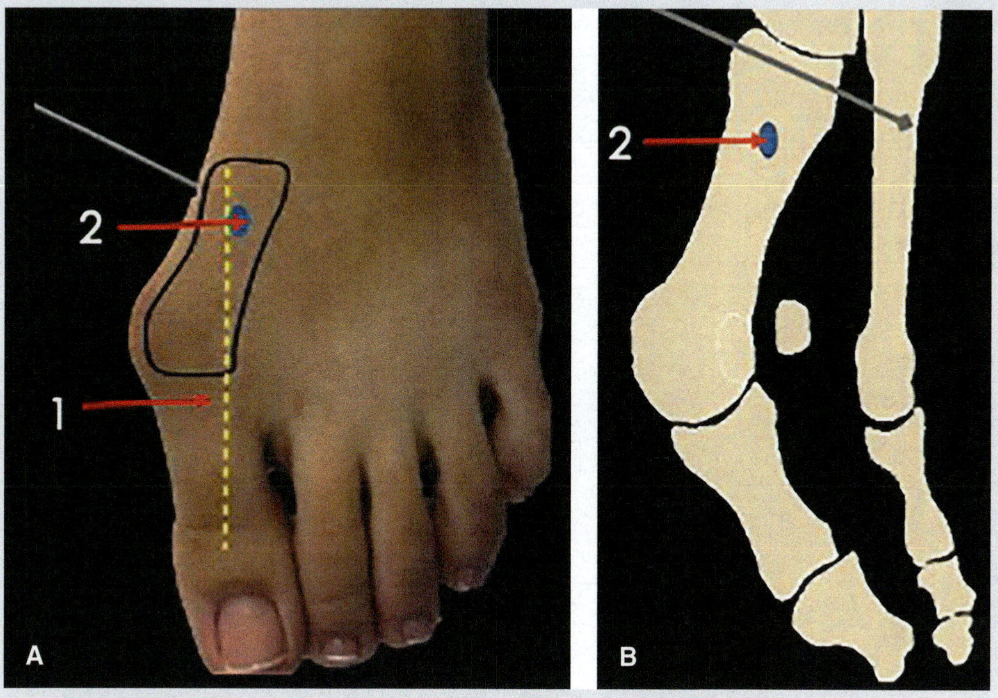

Figure 3.4 Dorsal approach lateral to the extensor hallucis longus (EHL) tendon. **A.** Clinical view. **B.** Schematic view. (*1*) EHL and (*2*) level of the approach.

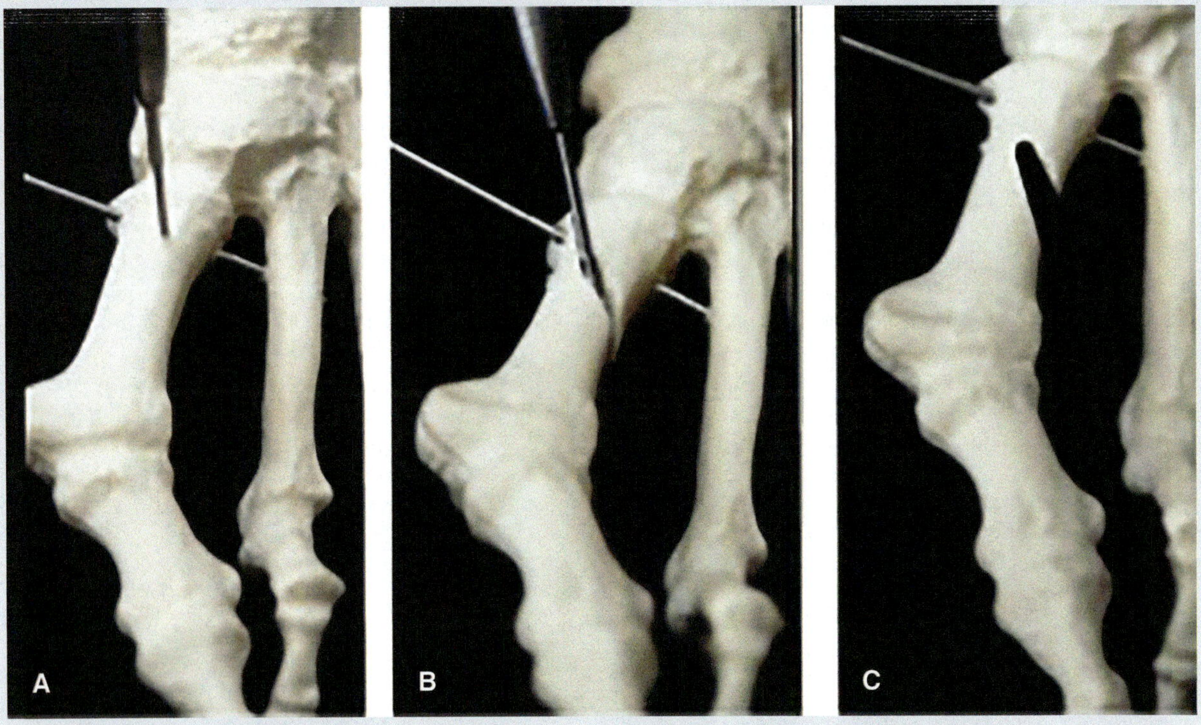

Figure 3.5 Schematic view of the osteotomy. **A.** Burr entry point. **B.** Osteotomy distal and lateral orientation. **C.** Lateral wedge removed.

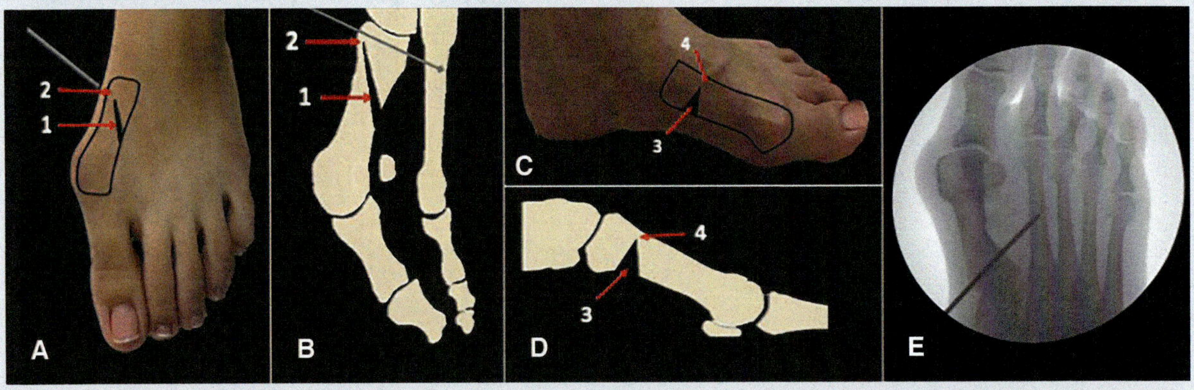

Figure 3.6 Lateral wedge removed from the base of the first metatarsal preserving the dorsomedial cortex. **A.** Anteroposterior clinical view. **B.** Anteroposterior schematic view. **C.** Sagittal clinical view. **D.** Sagittal schematic view. **E.** Fluoroscopic image after the basal osteotomy. (*1*) Medial wedge (*2*) Intact medial cortex (*3*) Plantar wedge (*4*) Intact dorsal cortex.

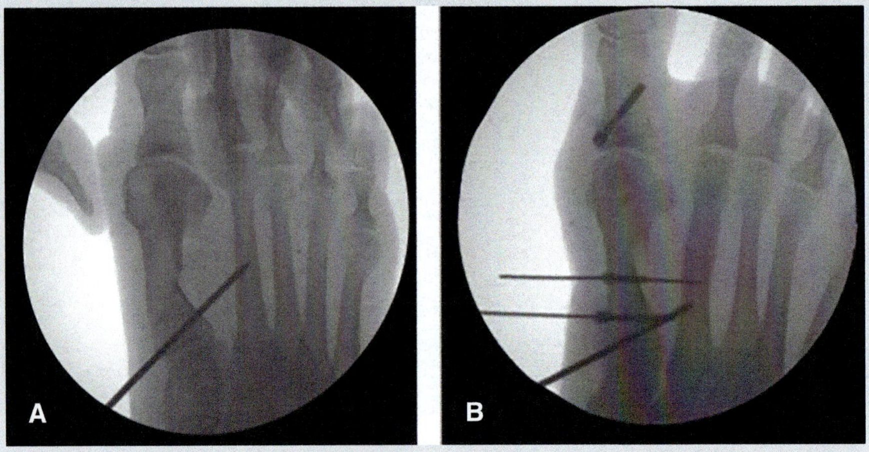

Figure 3.7 **A.** Fluoroscopic image after the reduction maneuver demonstrating correction of the deformity. **B.** Osteotomy fixation using two 3.0-mm cannulated screws.

7. The osteotomy reduction is temporally fixed with two 1.0-mm K-wires and then fixed with one or two 3.0-mm cannulated headless screws going from medial to lateral. If there is space to use two screws, the first one should be inserted at the level of the apex of the osteotomy and the other parallel and distally closing the osteotomy wedge (Figure 3.7B).
8. In cases where, even after correction of the deformity, there is still an incongruity of the 1MTPJ or the lateral sesamoid remains uncovered, the release of the lateral soft tissues (sesamoid-phalangeal ligament and lateral head of the flexor hallucis brevis) can be added.
9. An additional exostectomy of the medial eminence of the metatarsal head can also be performed as needed. Through an incision at the base of the flare of the medial eminence, a periosteal elevator is used to elevate the capsule from the bone. A 3.1-mm wedge burr is then advanced to perform the exostectomy. The bone debris is removed using the dedicated percutaneous rasps, and the joint is flushed with saline solution.
10. Finally, the Akin osteotomy is added in patients with residual deformity at the level of the hallux interphalangeal joint. It is undertaken by a midaxial portal on the medial aspect of the proximal phalanx. The 2 × 10 mm Shannon burr is inserted through this portal into the proximal metadiaphyseal junction and angled proximally. Said orientation of the osteotomy will make its fixation easier. The cut is completed both dorsally and plantarly while leaving the lateral cortex intact. The osteotomy is then manually reduced and stabilized with a 3.0-mm headless screw.
11. The procedure is completed with the closure of the surgical incisions and application of a padded dressing and adhesive tape. It is important to emphasize that the dressing must push the distal fragment laterally to help maintain the correction.

● PEARLS AND PITFALLS

- During the introduction of the burr, a mosquito clamp should be used to protect the soft tissues, especially the extensor hallucis longus tendon.
- A longer osteotomy facilitates fixation with two screws. Ideally, the osteotomy should be at approximately 45° angle to the metatarsal axis.
- Preservation of the dorsomedial cortex is essential to avoid dorsal malunion of the distal fragment.
- During the reduction maneuver, the 1MTPJ should be dorsiflexed to increase the plantarflexion forces on the distal fragment through a windlass mechanism.
- If it is not possible to close the medial wedge after the osteotomy with a 3.1-mm wedge burr, additional bone from the medial plantar cortex can be carefully removed using a 2 × 20 mm Shannon burr.
- In cases with pathological DMMA, it is mandatory to add a distal procedure together with the percutaneous BCWO.

◆ POSTOPERATIVE MANAGEMENT

At discharge, patients are allowed partial weight bearing in a heel wedge orthopedic shoe. During the first 14 days after surgery, they are instructed to keep their foot elevated above the level of the ipsilateral hip to minimize postoperative swelling. After the first week, the surgical dressing is replaced by an elastic bandage. Thereafter, the dressings are changed weekly until the 4th week. Gentle hallux range of motion exercises are recommended in the 2nd week and gradually progressed as deemed appropriate by the surgeon at the subsequent follow-up visits. After the 6th week, patients are allowed to wear regular shoes with a wide toe box and a rigid sole. Weight-bearing radiographs are ordered after 6 and 12 weeks of surgery (Figure 3.8). Low-impact sports such as cycling and swimming are allowed after the 6th week, whereas impact sports are allowed after the 3rd month.

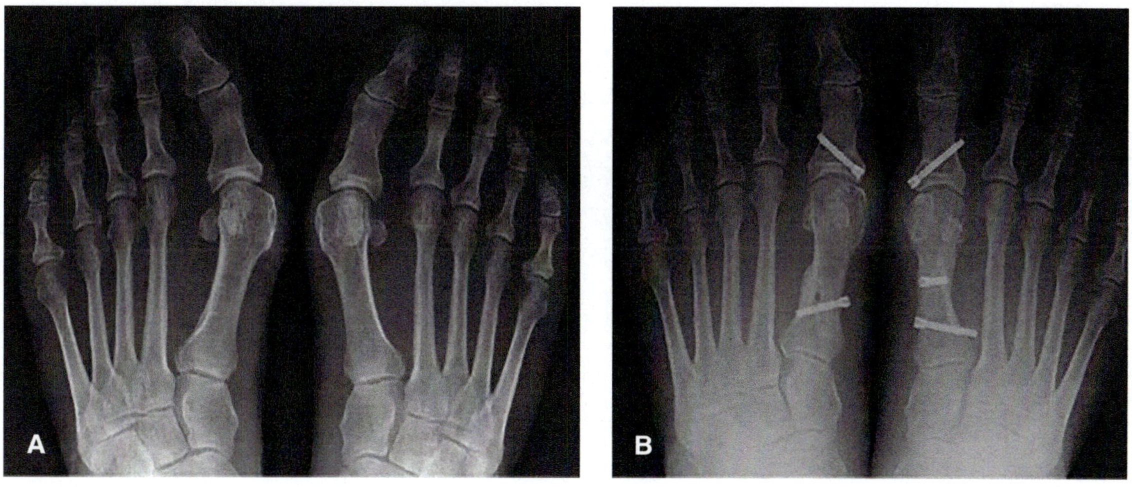

Figure 3.8 Bilateral severe hallux valgus treated with percutaneous basal closing wedge osteotomy and Akin osteotomy. **A.** Preoperative radiograph. **B.** Postoperative radiographic control showing bone consolidation.

◆ OUTCOMES

BCWO is a popular procedure used for correction of severe hallux valgus.[5] In relation to the percutaneous method, there are few studies in the literature analyzing its results.[21] With respect to radiographic outcomes, the percutaneous technique presents similar results to the open technique.[22] De Lavigne et al. described the first series of six patients affected by severe hallux valgus and treated with a double osteotomy, percutaneous BCWO fixed with screws and distal chevron. They reported an average decrease of the HVA and IMA of 27° and 11°, respectively.[23] In another study, Kurashige and Suzuki reported the 22-month postoperative radiographic outcomes of 17 feet with severe hallux valgus that underwent a percutaneous BCWO with Akin osteotomy. The authors observed a correction of the HVA and IMA of 27.8° and 8.7°, respectively.[22] Table 3.1 summarizes the radiographic outcomes of open and percutaneous BCWO.

Correcting severe deformities is challenging in light of the increased complication rates.[25] The largest series described by Vernois included 100 patients with a 1-year follow-up that described a 15% of complication rate. The most common complication was loss of reduction in 10 patients, of which three required surgical revision. There were also two cases of discomfort at the screw head, one infection, and two delayed unions.[13] Regarding the open BCWO, there is a concern about transfer metatarsalgia secondary to dorsal malunion of the proximal fragment and an excessive shortening of the first metatarsal. This complication is not commonly observed with the percutaneous method as the dorsomedial hinge is preserved, thus preventing elevation of the distal fragment. In addition, during the reduction maneuver, a slight plantarflexion of the distal fragment is also performed to mitigate said risk.[13,21]

Generally, there is concern about the recurrence of the deformity, especially in severe cases.[15] Unfortunately, there are no hallux valgus recurrence data in the literature with the percutaneous BCWO. Another concern with the percutaneous BCWO is the impossibility to address rotational deformities of the first metatarsal.[18] In fact, the preservation of the dorsomedial hinge prevents full freedom of movement of the distal fragment.[13] Although two case series demonstrated an improvement of the sesamoid coverage postoperatively—an indirect sign of correction of the first ray pronation—no study in the literature has ever directly assessed this variable.[13,21]

In the authors' hands, the percutaneous BCWO demonstrated to be a safe and effective procedure to correct moderate to severe hallux valgus.[13,21,22] However, the reader should be reminded that surgeon experience is paramount to the success of the technique, and therefore, beginners are discouraged from using said approach until very comfortable with percutaneous surgery.

Table 3.1

Radiographic Results of Percutaneous and Open First Metatarsal Basal Close Wedge Osteotomy

Study	Method	Mean Preoperative HVA (°)	Mean Postoperative HVA (°)	Mean Improvement in HVA (°)	Mean Preoperative IMA (°)	Mean Postoperative IMA (°)	Mean Improvement in IMA (°)
Trnka et al.[5]	Open	38.9	19.9	19	16.1	6.7	9.4
Wagner et al.[6]	Open	35.6	12.3	23.3	15.3	4.8	10.5
Day et al.[24]	Open	31	11	20	13.2	4.4	8.8
De Lavigne et al.[23]	PERC	43	16	27	22	11	11
Chan and Yeung[21]	PERC	46.4	17.9	27.8	18.6	9.9	8.7
Kurashige and Suzuki[22]	PERC	39.4	14.7	24.7	14.9	6.6	8.3

Abbreviations: PERC, percutaneous; HVA, hallux valgus angle; IMA, first intermetatarsal angle.

References

1. Lee M, Walsh J, Smith MM, Ling J, Wines A, Lam P. Hallux valgus correction comparing percutaneous chevron/Akin (PECA) and open scarf/Akin osteotomies. *Foot Ankle Int.* 2017;38(8):838-846.
2. Siddiqui NA, LaPorta G, Walsh AL, Abraham JS, Beauregard S, Gdalevitch M. Radiographic outcomes of a percutaneous, reproducible distal metatarsal osteotomy for mild and moderate bunions: a multicenter study. *J Foot Ankle Surg.* 2019;58(6):1215-1222.
3. Robinson AH, Limbers JP. Modern concepts in the treatment of hallux valgus. *J Bone Joint Surg Br.* 2005;87(8):1038-1045.
4. Bia A, Guerra-Pinto F, Pereira BS, Corte-Real N, Oliva XM. Percutaneous osteotomies in hallux valgus: a systematic review. *J Foot Ankle Surg.* 2018;57(1):123-130.
5. Trnka HJ, Mühlbauer M, Zembsch A, Hungerford M, Ritschl P, Salzer M. Basal closing wedge osteotomy for correction of hallux valgus and metatarsus primus varus: 10- to 22-year follow-up. *Foot Ankle Int.* 1999;20(3):171-177.
6. Wagner E, Ortiz C, Gould JS, et al. Proximal oblique sliding closing wedge osteotomy for hallux valgus. *Foot Ankle Int.* 2013;34(11):1493-1500.
7. Loison M. Note sur le traitement chirugical de hallux valgus d'apres l'étude radiographique de la deformation. *Bull Mem Soc Chir Paris.* 1901;27:528Y531.
8. Haas Z, Hamilton G, Sundstrom D, Ford L. Maintenance of correction of first metatarsal closing base wedge osteotomies versus modified Lapidus arthrodesis for moderate to severe hallux valgus deformity. *J Foot Ankle Surg.* 2007;46(5):358-365.
9. Lian GJ, Markoff K, Cracchiolo A III. Strength of fixation constructs for basilar osteotomies of the first metatarsal. *Foot Ankle.* 1992;13:509Y514.
10. Kirchwein WW. Cross screw compression fixation technique in proximal osteotomies of the first metatarsal for correction of hallux abductor valgus. *J Foot Surg.* 1988;27:211Y218.
11. De Prado M, Ripoll PL, Golano P. *Minimally Invasive Foot Surgery.* About Your Health; 2009
12. Vernois J, Redfern DJ. Percutaneous surgery for severe hallux valgus. *Foot Ankle Clin.* 2016;21(3):479-493.
13. Vernois J, Redfern D, Amouyel T. Percutaneous basal closing wedge osteotomy for hallux valgus deformity. *Oper Orthop Traumatol.* 2021;33(4):358-363. English.
14. Al-Nammari SS, Christofi T, Clark C. Double first metatarsal and Akin osteotomy for severe hallux valgus. *Foot Ankle Int.* 2015;36(10):1215-1222.
15. Nunes GA, Ferreira GF, Baumfeld T, Filho MVP, Baumfeld D, Lam P. Minimally invasive chevron Akin: locking the metatarsal-cuneiform joint. *Foot Ankle Spec.* 2022;19386400221079155.
16. Walker R, Redfern D. Experience with a minimally invasive distal lesser metatarsal osteotomy for the treatment of metatarsalgia. *J Bone Joint Surg Br.* 2012;94-B(suppl XXII):39.
17. Doty JF, Harris WT. Hallux valgus deformity and treatment: a three-dimensional approach. *Foot Ankle Clin.* 2018;23(2):271-280.
18. Mahmoud K, Metikala S, Mehta SD, Fryhofer GW, Farber DC, Prat D. The role of weightbearing computed tomography scan in hallux valgus. *Foot Ankle Int.* 2021;42(3):287-293.
19. Hecht PJ, Lin TJ. Hallux valgus. *Med Clin North Am.* 2014;98(2):227-232.
20. Welck MJ, Al-Khudairi N. Imaging of hallux valgus: how to approach the deformity. *Foot Ankle Clin.* 2018;23(2):183-192.
21. Chan KB, Yeung R. Percutaneous basal closing wedge osteotomy of the first metatarsal in the treatment of moderate to severe hallux valgus and its short-term clinical outcomes. *Foot Ankle Orthop.* 2018;3(1):1-6.
22. Kurashige T, Suzuki S. Effectiveness of percutaneous proximal closing wedge osteotomy with Akin osteotomy to correct severe hallux valgus determined by radiographic parameters. *Foot Ankle Spec.* 2017;10(2):170-179.
23. De Lavigne C, Rasmont Q, Hoang B. Percutaneous double metatarsal osteotomy for correction of severe hallux valgus deformity. *Acta Orthop Belg.* 2011;77(4):516-521.
24. Day T, Charlton TP, Thordarson DB. First metatarsal length change after basilar closing wedge osteotomy for hallux valgus. *Foot Ankle Int.* 2011;32:513-518.
25. Malagelada F, Sahirad C, Dalmau-Pastor M, et al. Minimally invasive surgery for hallux valgus: a systematic review of current surgical techniques. *Int Orthop.* 2019;43(3):625-637.

4 Percutaneous Scarf

Eduard Rabat and Josep Torrent

◆ INTRODUCTION

The open scarf osteotomy is an effective and reproducible technique that allows for the correction of the hallux valgus angle (HVA), intermetatarsal angle (IMA), and distal metatarsal articular angle (DMAA) and provides postoperative pain relief.[1,2]

Burutaran in 1976 was the first to describe a Z-shaped osteotomy. The technique's main indication was for lengthening the first metatarsal in pediatric patients with brachymetatarsia (Morton syndrome).[3]

Weil named the Z-shaped first metatarsal osteotomy the scarf osteotomy. They performed the first study on local vascularization, modified the bony cuts, and increased the length of the osteotomy.[4] Finally, Barouk popularized the technique globally, particularly in Europe.[5] Influenced by Barouk, we began implementing the scarf procedure in the 1990s, and it has since become the authors' gold standard procedure for hallux valgus correction.

The three cuts of the scarf osteotomy provide good inherent postoperative stability.[6] The main displacements of the osteotomy are in the transverse plane, mainly lateral shift, with medial rotation (DMAA correction) if necessary. In the frontal plane, it is possible to rotate and lower the metatarsal head, while in the sagittal plane, shortening or lengthening can be performed if required.

The great versatility of the scarf osteotomy was the reason we chose this technique as the first option for hallux valgus treatment, apart from the natural evolution toward a minimally invasive procedure. We perform the osteotomy percutaneously with burrs and the use of internal fixation in the form of headless compression screws, also introduced via a minimally invasive approach.

Main Characteristics of the Percutaneous Scarf

- Distal and extra-articular metatarsal osteotomy
- Mild bunionectomy if required
- Three cuts: distal dorsal, diaphyseal, and plantar proximal
- Two apexes of the osteotomy: proximal and distal
- Osteosynthesis: one or two cannulated headless 3-mm screws
- Soft-tissue procedures: lateral release in most cases
- Akin osteotomy[7] is performed in 95% of cases, without osteosynthesis
- Akin osteotomy is incomplete preserving the dorsolateral cortex

◆ INDICATIONS AND CONTRAINDICATIONS

The indications for the scarf osteotomy are wide-ranging, from mild to severe deformities.[8-10] The indications for the percutaneous scarf osteotomy are the same as those applicable to the open scarf procedure.

Specific contraindications are severe first tarsometatarsal instability, osteoarthritis of the first metatarsophalangeal (MTP) joint, and severe osteoporosis.[6]

◆ PREOPERATIVE PLANNING AND PREPARATION

Weight-bearing radiographs of both feet are taken in anteroposterior and lateral projection, preoperatively and during long-term follow-up. The factors evaluated included HVA, I/II IMA, the congruence of the first MTP joint, the presence of arthritis of the first MTP joint, and the position of the medial sesamoid.

Arthritis was graded according to Coughlin and Shurnas' classification.[11] The position of the medial sesamoid was assessed in relation to a line drawn along the longitudinal axis of the first metatarsal on the dorsoplantar weight-bearing radiograph according to the measurement system proposed by Hardy and Clapham.[12]

We also recorded the metatarsal shortening point (MS point) as described by Barouk.[5] The MS point is the proximal location of the first phalanx basis. The MS point determines the need of the lateral release and shortening of the first metatarsal. The MS point becomes more proximal when there is retraction of the structures on the lateral part of the first MTP joint.

Materials

Specific instruments include a 3-mm Beaver blade, a large Shannon burr (20 mm × 2 mm), and a short Shannon burr (12 mm × 2 mm). A wedge burr (13 mm × 3.1 mm) is used in case medial eminence excision is needed. A specific handpiece system set at high torque and low speed is required.

Osteosynthesis is performed with headless compression screws of 3 mm diameter. As the aim of the fixation is stabilization, not compression, fully threaded screws are recommended.

Surgical Approach

Patients are placed in the supine position. A single intravenous dose of antibiotic prophylaxis (2 g of cefazolin) is indicated for all patients just before surgery.

The procedure is performed under an ankle nerve block without a tourniquet assisted by intraoperative fluoroscopy. The ankle block includes the block of the tibialis posterior nerve, deep peroneal nerve, superficial peroneal nerve, saphenous nerve, and sural nerve, for which 30 mL of equal parts 0.25% bupivacaine and 1% lidocaine without epinephrine is used.

Scarf is performed on an outpatient basis. After the procedure, patients spend 2 to 5 hours in the ambulatory area before being discharged.

SURGICAL TECHNIQUE

The scarf osteotomy can correct the 1-2 IMA and the DMAA and allows for rotation of the metatarsal head and big toe, elevation and lowering of the metatarsal head, as well as lengthening or shortening of the first metatarsal. First, the amount of lateral displacement of the metatarsal head required to correct the IMA is estimated. Then, the need for metatarsal shortening or lengthening is assessed based on the Barouk technique[3] of calculating the MS point.

STEP 1: Incision and Creation of the Working Space

1. The patient is placed in a supine position without a tourniquet. A horizontal 0.5- to 1-cm wound is made in the medial side of the foot, approximately 0.5 cm proximal and centered just below the hypertrophic medial eminence on the first metatarsal head and parallel to its long axis (Figure 4.1). Then, a gentle dissection is performed between the metatarsal head and the articular capsule to create the working space. Thereafter, with the elevator, the most dorsal aspect of the metatarsal bone is reached. The distal apex is positioned at the midpoint of the dorsal cortex and the plantar cortex.

STEP 2: Distal Apex

The distal apex is present at the midpoint of the dorsal and plantar aspects of the metatarsal bone. This surgical point is the reference for the scarf osteotomy. Once the exact point is decided, the metatarsal is drilled in a medial to lateral direction with the burr.

The large Shannon burr (20 mm × 2.2 mm) is inserted through the percutaneous incision, and fluoroscopy is used to verify that the tip of the burr is centered at the distal apex of the planned osteotomy (Figure 4.2).

According to the preoperative plan, the length of the metatarsal bone can be modified with the transverse cuts of the scarf osteotomy. As a burr is used instead of a saw to perform the osteotomy, the unavoidable shortening produced by the burr must be considered, meaning that a minimum of 2 mm and an additional 1 mm due to the vibration is shortened as the osteotomy progresses.

Direction of the Distal Apex

The reference is the long axis of the second metatarsal. The length of the first metatarsal can be modified according to this reference. The direction of the proximal transverse cut must be the same.

A proximal inclination cut relative to the long axis of the second metatarsal will shorten the first metatarsal. A perpendicular cut relative to the long axis of the second metatarsal maintains the length, and when the cut is directed distally, the metatarsal bone is lengthened. Nevertheless, considering the extra shortening because of the burr, the direction of the transverse cut must always be designed to be slightly more distal than planned (Figure 4.3).

1. **Perpendicular cut**
   This direction will shorten the first metatarsal by about 3 mm considering that the cut is performed with a burr instead of a saw. This design is indicated for patients with mild index plus, where it is only necessary for a slight shortening of the first metatarsal.
2. **Proximal inclination**
   The proximal inclination of the cut shortens the metatarsal bone. This shortening is necessary for severe hallux valgus with an increased IMA in order to create enough space to shift the fragment laterally enough. It is possible to achieve shortening of up to 1 cm with the proximal inclination of the burr.

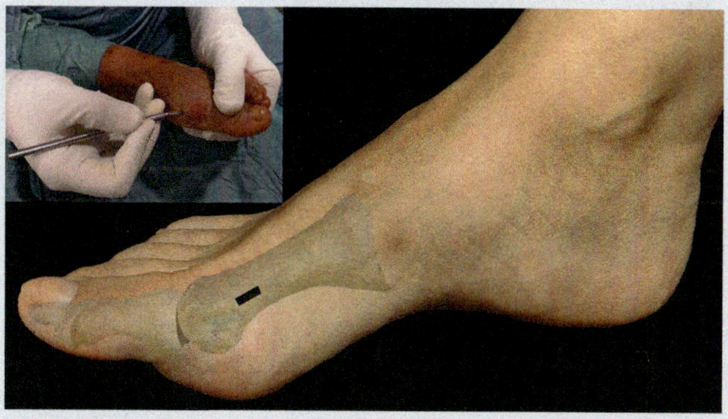

Figure 4.1 Medial view of the foot showing the metatarsophalangeal joint. Percutaneous approach to perform the scarf osteotomy.

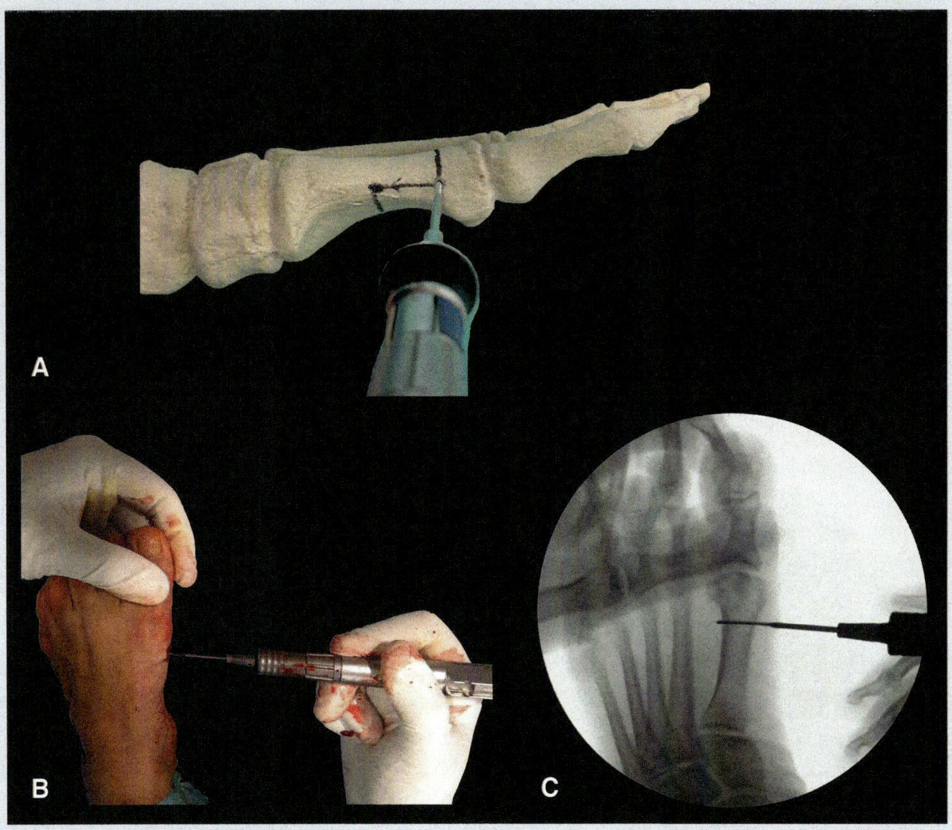

Figure 4.2 **A.** Distal apex of the osteotomy. **B.** Clinical view of the introduction of the percutaneous burr at the starting point. **C.** Fluoroscopic view of the location of the starting point once both cortexes of the first metatarsal bone have been pierced.

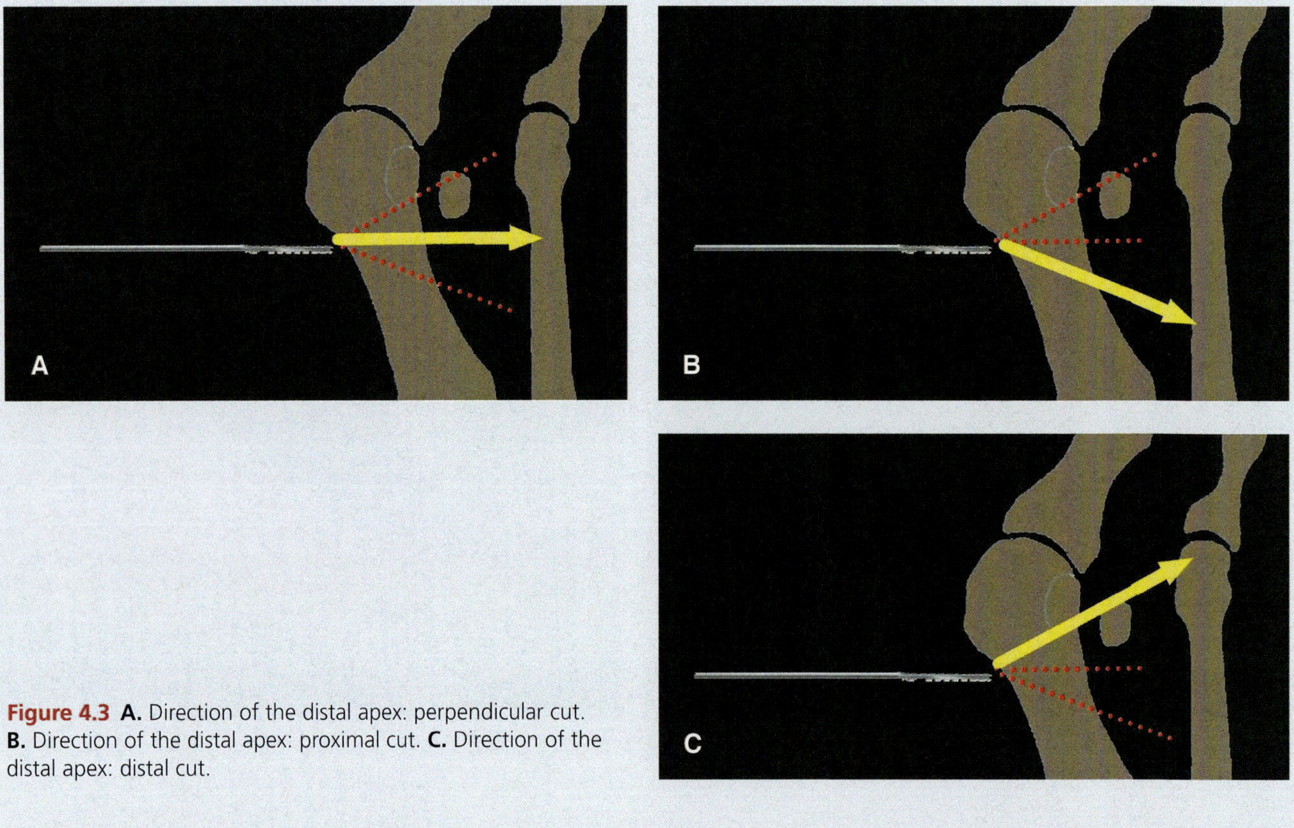

Figure 4.3 **A.** Direction of the distal apex: perpendicular cut. **B.** Direction of the distal apex: proximal cut. **C.** Direction of the distal apex: distal cut.

3. **Distal inclination**
   The 3 mm of unavoidable shortening because of the burr must be considered. If the length of the first metatarsal is to be retained, the direction of the transverse cut should always be designed to be slightly distal. The main indication here is hallux valgus with index minus to avoid transfer metatarsalgia.
4. **Plantarization of the metatarsal head**
   In some cases, plantarization of the head of the first metatarsal bone may be required, for which the apex could be directed from medial-dorsal to lateral-plantar. This maneuver could be useful to avoid secondary metatarsalgia.

STEP 3: Distal Transverse Cut

The distal cut is performed following the direction of the apex exactly (Step 2; Figure 4.4). The first cut begins under constant irrigation at the distal apex of the osteotomy. It is directed following the planned direction straight to the lateral cortex. The position must be checked via fluoroscopy in the anteroposterior and lateral views. Then, the burr is directed dorsally until entirely through the dorsal cortex. By touching the skin, the burr can be felt by the surgeon as it fully completes the osteotomy, avoiding damage of the extensor tendons.

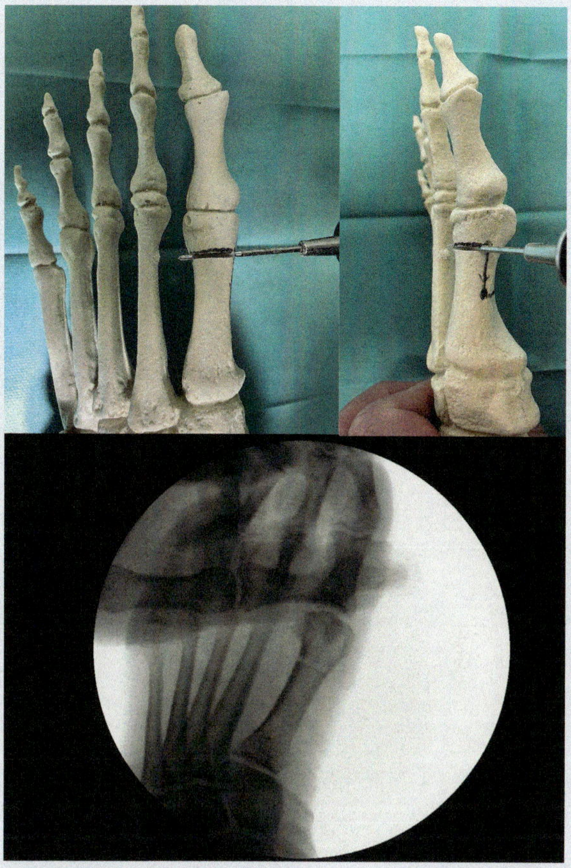

Figure 4.4 Distal transverse cut of the scarf osteotomy.

STEP 4: Longitudinal Cut

Under constant irrigation, the second cut originates from the same distal apex and is directed proximally following the longitudinal axis of the first metatarsal (Figure 4.5). The dorsoplantar inclination should be parallel to the dorsal cortex to facilitate the displacement. The osteotomy should not be less than 2 cm in length. This segment of the osteotomy could be extended, depending on the case. As the standard technique of the scarf, a more extended osteotomy is required to correct a bigger 1-2 IMA.

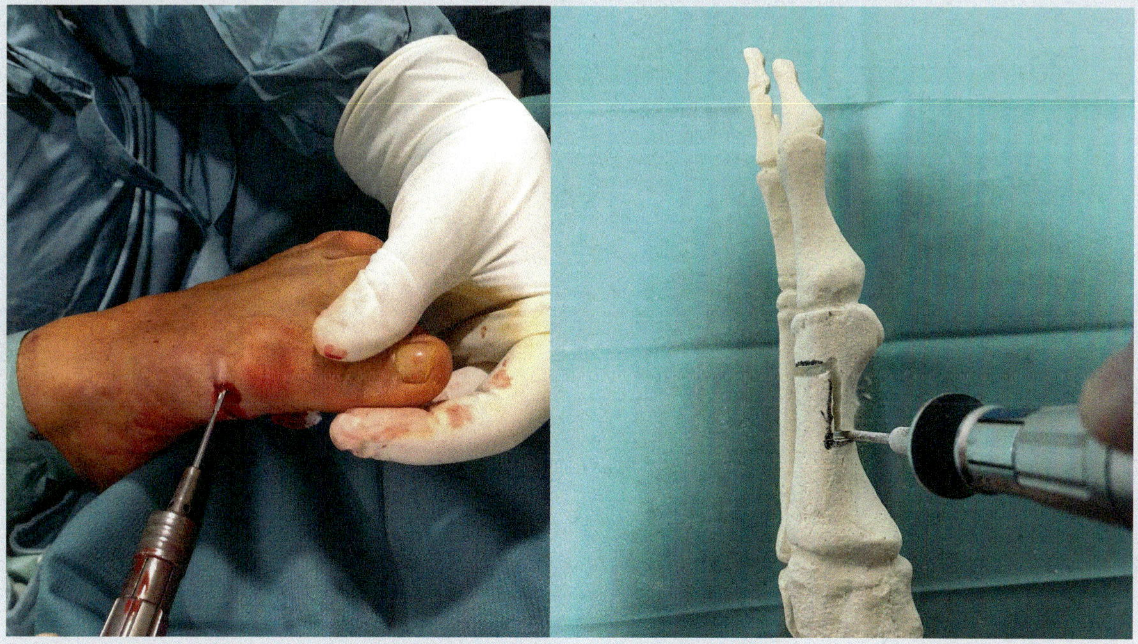

Figure 4.5 Longitudinal cut of the scarf osteotomy.

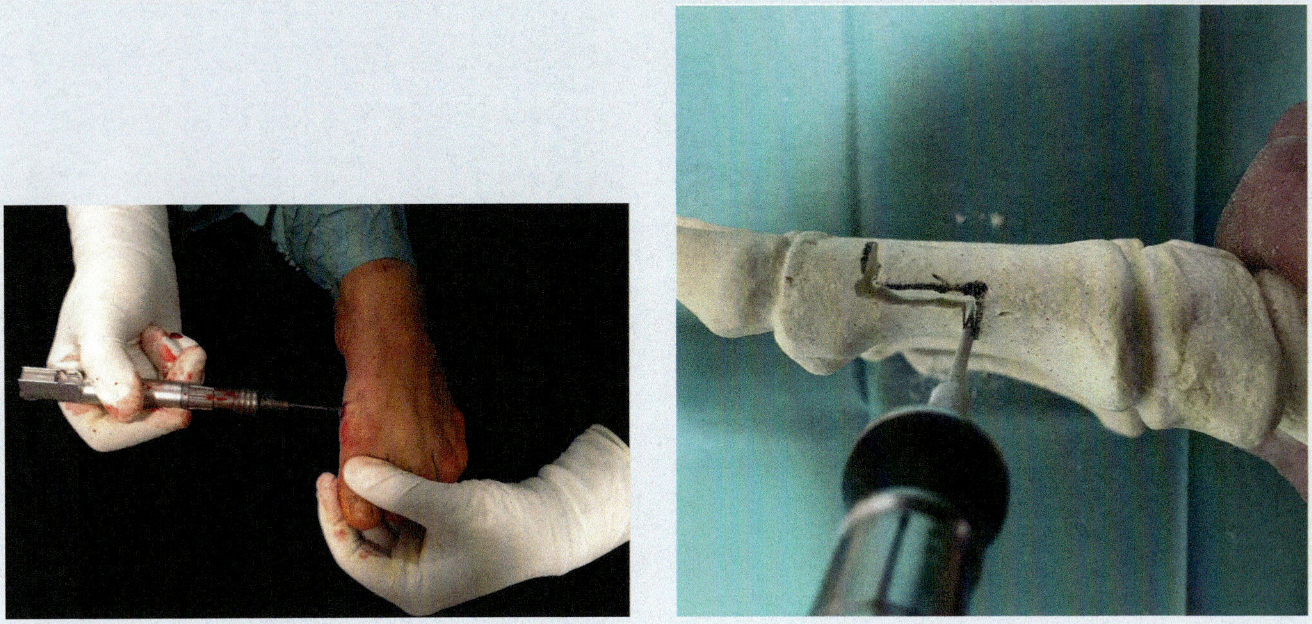

Figure 4.6 Proximal transverse cut of the scarf osteotomy.

The proximal ending point of the longitudinal cut will be the proximal apex of the osteotomy and must be parallel with the distal apex.

STEP 5: Proximal Transverse Cut

The third cut begins at the proximal apex of the osteotomy and is directed plantarly until the plantar cortex has been completely osteotomized, completing the scarf "Z" osteotomy (Figure 4.6). Under fluoroscopy, the distal segment of the metatarsal is moved by hand to verify that a complete osteotomy has been achieved.

Once the osteotomy is performed, the lateral displacement of the head is performed. Under fluoroscopic control, the head is pushed laterally with the thumb. This maneuver is used to ensure that the osteotomy is complete, and the metatarsal head is free of attachments (Figure 4.7).

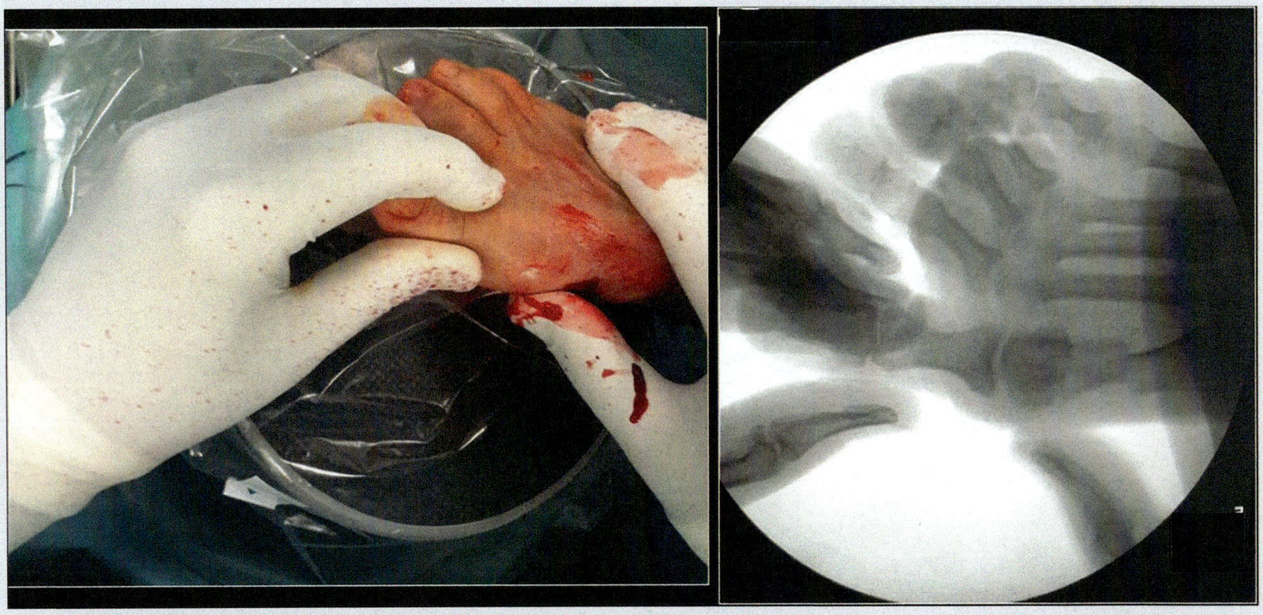

Figure 4.7 Check of the lateral displacement of the head after the osteotomy is completed, under fluoroscopic control.

STEP 6: Lateral Displacement

Lateral displacement of the distal segment is achieved by inserting a Kirschner wire (K-wire) of 2.0 to 2.5 mm diameter through the percutaneous incision and drilling it proximally 2 to 3 cm into the first metatarsal without crossing the tarsometatarsal joint (Figure 4.8).

Lateral leverage on the K-wire is applied until the head is shifted into the desired position. Once final positioning has been achieved, the K-wire is advanced temporarily across the tarsometatarsal joint to provide stability to the osteotomy.

Excessive plantarization of the metatarsal head with this procedure must be avoided. When the head is pushed laterally, it must simultaneously be pushed dorsally to avoid this potential complication.

STEP 7: Restoring DMAA and Metatarsal Head Rotation

Once the 1-2 intermetatarsal is corrected, the DMAA and the rotation of the metatarsal head can be addressed. Considering the integrity of the abductor tendon, as the big toe is manually abducted against the K-wire, internal rotation of the head can be achieved, correcting the DMAA. Simultaneously, the metatarsal head can be rotated with the other hand as planned. Once the desired correction is observed via fluoroscopy, the exact position is maintained, retaining the tension with a gauze lace around the K-wire and the big toe (Figure 4.9). Once the osteotomy is stabilized in the planned position, osteosynthesis can be performed.

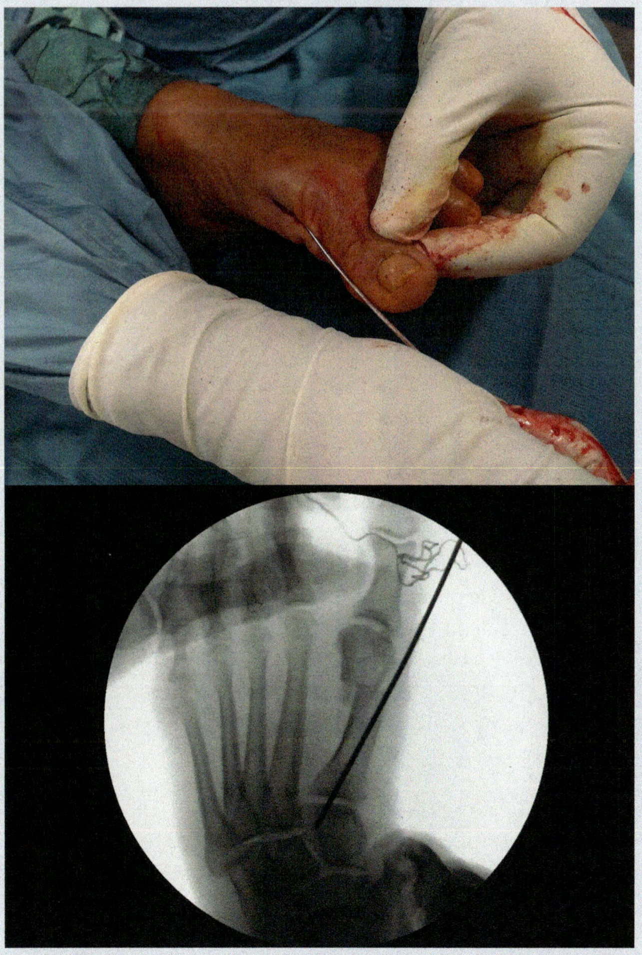

Figure 4.8 The lateral displacement of the distal segment is achieved by inserting a 2.0- to 2.5-mm-diameter K-wire through the percutaneous incision.

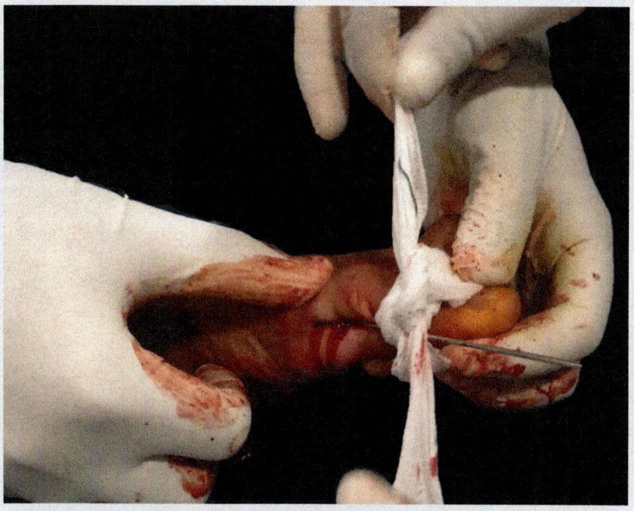

Figure 4.9 A gauze lace around the K-wire and the big toe fix the achieved correction of the rotation and distal metatarsal articular angle.

STEP 8: Osteosynthesis of the Osteotomy and Medial Eminence Removal

Osteosynthesis must only be performed once the planned correction is obtained. Internal fixation of the osteotomy is achieved using a 3.0-mm cannulated headless screw. Fully threaded screws are used to ensure the stabilization of the fragments while avoiding excessive compression. Osteosynthesis can be performed with one or two screws.

Osteosynthesis With One Screw

The K-wire guide is positioned approximately 1 cm proximal to the distal vertical cut in the center of the dorsal metatarsal surface and drilled at a 45° angle (proximal dorsal to distal plantar) to the longitudinal axis of the first metatarsal (Figure 4.10).

Under fluoroscopy, verify that the metatarsal head cartilage or MTP joint has not been violated by the tip of the K-wire for correct measurement of the length.

After the measurement, the K-wire is introduced further into the cartilage. This prevents its accidental removal during the drilling maneuver.

With a scalpel, a small incision (~0.5 cm or less) is created around the K-wire. The selected cannulated 3.0-mm headless compression screw is inserted over the K-wire to stabilize the osteotomy and until the screw is level with the dorsal cortex of the osteotomy.

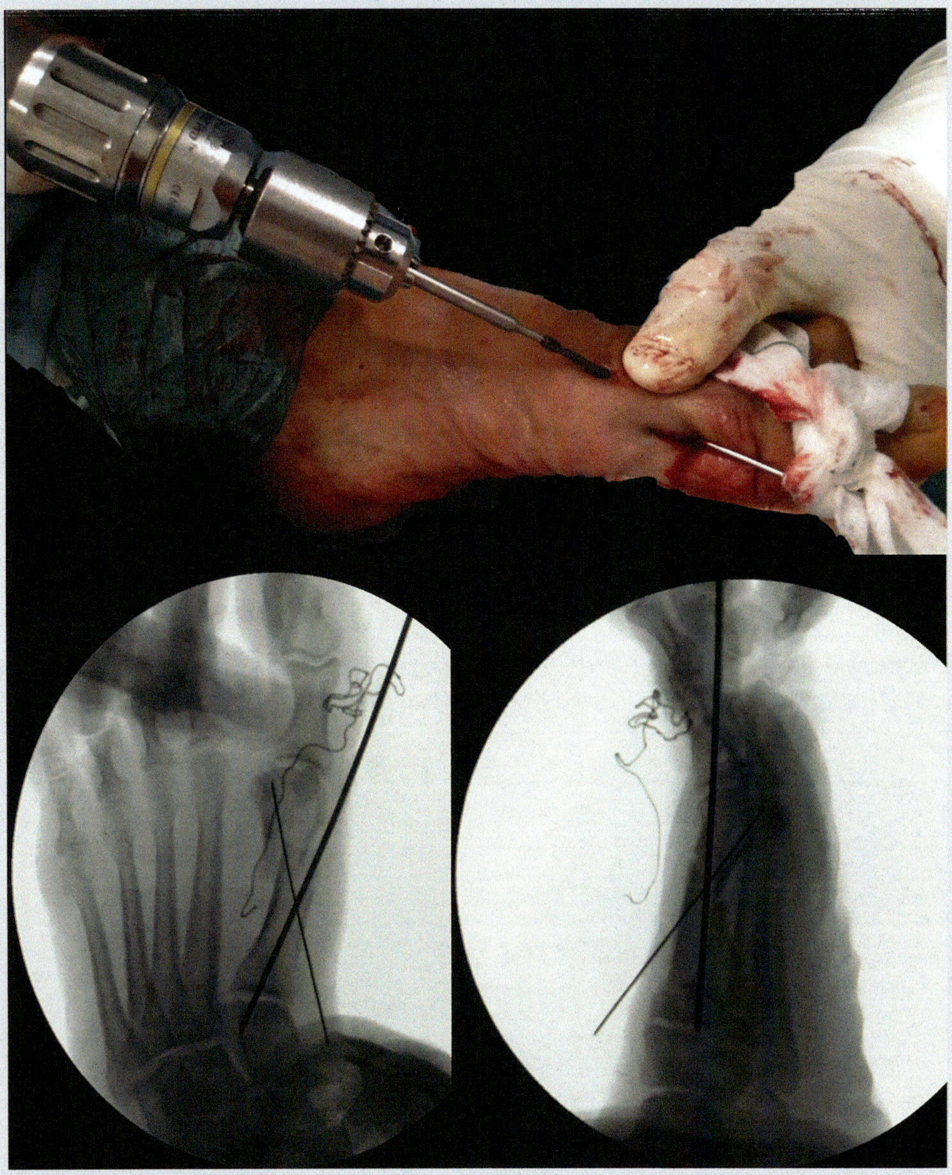

Figure 4.10 Osteosynthesis of the osteotomy with one screw.

Final tightening of the screw is performed simultaneously as the 2.5-mm K-wire is removed by an assistant. The introduction of the screw is completed at the same time as the removal of the K-wire. With this maneuver, the potential gap created by the space occupied by the K-wire is avoided, and total contact of the osteotomy parts is achieved. A possible plantarization of the head can also be corrected (Figure 4.11).

Note: With an obliquity of approximately 45°, it is recommended to subtract 2 mm from the measured depth of the screw. This way, the penetration of the screw in the plantar aspect can be avoided.

Osteosynthesis With Two Screws

It is possible to insert a second screw to fix the osteotomy (Figure 4.12). Although most of the time, osteosynthesis is sufficiently stabilized with only one screw, in some cases, this stability is not confirmed. To solve this issue or at the discretion of the surgeon, a second screw can be inserted proximally.

Before the introduction of the first screw, the second K-wire guide is placed in the midpoint of the medial cortex, 1 cm proximal to the proximal transverse cut and directed toward the metatarsal head. The screw may be bicortical when it exits though the lateral aspect of the metatarsal head, also depending on the preferences of the surgeon.

Medial Eminence Removal

Decisions about performing medial eminence removal are always made after osteosynthesis as it is easier to achieve a good lateral displacement without any previous bunionectomy. This procedure is especially useful when there is a sharp or large eminence of the metatarsal head.

This technique requires a high-speed burr. The wedge burr of 4.3 mm diameter is connected and inserted through

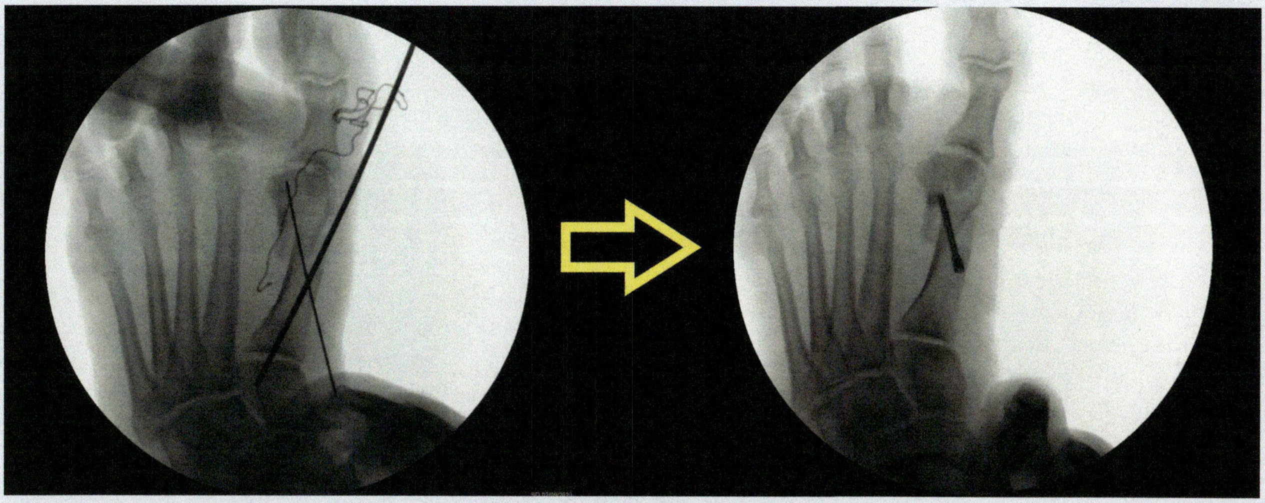

Figure 4.11 Compression of the osteotomy once the 2-mm Kirschner wire is removed.

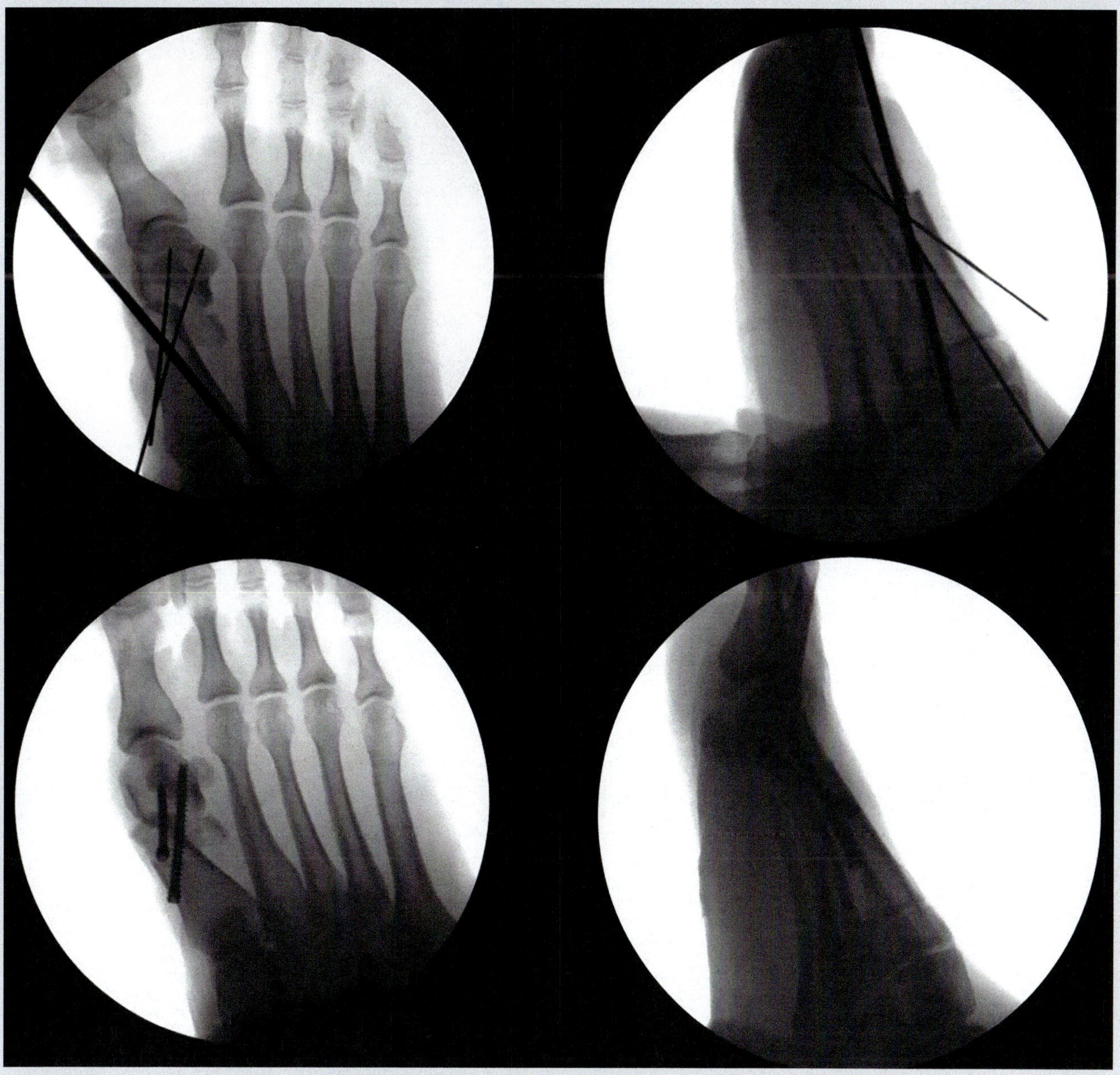

Figure 4.12 Osteosynthesis of the osteotomy with two screws.

the percutaneous medial incision. The burr should be irrigated constantly to combat excessive heat generation. Then, under power, the burr is moved around the medial eminence until the bony prominence has been removed, with periodic checks via fluoroscopy.

STEP 9: Lateral Release

The percutaneous lateral release can be performed at the discretion of the surgeon (Figure 4.13).[13,14] The authors' indication for the lateral release is a subluxated (noncongruent) MTP joint on a weight-bearing anteroposterior radiograph. Through a small dorsal incision using a Beaver blade, the MTP joint is accessed. The approach of the percutaneous lateral release is just lateral to the extensor hallucis longus at the level of the MTP joint.

After checking the position via fluoroscopy and directing the Beaver blade laterally and perpendicular to the long axis, the blade is then externally rotated to reach the adductor tendon, which is then sectioned with a distal movement of the blade, tensioning the first toe into varus until the tendon is released. For its plantar position, care must be taken not to damage the lateral collateral ligament that it is more dorsal than the abductor expansion.

The effectiveness of the tenotomy can be assessed via fluoroscopy. The lateral sesamoid should not move with the adduction of the big toe.

STEP 10: Akin Osteotomy

The Akin osteotomy is a medially based closing wedge osteotomy of the proximal phalanx (Figure 4.14). In 95% of cases, we combine the scarf osteotomy with an Akin procedure after hallux valgus correction. The procedure is performed percutaneously and under radiograph control, as described by De Prado et al.[15]

- The osteotomy is performed with a 12 × 2 mm Shannon burr at the dorsal aspect of the proximal phalanx. The osteotomy starts in the medial junction of the proximal metaphysis and the diaphysis of the phalanx.
- The working space is created with an elevator or mosquito clamp.

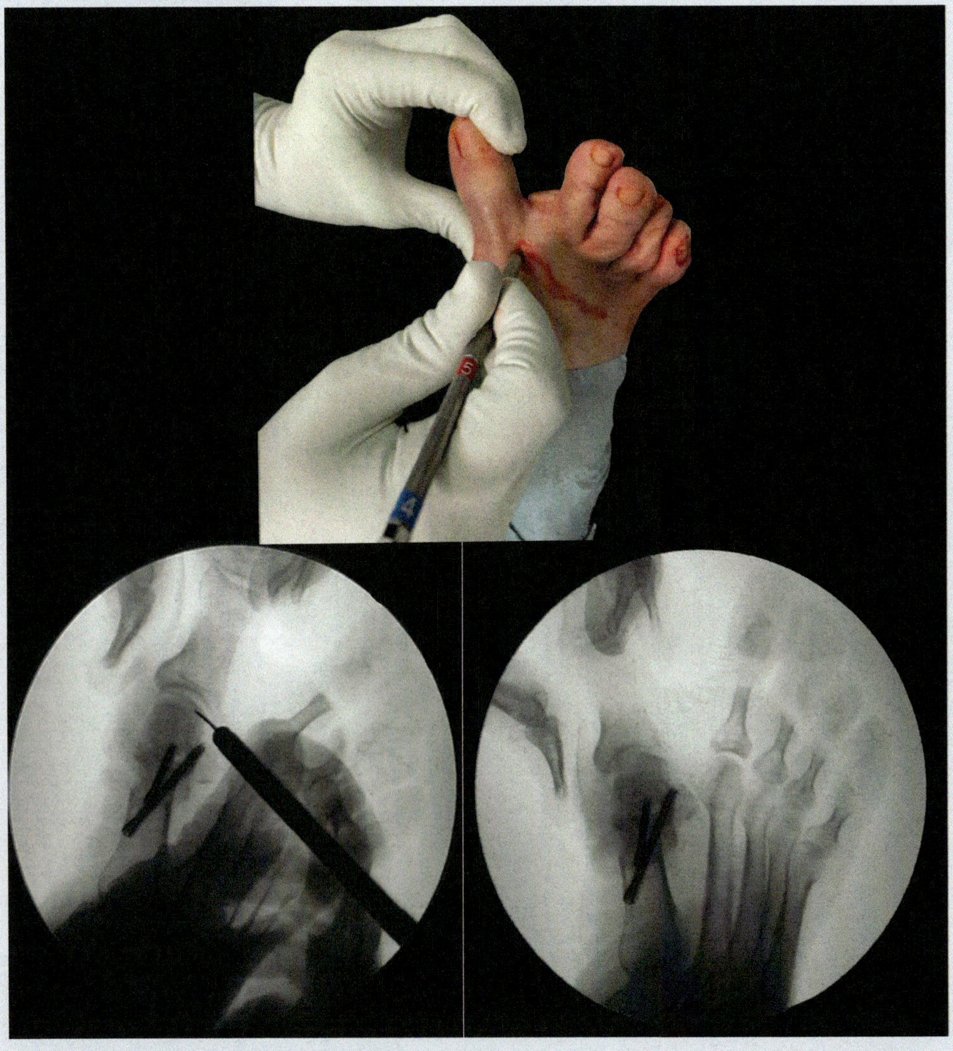

Figure 4.13 Percutaneous lateral release. The lateral sesamoid does not move with the adduction of the big toe, as the hallux abductor tendon has been cut.

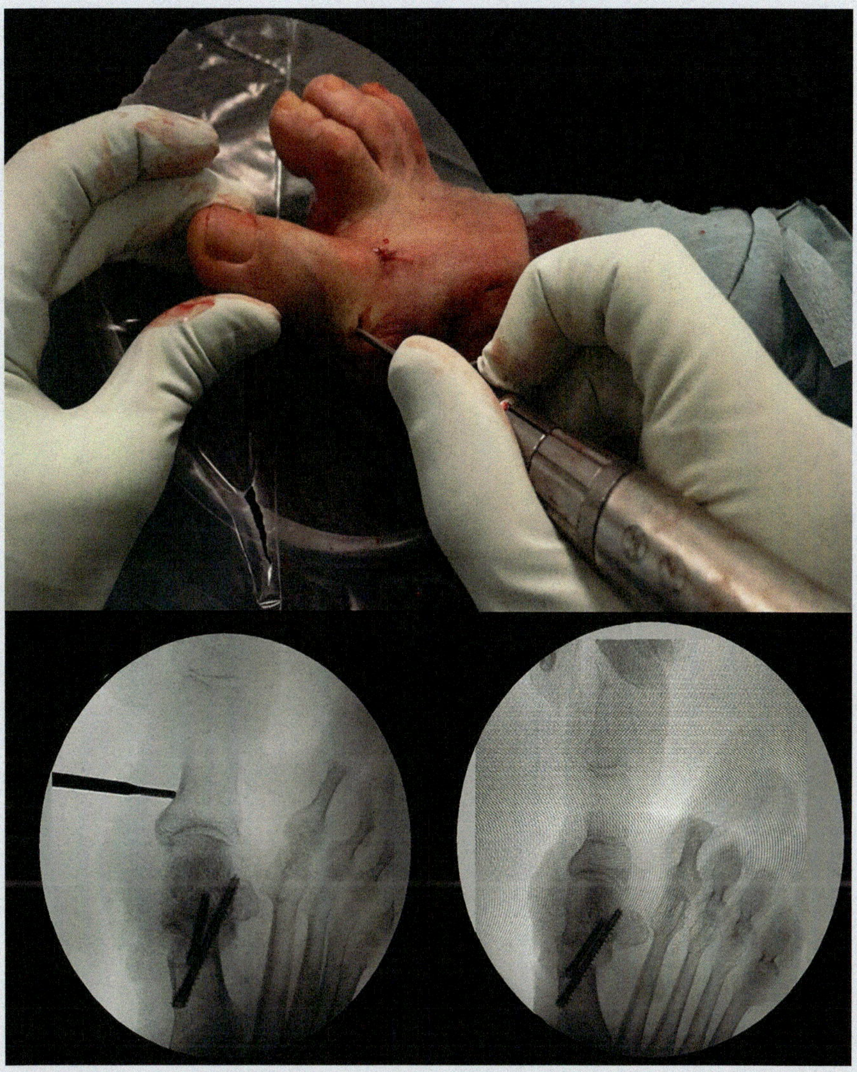

Figure 4.14 Akin osteotomy.

- The osteotomy begins medial-plantar and is directed toward the lateral cortex. The lateral cortex must be preserved, creating a bone hinge. The burr creates a medial-based wedge that could be increased, depending on the case.
- The hallux is then forced in adduction, closing the Akin osteotomy. The bony hinge provides stability, and in most cases, osteosynthesis is not necessary.

PEARLS AND PITFALLS

- As we perform the osteotomy with a burr instead of a saw, we always remove at least 3 mm of bone. Take care during the preoperative plan to avoid undesirable shortening.
- The direction of the medial incision must follow the metatarsal shaft. This orientation will make easier to follow the axis of the longitudinal cut.
- One of the main concerns is the excessive plantarization of the head. We must ensure, in the AP radiograph view, that there is a gap between the 2-mm K-wire and the metatarsal head. If the wire appears directly abutting the metatarsal head, this means the head is displaced plantarly. A gap indicates that soft tissue, the medial capsular tissue, is between the wire and metatarsal head, indicating the head is directed in proper position by the wire (Figure 4.15).
- During the learning curve of the percutaneous scarf, if the plantar cortex is breached during the longitudinal cut a chevron osteotomy is created. This osteotomy is less stable. This would be a kind of accidental "chevron." This osteotomy would be less stable, but one could complete the procedure by fixing the osteotomy. In this case, we recommend a closer postoperative control and avoid weight bearing for 2 to 3 weeks.

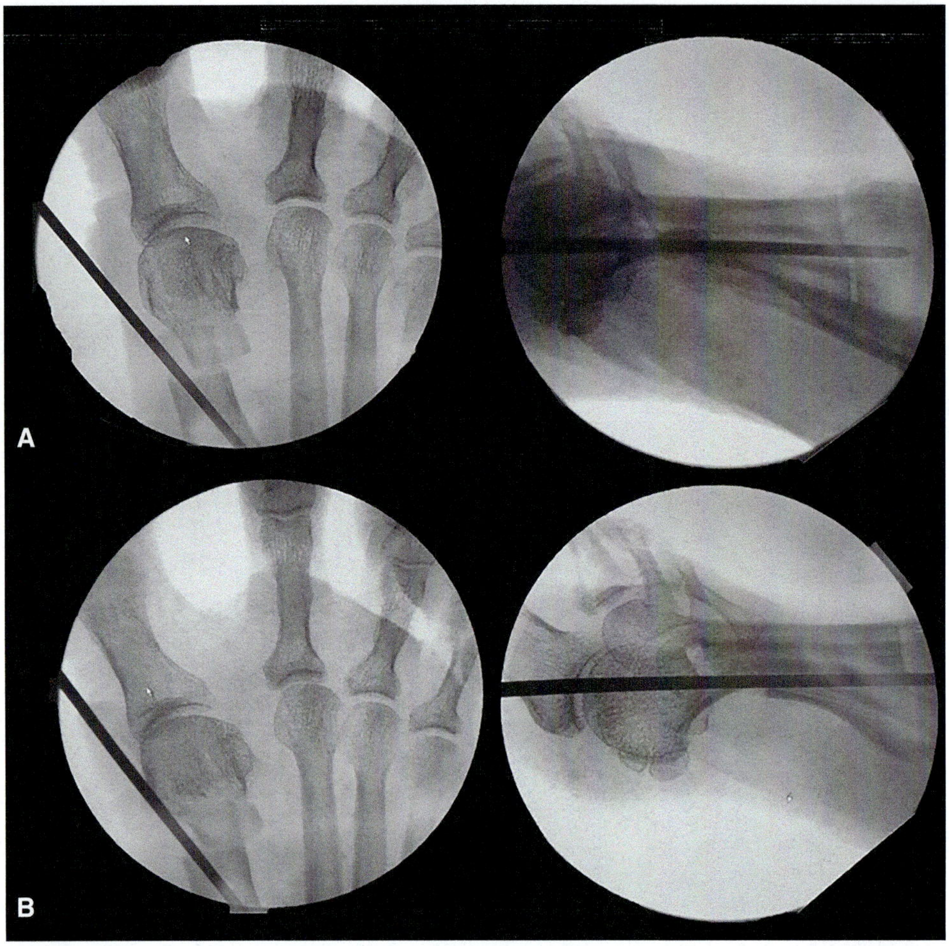

Figure 4.15 **A.** Correct position of the Kirschner and the metatarsal head. **B.** Plantarization of the metatarsal head; there is no gap between the Kirschner and the metatarsal head.

◆ POSTOPERATIVE MANAGEMENT

The patient is allowed to weight bear immediately in a postoperative flat shoe. Soft dressings are applied; we use gauzes just to avoid the direct contact of the toes. The wounds and dressing are checked each week, and after 5 weeks, a radiograph is taken when the postoperative shoe is removed to verify that the osteotomy is consolidated.

◆ OUTCOMES

In 2021, the authors team published a paper[16] comparing the clinical and radiological outcomes of patients who underwent open or percutaneous scarf osteotomies.

Fifty-eight patients were randomized to either open or minimally invasive scarf to treat hallux valgus deformities. Prospective patient-reported outcome measures and weight-bearing radiographs were obtained.

The minimally invasive procedure (Table 4.1) was statistically significantly faster than the open procedure. From the time of skin incision to the time of finalizing closure, mean procedure times were 16.7 (range, 12 to 25) minutes in the minimally invasive group and 26.1 (range, 21 to 34) minutes in the open group.

Intraoperative fluoroscopy use was clearly higher in the minimally invasive group. The mean intraoperative fluoroscopy dose was 34 (range, 19.2 to 52.8) mGy/cm^2 in the minimally invasive group and 2.4 (range, 0.7 to 4.2) mGy/cm^2 in the open group ($P < .001$).

The mean postoperative visual analog scale (VAS) for pain at 24 hours postoperatively was 2.33 (range, 0 to 6) in the minimally invasive group and 3.68 (range, 0 to 8) in the open group. The postoperative VAS was statistically significantly lower in the minimally invasive group.

Tramadol (pills of 50 mg) use in the first 24 hours postoperatively did not differ between groups. In the minimally invasive group, 4 patients needed two pills (13.3%), 1 patient one pill (3.3%), and 25 patients no pills (83.3%). In the open group, 3 patients needed two pills (10.7%), 8 patients one pill (28.6%), and 17 patients no pills (60.7%) (Table 4.2).

Postoperative hallux valgus, IMA, and DMAA were similar in both groups (Table 4.2), and significant improvements compared to preoperative values were observed at final follow-up (Figure 4.16).

Table 4.1

Intraoperative and Postoperative Characteristics

	MI Scarf Group (*n* = 30)	Open Scarf Group (*n* = 28)	*P* value
Procedure duration	16.70 ± 3.74 (12-25) min	26.13 ± 3.56 (21-34) min	**.0001**
Intraoperative radiographs	33.98 ± 9.42 (19.2-52.76) mGy/cm²	2.36 ± 1.93 (0.66-4.25) mGy/cm²	**.0001**
Rescue medication—tramadol	15 ± 35 (0-100) mg	25 ± 34.5 (0-100) mg	.280
24-h postoperative VAS	2.33 ± 2.04 (0-7)	3.68 ± 2.54 (0-8)	**.030**

Complications: Screw removal (one patient in MI group); Hypertrophic scar (two patients in Open group).

MI, minimally invasive; VAS, visual analog scale.

Boldface indicates significance.

The mean AOFAS score improved from 41 (inter quartile range [IQR], 10) preoperatively to 84 (IQR, 16) at follow-up ($P < .001$) in the minimally invasive group. In the open group, the mean AOFAS score improved from 39 (IQR, 14) preoperatively to 82 (IQR, 15) at follow-up ($P < .001$). In both groups, the AOFAS score showed a significant improvement at the latest follow-up compared to preoperative scores, without significant differences between groups ($P < .001$).

All osteotomies showed radiological bony healing at final follow-up. There were no major complications in either group.

Table 4.2

Radiological Outcome

	MI Scarf Group (*n* = 30)	Open Scarf Group (*n* = 28)	*P* value
HVA			
Preoperative	32.87 ± 6.323°	33.34 ± 5.56°	.764
Last follow-up	12.69 ± 4.38°	10.49 ± 5.02°	.08
IMA			
Preoperative	15.27 ± 1.64°	14.66 ± 2.06°	.212
Last follow-up	7.31 ± 2.60°	7.50 ± 2.83°	.793
DMAA			
Preoperative	10.73 ± 6.54°	10.71 ± 5.58°	.991
Last follow-up	2.83 ± 2.13°	3.00 ± 2.89°	.803

DMAA, distal metatarsal articular angle; HVA, hallux valgus angle; IMA, intermetatarsal angle 1-2 metatarsal; MI, minimally invasive.

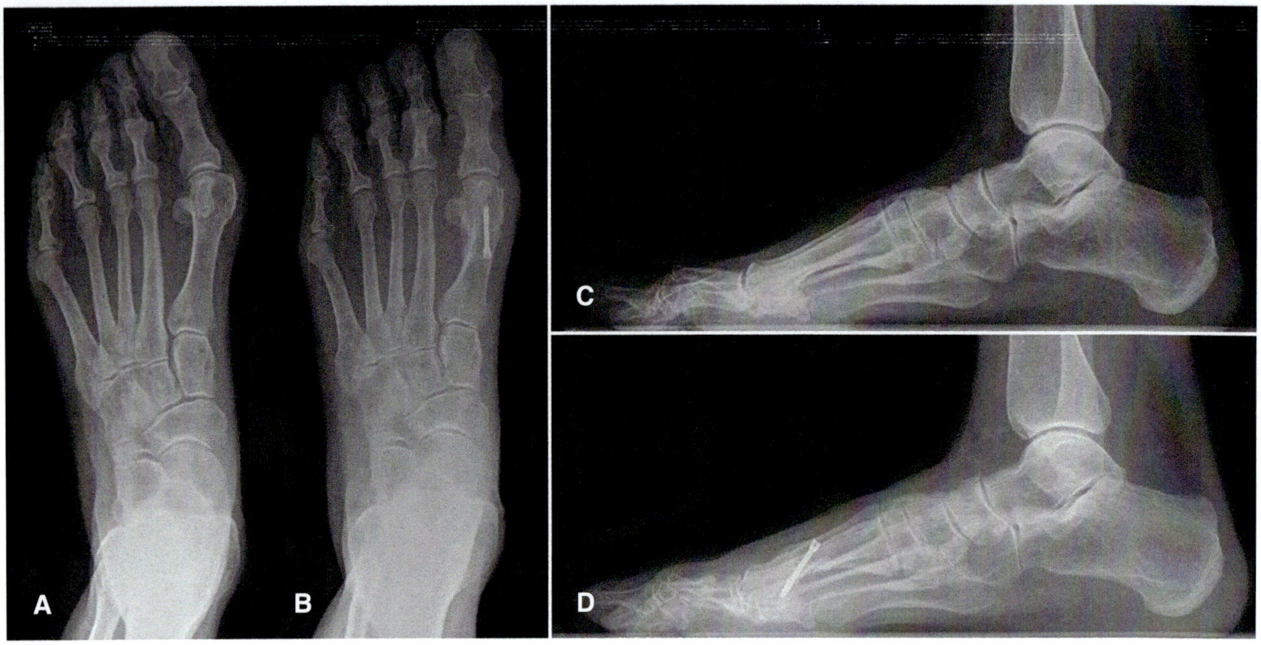

Figure 4.16 Preoperative **(A, C)** and postoperative **(B, D)** dorsoplantar and lateral radiographs of the percutaneous scarf.

◆ CONCLUSION

In conclusion, the minimally invasive scarf osteotomy is a reproducible, safe, and effective technique to treat hallux valgus. The minimally invasive scarf osteotomy shows comparable outcomes to open scarf osteotomy, with shorter operative times and lower postoperative pain levels.

Acknowledgments

We would like to thank Dr. Albert Baduell and Dr. Julieta Porta for their help with the figures in this chapter.

References

1. Lenz CG, Niehaus R, Knych I, Eid K, Borbas P. Scarf osteotomy for hallux valgus deformity: radiological outcome, metatarsal length and early complications in 118 feet. *Foot Ankle Surg.* 2020;27(1):20-24.
2. Aminian A, Kelikian A, Moen T. Scarf osteotomy for hallux valgus deformity: an intermediate followup of clinical and radiographic outcomes. *Foot Ankle Int.* 2006;27(11):883-886.
3. Burutaran J. Hallux valgus y cortedad anatómica del primer metatarso (corrección quirúrgica). *Actual Med Chir Pied.* 1976;13:261-266.
4. Weil LS. Scarf osteotomy for correction of hallux valgus. Historical perspective, surgical technique, and results. *Foot Ankle Clin.* 2000;5(3):559-580.
5. Barouk LS. Scarf osteotomy for hallux valgus correction. Local anatomy, surgical technique, and combination with other forefoot procedures. *Foot Ankle Clin.* 2000;5(3):525-558. http://www.ncbi.nlm.nih.gov/pubmed/11232396
6. Trnka HJ, Parks BG, Ivanic G, et al. Six first metatarsal shaft osteotomies: mechanical and immobilization comparisons. *Clin Orthop Relat Res.* 2000;381:256-265. http://www.ncbi.nlm.nih.gov/pubmed/11127663
7. Vernois J, Redfern DJ. Percutaneous surgery for severe hallux valgus. *Foot Ankle Clin.* 2016;21(3):479-493.
8. Coetzee JC, Rippstein P. Surgical strategies: scarf osteotomy for hallux valgus. *Foot Ankle Int.* 2007;28(4):529-535.
9. Molloy A, Widnall J. Scarf osteotomy. *Foot Ankle Clin.* 2014;19(2):166-180.
10. Castioni D, Fanelli D, Gasparini G, Iannò B, Galasso O. Scarf osteotomy for the treatment of moderate to severe hallux valgus: analysis of predictors for midterm outcomes and recurrence. *Foot Ankle Surg.* 2020;26(4):439-444.
11. Coughlin MJ, Shurnas PS. Hallux rigidus. Grading and long-term results of operative treatment. *J Bone Joint Surg Am.* 2003;85(11):2072-2088.
12. Hardy RH, Clapham JCR. Observations on hallux valgus; based on a controlled series. *J Bone Joint Surg Br.* 1951;33-B(3):376-391.
13. Del Vecchio JJ, Cordier G, Dealbera ED, et al. Correction power of percutaneous adductor tendon release (PATR) for the treatment of hallux valgus: a cadaveric study. *J Foot Ankle Surg.* 2021;60(6):1103-1109.
14. Del Vecchio JJ, Dalmau-Pastor M. Percutaneous lateral release in hallux valgus: anatomic basis and indications. *Foot Ankle Clin.* 2020;25(3):373-383.
15. De Prado M, Ripoll PL, Golano P. *Minimally Invasive Foot Surgery.* Masson; 2009.
16. Torrent J, Baduell A, Vega J, Malagelada F, Luna R, Rabat E. Open vs minimally invasive scarf osteotomy for hallux valgus correction: a randomized controlled trial. *Foot Ankle Int.* 2021;42(8):982-993.

5 Lapidus

Conor I. Murphy, Akshay Jain, and A. Holly Johnson

◆ INTRODUCTION

There is a growing application for percutaneous techniques in orthopedic foot and ankle surgery and a trend toward incorporation of minimally invasive procedures in practice today. Many minimally invasive procedures such as percutaneous bunionectomy and lesser toe corrective surgery have demonstrated sustained success and outcomes with minimal complications.[1,2] While the literature pertaining to percutaneous Lapidus surgery is limited, the authors have found reliable and predictable outcomes in the appropriately indicated patient.

The Lapidus procedure was first reported in 1934 and is a versatile procedure used to treat a wide array of first ray deformities.[3,4] The Lapidus procedure aims to treat pathologies including but not limited to tarsometatarsal (TMT) joint instability, hallux valgus deformity, flatfoot deformity, as well as TMT arthritis with the primary goal of surgery to obtain a fusion of the first TMT joint in appropriate alignment. The open Lapidus procedure has increased in popularity as surgeons have recognized the powerful ability to correct the multiple planes of hallux valgus deformity using this midfoot fusion.[5] The percutaneous method to the Lapidus procedure was first introduced in Europe by Dr. Mariano do Prado in the 1990s and further substantiated by the international minimally invasive foot and ankle society, MIFAS by GRECMIP international society over the last two decades. In a recent study published by Vernois et al., the investigators followed and reviewed 75 feet treated with a percutaneous Lapidus procedure by a single surgeon.[6] An Akin osteotomy was routinely performed, and the procedure was performed for a flatfoot correction in 10 of the cases. The satisfaction rate was found to be good or excellent in 95% of the cases with no complications involving metatarsalgia transfers or infections. While further long-term outcome studies are needed, the authors have found similarly encouraging outcomes and remain optimistic about the evolution of the percutaneous Lapidus using the described technique in treating first ray deformities minimally invasively moving forward.

◆ INDICATIONS AND CONTRAINDICATIONS

As with many preferred hallux valgus correction surgical techniques, indications for Lapidus can vary from surgeon to surgeon. Traditionally, any break in Meary angle on lateral radiograph signals first TMT hypermobility and instability, which warrants correction through this joint as opposed to a more distal procedure. Intermetatarsal angle measurements greater than 15° warrant consideration for Lapidus. Patients with a bunion deformity and arthritis at the first TMT should be treated with a Lapidus to correct the deformity and symptomatic arthritis simultaneously. Patients prone to recurrent hallux valgus, such as those with hyperligamentous laxity and connective tissue diseases, can be treated successfully with a first TMT fusion. Lastly, revision hallux valgus surgery after a prior failed distal procedure is often an indication for a Lapidus as well.

Most contraindications are not unique to Lapidus when compared to other hallux valgus correction techniques. However, care must be taken in those at high risk for nonunion. With newer minimally invasive techniques, there is less soft-tissue dissection and presumably less vascular disruption to the bone theoretically lowering the risk for nonunion.

◆ PATIENT HISTORY AND PHYSICAL EXAMINATION

Patients typically present with a painful bunion deformity that has failed prior nonsurgical treatment options and lifestyle modifications. Many will have already tried toe spacers, bunion splints, custom orthotics, and other various shoe wear alterations to accommodate the deformity and alleviate discomfort. The primary site of discomfort may be along the medial eminence, plantarly in line with the sesamoids, or more global pain across the entire first metatarsophalangeal (MTP) joint in cases of early-stage hallux rigidus. Family history usually demonstrates a lineage of bunion deformity.

On physical examination, the bunion deformity is obvious and easily visualized. But, it is important to perform a comprehensive lower extremity examination before all attention is drawn to the forefoot. Initial visual inspection of the gait, calcaneal alignment, ankle alignment, arch, and skin elucidate other associated pathologies. It is important to identify concomitant malalignment such as progressive collapsing flatfoot deformity or metatarsus adductus. Performing a Silverskiöld test to assess gastrocnemius and Achilles tightness helps to prevent forefoot overload or over plantarflexion of the first ray during surgical correction.

Mobility of the first TMT joint helps with presurgical planning and decision-making. Lastly, a thorough neurovascular examination should be documented.

◆ IMAGING STUDIES

The primary imaging study is plain radiography. Anteroposterior, oblique, and lateral radiographs of the foot allow for the evaluation of the deformity, position of the sesamoids relative of the first metatarsal head, as well as other associated deformity such as hallux interphalangeus or metatarsus adductus. Anteroposterior views allow for measurement of the hallux valgus angle and more importantly, the intermetatarsal angle. Lateral radiographs evaluate for first TMT joint instability, noted by plantar gapping or subluxation of the metatarsal cuneiform joints, as well as associated flatfoot deformity. Oblique radiographs visualize the lesser metatarsal shafts in finer detail, which may show evidence of cortical hypertrophy in cases of chronic overload due to abnormal force distribution attributable to the hallux valgus deformity.

There is a growing role for the utility of CT, especially weight-bearing CT scans in hallux valgus deformity. This allows for better visualization and quantification of the pronation deformity of the first metatarsal and the relative position of the sesamoids to the crista of the plantar first metatarsal head. CT may also reveal degenerative changes in the first MTP joint that dissuade the surgeon from choosing the Lapidus to correct the deformity. These studies are not vital for surgical planning and can be financially burdensome. There is no defined role for MRI in the evaluation of isolated hallux valgus deformity unless the presentation is atypical and the surgeon is seeking an alternative reason for pain.

◆ PREOPERATIVE PLANNING AND PREPARATION

Preoperative planning begins with the history and physical examination. The severity of the deformity, flexibility of the first TMT, and associated pathologies such as concomitant hammertoes or metatarsus adductus help to determine the surgical and postoperative plan. Radiographic assessment and planning are paramount. Measuring the intermetatarsal angle, hallux valgus angle, and metatarsal length creates an objective assessment of the amount of planned correction to use as reference.

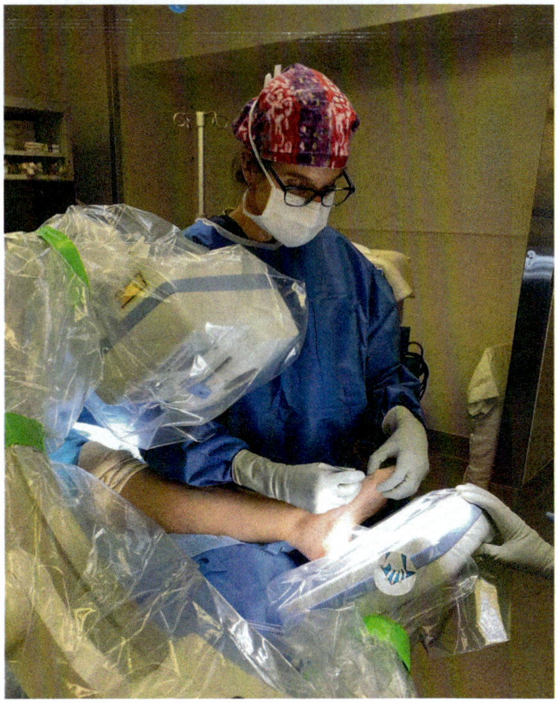

Figure 5.1 Patient setup and surgeon positioning for a right-handed surgeon operating on a right foot.

Setup is unique to the surgeon's handedness and the laterality of the operative extremity. The patient is positioned with the operative foot hanging off the end of the bed just proximal to the level of the malleoli. For a right-handed surgeon, the fluoroscopy will be on the right side of the patient regardless of the laterality of the operative extremity. For a left foot, the surgeon will stand on the left side of the operating room table, proximal to the foot while the assistant will stand at the foot of the bed. For a right foot, the surgeon will stand at the foot of the bed and the assistant on the right side of the bed. This positioning allows for unimpeded access to the foot during fluoroscopy, maneuverability of the handpiece, and it avoids the need to use the burr ambidextrously (Figure 5.1). Naturally, this setup is reversed for a left-handed surgeon.

SURGICAL TECHNIQUE

Lateral Release

The lateral release is performed first and routinely for all Lapidus cases. Using a Beaver blade, identify the lateral aspect of the first MTP joint using fluoroscopy. Then, insert the Beaver blade and release the lateral joint capsule from the base of the proximal phalanx (Figure 5.2A and B). If needed, the adductor tendon can be released from the fibular sesamoid to allow for greater correction.

Medial Eminence Resection

The medial eminence resection can be performed before or after the TMT joint is fused. It is the authors' preference to begin with the medial eminence resection prior to moving proximally. Care must be taken to avoid overresection of the eminence before the bony correction is achieved in order to avoid hallux varus overcorrection.

The medial eminence resection is performed through a small medial incision just proximal to the metaphyseal flare (Figure 5.3). A 2- to 3-mm incision is made, and blunt dissection is made down to the bone. The capsule is then released from the medial first metatarsal head with a sharp elevator, creating a working space for the burr. The 3.1 × 13 mm wedge burr is then used to morselize the prominent medial eminence. Care is taken to copiously irrigate all bony debris from the wound.

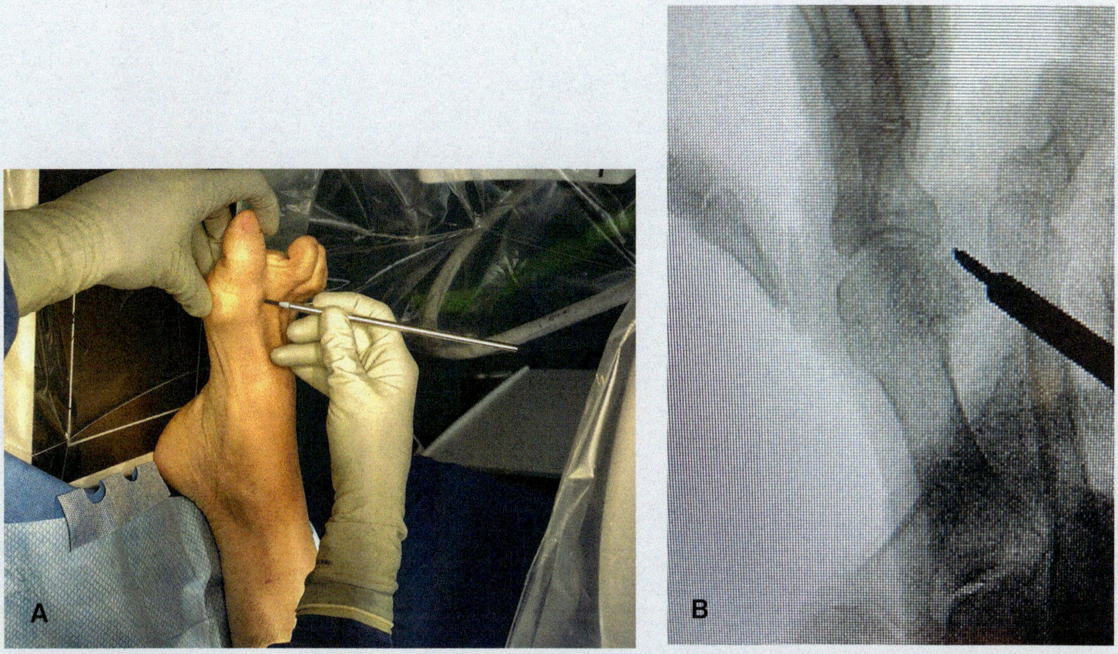

Figure 5.2 A, B. Insertion of the Beaver blade into the first webspace to perform a lateral release of the first metatarsophalangeal.

First TMT Fusion

First, identify via fluoroscopy and then mark out the joint line on the skin to help guide the percutaneous joint preparation (Figure 5.4A and B). Make a 5-mm incision just above the anterior tibial tendon medially at the joint. Carefully spread down to bone with a dull hemostat and perforate the medial joint capsule, using fluoroscopy as needed to ensure proper position. Use an elevator to distract the joint and open the space within the first TMT to accommodate the burr (Figure 5.5). Using the 3.1 × 13 mm, remove the cartilage from the first TMT in a gentle sweeping motion, using fluoroscopy to prevent deviation into the metatarsal or medial cuneiform (Figure 5.6A and B). Because the length of the burr does not span the width of the joint, the authors remove the cartilage systematically in quartiles, starting with the medial aspect of the metatarsal, then the lateral metatarsal, then medial cuneiform, and then lateral cuneiform. After preparing the joint, larger pieces of loose cartilage may be removed using a narrow pituitary rongeur. The morselized cartilage is then flushed out the incision using irrigation through a 14-gauge angiocatheter with a 30-mL syringe. An additional small dorsal incision may be made directly over the TMT joint laterally adjacent to the extensor hallucis longus (EHL) tendon to allow outflow of the irrigation and ensure that all cartilage and bony debris is removed from the space (Figure 5.7). Flush the joint at least 10 cycles. Any remaining cartilage on the joint surface can be removed with the burr, small curette, or pituitary rongeur (Figure 5.8A and B). Confirm that the joint surfaces are smooth and all bone has been removed using fluoroscopy (Figure 5.9A and B). A small arthroscope can be placed through the medial portal to examine the joint for remaining cartilage as well.

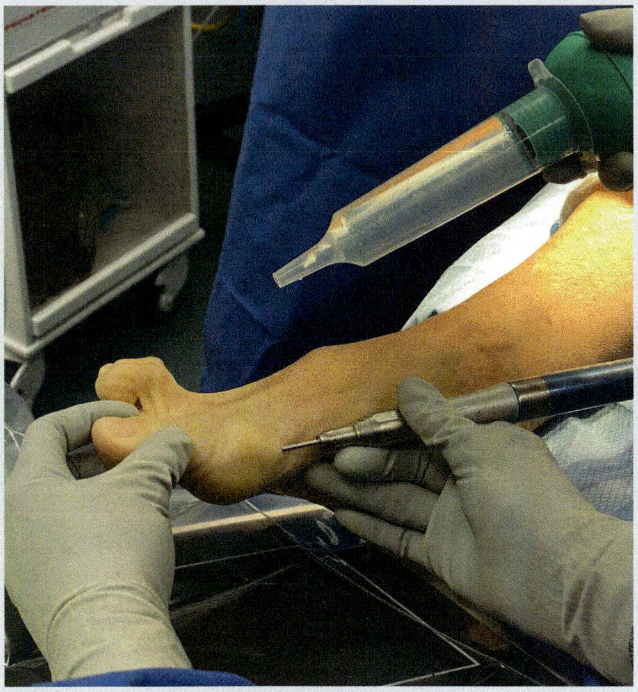

Figure 5.3 Medial eminence resection.

Bone graft or other biologic adjuvants may be placed in the joint if the patient is at higher risk for nonunion. Position two to three crossing wires provisionally at the TMT joint (Figure 5.10A and B). The lateral wire should travel from proximal to distal, and the medial wire is placed distal to proximal. Manually derotate, reduce, and compress the TMT joint while the assistant drives the wires across the joint. Confirm the alignment and wire position on radiograph. Simulate the weight-bearing position of the foot using a flat plate to assess clinical

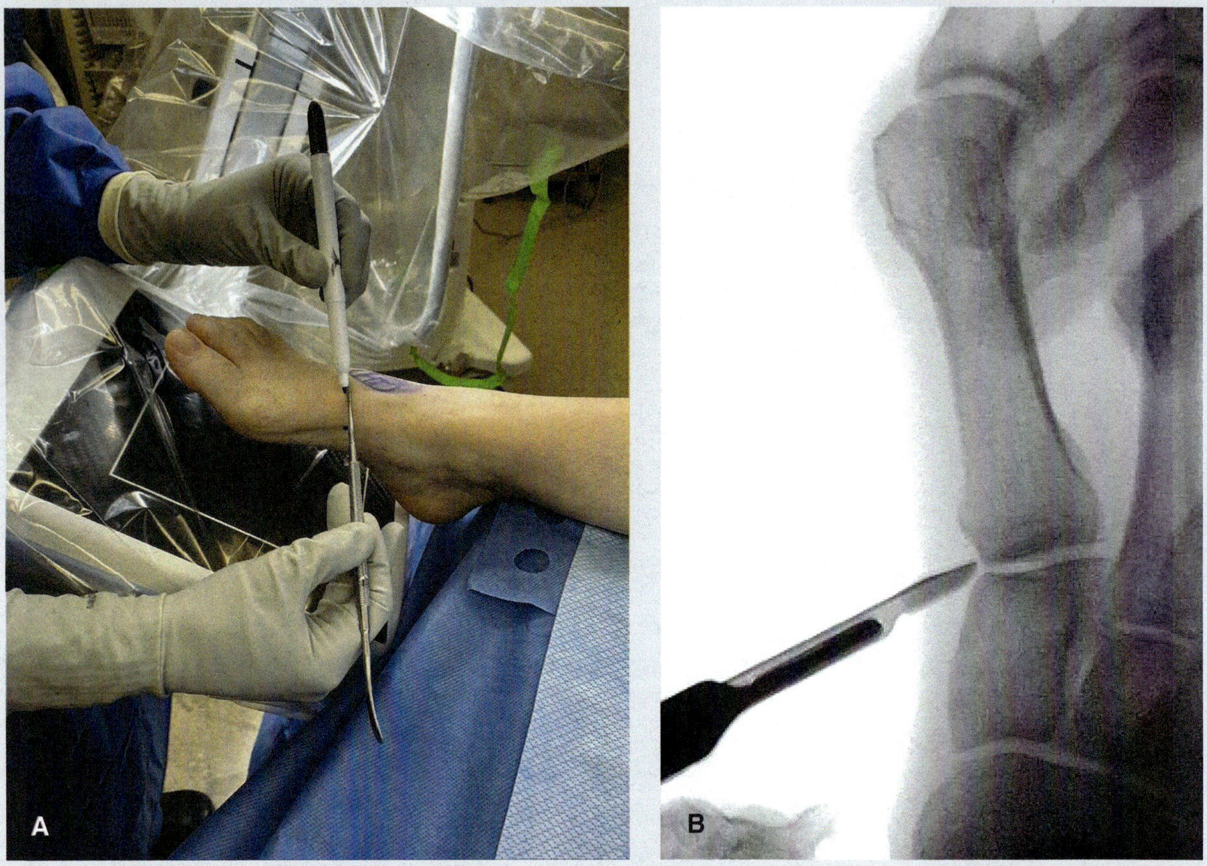

Figure 5.4 **A, B.** Marking the first tarsometatarsal joint on fluoroscopy prior to skin incision.

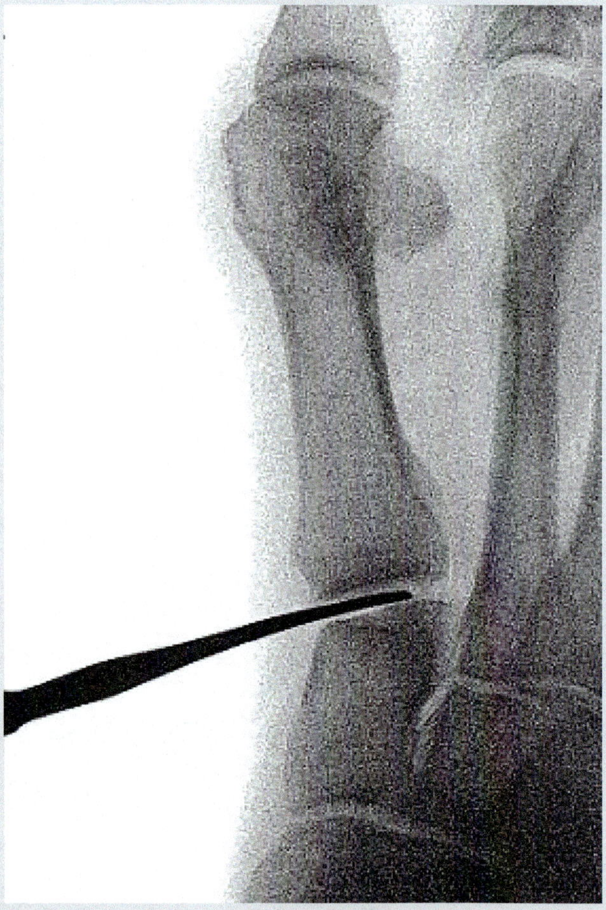

Figure 5.5 Mobilization of the first tarsometatarsal joint using a freer elevator under fluoroscopy.

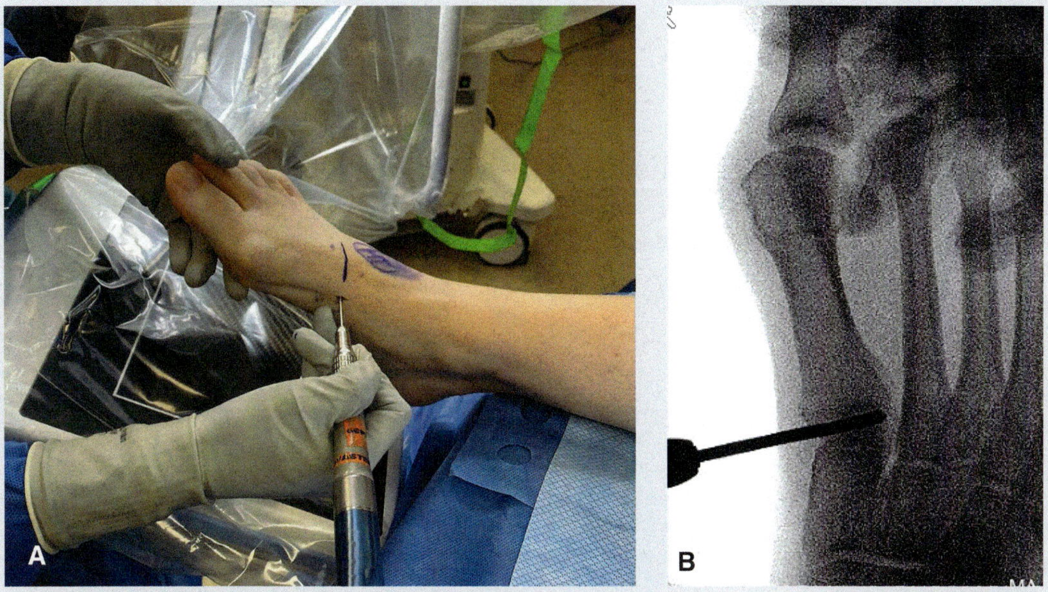

Figure 5.6 **A, B.** Resection of the cartilage within the first tarsometatarsal joint and corrective cut along the cuneiform.

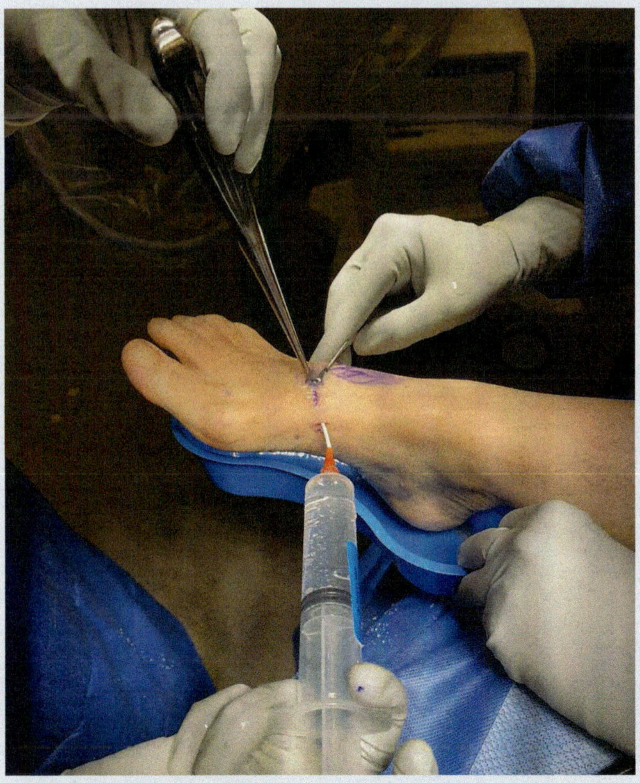

Figure 5.7 Outflow incision for irrigation along the lateral border of the extensor hallucis longus tendon.

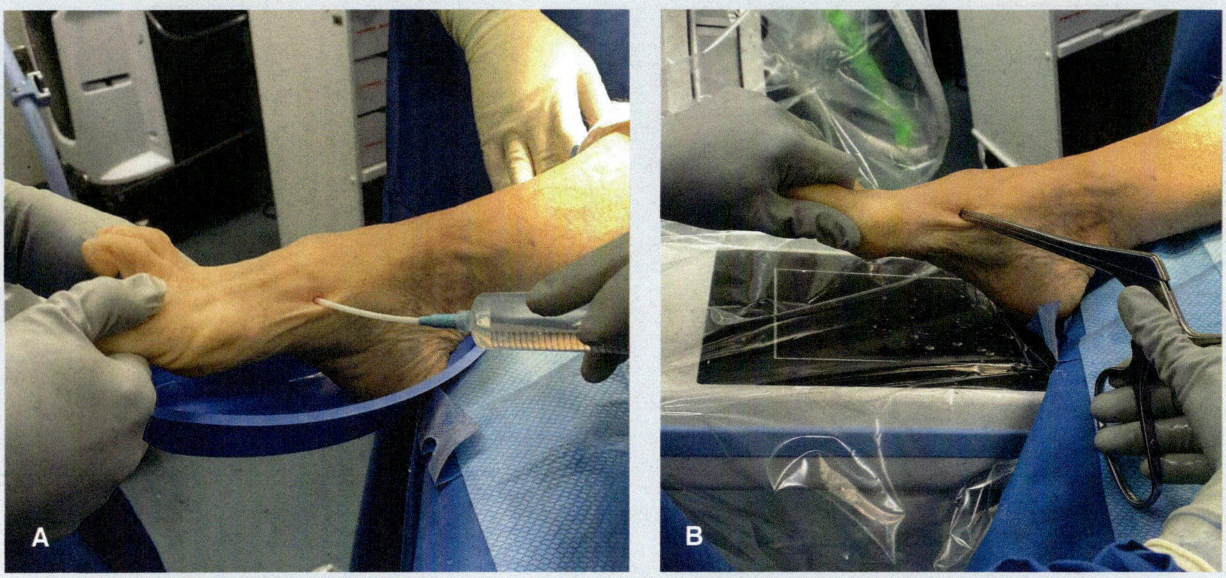

Figure 5.8 A, B. Irrigation of the first tarsometatarsal joint to remove debris using a 14-gauge angiocatheter.

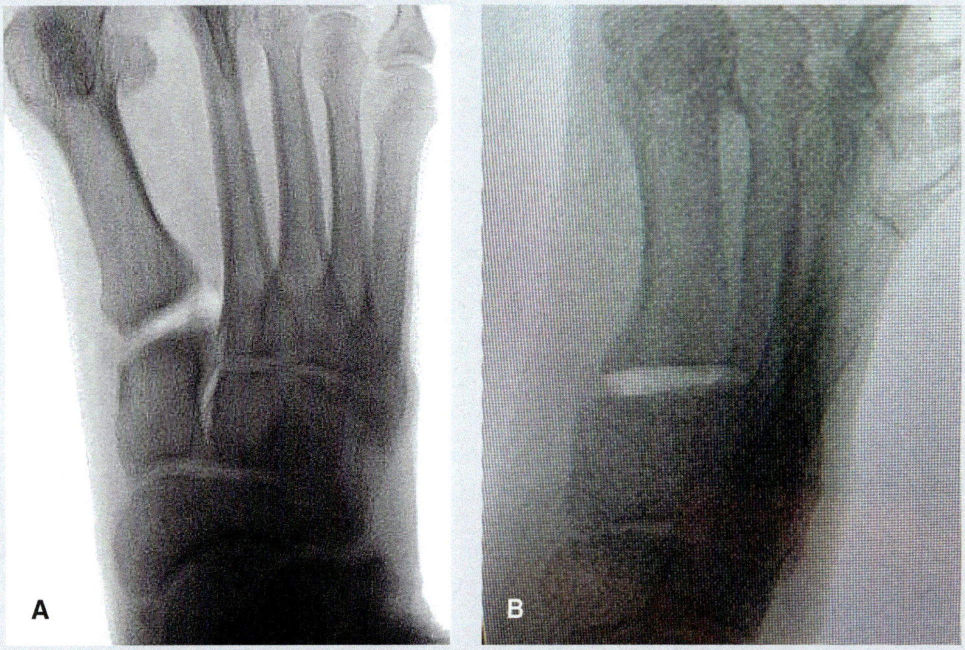

Figure 5.9 A, B. Ensure that joint space is clear of debris and joints surfaces are flat.

reduction as well as plantarflexion and dorsiflexion of the joint (Figure 5.11A-C). If the joint position is well-reduced, each wire is measured using an indirect depth gauge and then overdrilled. A partially threaded, headless, 4.0-mm compression screw is placed over the lateral wire to secure the correction. The medial screw is placed next (Figure 5.12A-C). A K-wire is placed under fluoroscopic guidance from the midportion of the medial cuneiform into the base of the second metatarsal to stabilize the intercuneiform joint (Figure 5.13). The final screw is placed over this wire. Repeat the simulated weight-bearing assessment with the flat plate to ensure the correction and fixation.

In almost every case, a percutaneous Akin osteotomy is performed for further correction. Under fluoroscopic guidance, a 2-mm incision is made just distal to the medial midline of the proximal phalanx. A 2 × 12 mm Shannon burr is used to make an oblique osteotomy angled toward the proximal lateral metaphysis, taking care to maintain the lateral hinge. The osteotomy is then closed down and held with a 1.0 wire placed percutaneously from the base of the medial proximal phalanx perpendicular to the cut. After fluoroscopy confirms correct placement of the wire, a small incision is made over wire, the wire is measured using an indirect guide, and a 3.0-mm screw is placed over the wire. Care is taken to hold the reduction as the screw is placed to maintain correction. Final assessment using flat plate weight-bearing simulation is performed again to confirm adequacy of the reduction. All incisions are then copiously irrigated again and closed with 4-0 nylon suture. Bacitracin ointment followed by a nonadherent dressing is then placed on the wounds (Figure 5.14A-C).

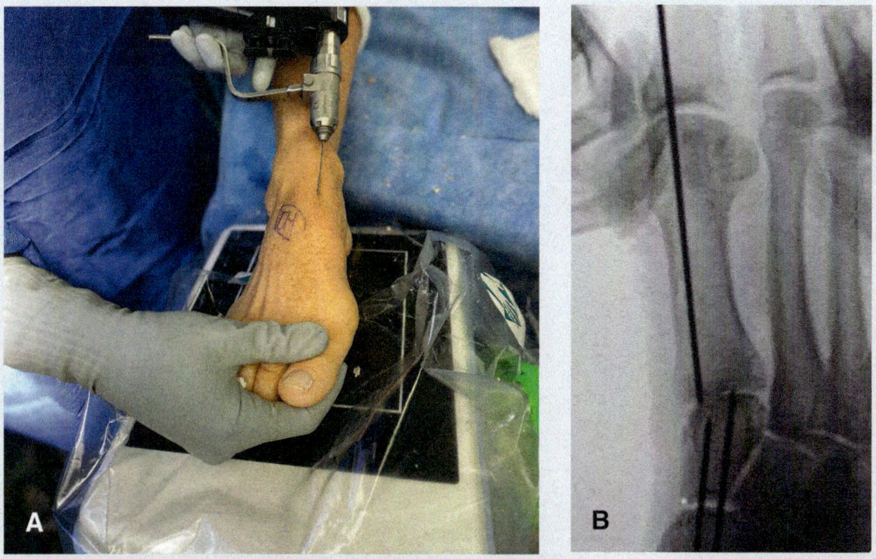

Figure 5.10 A, B. Provisional placement of the K-wire for joint reduction and fixation.

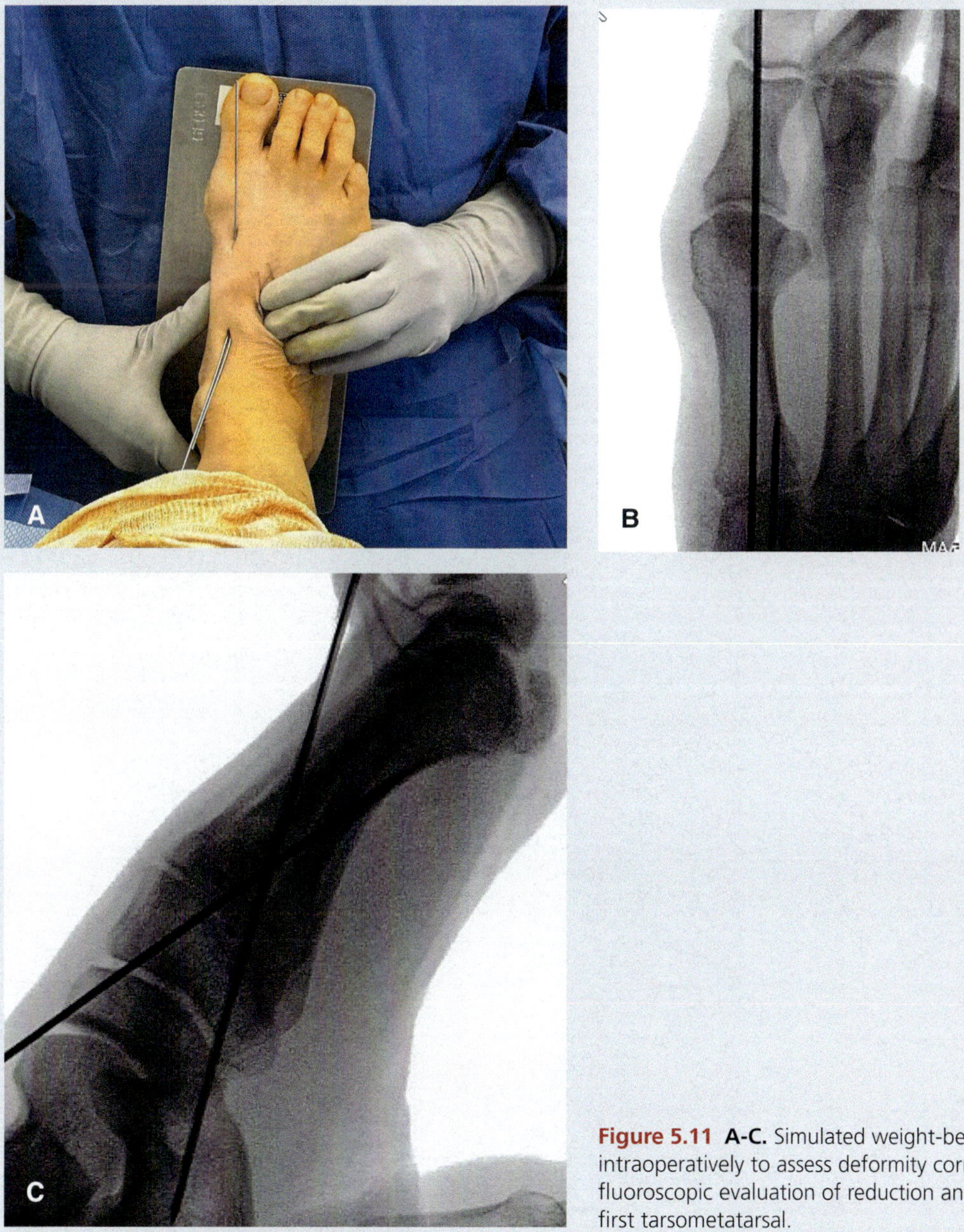

Figure 5.11 A-C. Simulated weight-bearing evaluation of the foot intraoperatively to assess deformity correction using a flat plate with fluoroscopic evaluation of reduction and K-wire placement across the first tarsometatarsal.

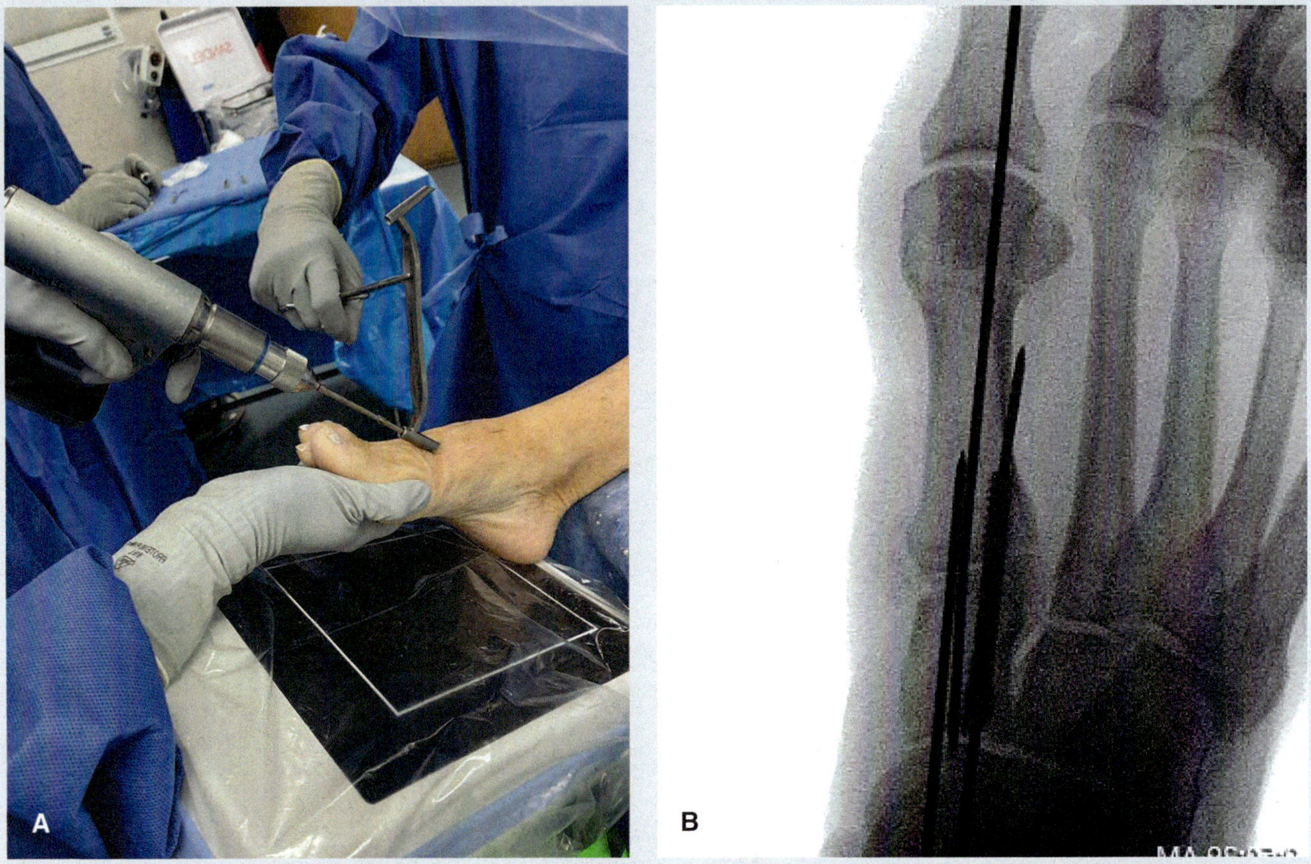

Figure 5.12 A, B. Placement of screws over the wires.

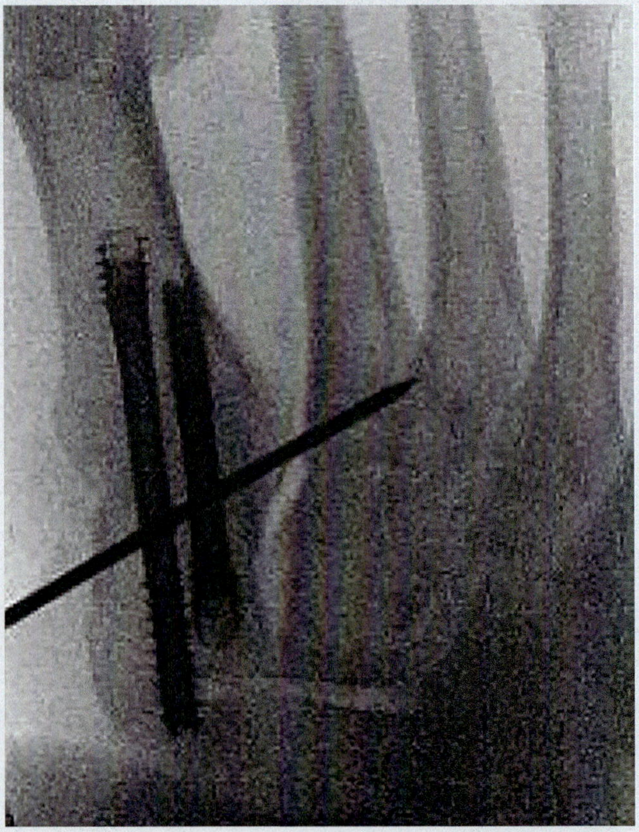

Figure 5.13 Placement of the C1-M2 wire.

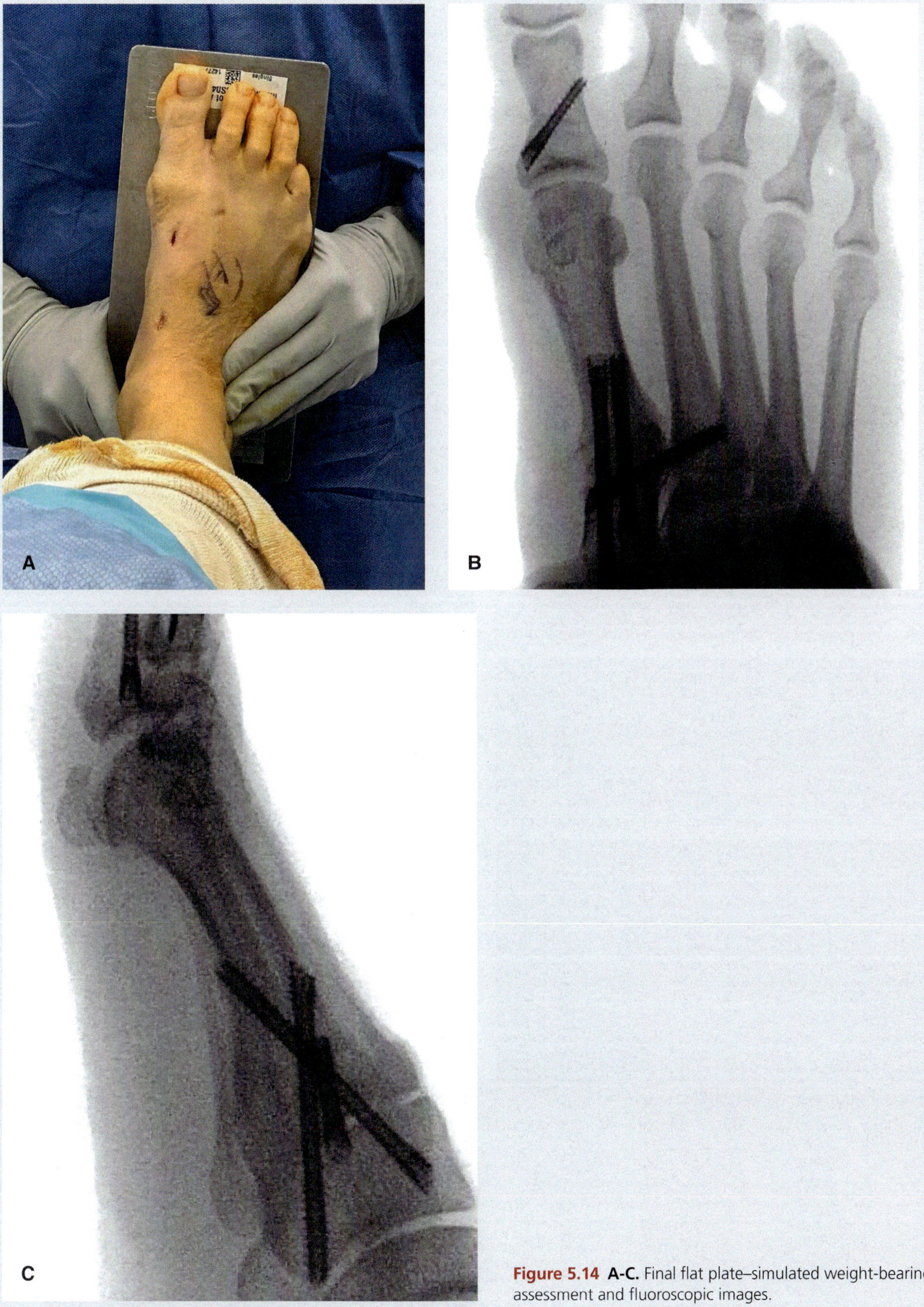

Figure 5.14 A-C. Final flat plate–simulated weight-bearing assessment and fluoroscopic images.

◆ POSTOPERATIVE MANAGEMENT

After the incisions have been closed, gauze moistened in saline is placed as a spica bunion dressing around the forefoot. The patient is then placed into a short leg splint in the operating room and is been non–weight bearing for the first 2 weeks after surgery. Pain is managed with ibuprofen and acetaminophen after the 24-hour popliteal block wears off. At the first postoperative visit in 2 weeks, the patient is transitioned into a walker boot where they begin progressive weight bearing over the next 2 weeks. Physical therapy is initiated to work on range of motion, strengthening, and soft-tissue management. At 4 weeks postoperatively, the patient will be allowed to weight bear as tolerated in the boot until 6 to 8 weeks at which point they will transition into a regular sneaker. Serial, weight-bearing radiographs are obtained at 2 weeks, 6 weeks, 3 months, and 6 months. Patients are released to resume all physical activity without restrictions at 3 months. Follow-up is encouraged to 1 year (Figure 5.15A-F).

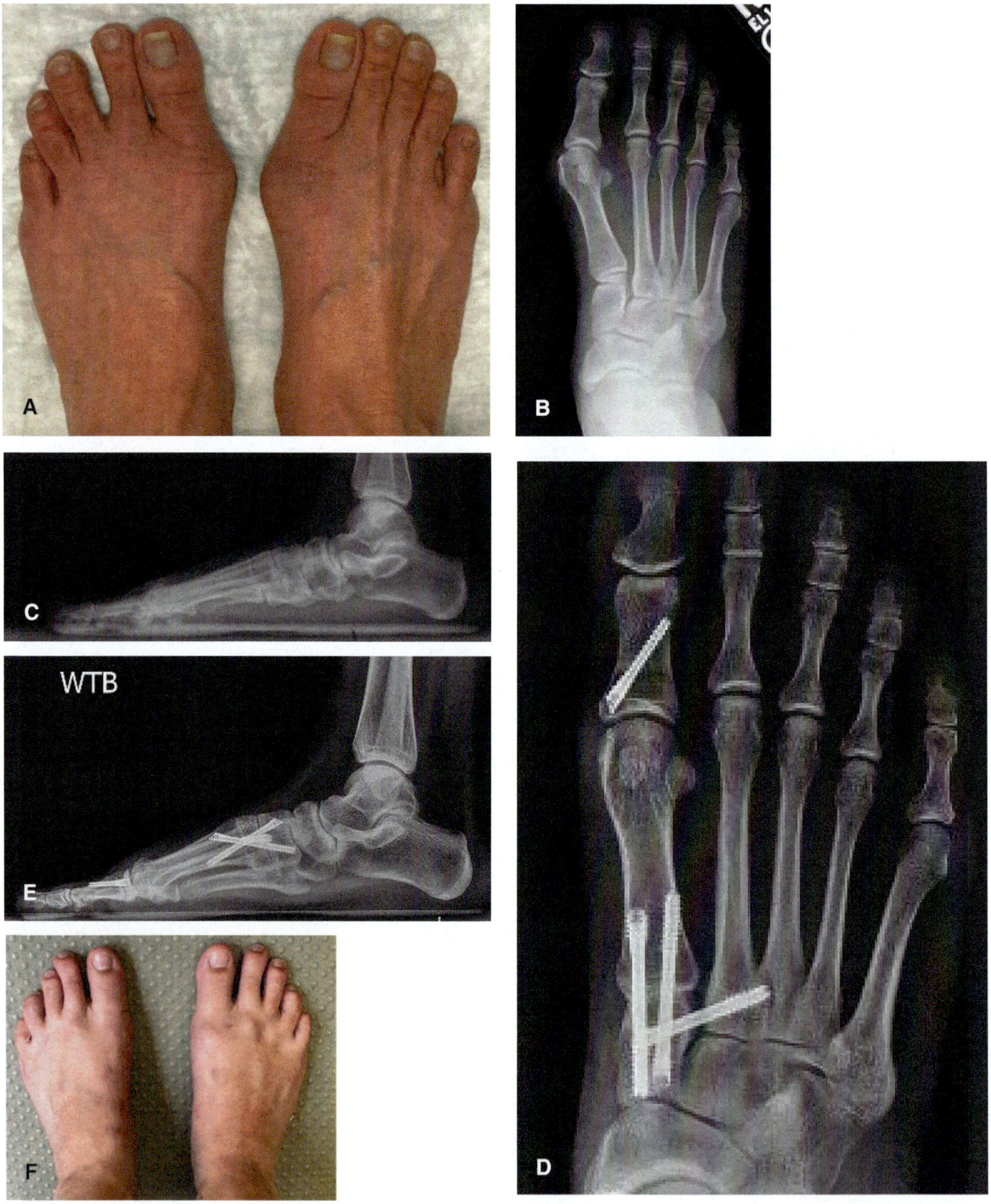

Figure 5.15 A-F. Bilateral hallux valgus deformities preoperatively. One year postoperative images on the left foot. Clinical image of both feet postoperatively, left side 12 months and right side 9 months.

◆ OUTCOMES

There are relatively few literature reports on outcomes of the minimally invasive (MI) Lapidus procedure at this time. The Lapidus procedure has undergone numerous iterations over time, mostly involving changes to hardware and fixation technique. The procedure has been relied upon by many because of its ability to address severe deformities with reliable stability and also correct deformity in multiple planes, which has been an issue for other operations. The belief is that because the TMT joint is fused, the risk of recurrence is lower. Complications of the Lapidus operation have been a concern for surgeons, however, with delayed healing and higher malunion and nonunion rates being reported. A recent systematic review cited the most complications of Lapidus to be nonunion or delayed union (4.4%), hardware-related pain (2.8%), recurrence (2%), hallux varus (1.4%), postoperative wound complication (1.3%), and transfer metatarsalgia (1.1%).

In light of this, minimally invasive techniques have been developed in an effort to minimize these complication rates while improving outcomes. In 2005, Lui et al. described the arthroscopic first TMT fusion technique and reported that by allowing for a more accurate joint preparation under direct visualization, shortening, dorsiflexion, and adduction could be minimized. The less invasive technique also allowed for less soft-tissue damage, postoperative pain, increased bone blood supply, better cosmesis, and less wound complications. In a study done by Michels et al. using this technique in five patients, radiographic evaluation confirmed fusion in all the patients without any major complications.[7] The hallux valgus angle improved by 25.68, and the intermetatarsal angle improved by 10.68. The shortening of the first ray was limited to 2.7 mm.

There have been few comparison studies involving the MI Lapidus procedure thus far. A recent study performed by Cardoso et al. is the first article reporting comparative outcomes between MI and open first TMT fusion.[8] Their group reported on 91 patients (47 MI vs 44 open) and found that in both techniques, postoperative measures (intermetatarsal angle [IMA], hallux valgus angle, distal metatarsal articular angle, and sesamoid station) were significantly improved from preoperative measures. When comparing postoperative measures between both groups, the IMA was significantly lower in the open group. The open group was associated with more correction than the MI group for IMA and hallux valgus angle. Wound complication and nonunion rates trended higher in the open group with four complications in the open group and zero in the minimally invasive group.

A review of patients undergoing the MI Lapidus procedure at the authors' institution by a single surgeon was performed with the advent of this technique in 2020. Sixty patients underwent the operation and were eligible for analysis. There were found to be four nonunions (two requiring revision and two stable managed nonoperatively), four recurrences requiring a revision, three hardware removals for painful hardware, and one reoperation for medial eminence resection. There were no infections reported. Currently, pre- and postoperative radiographic results and patient-reported outcome scores are being collected to report formally on these outcomes.

◆ CONCLUSION

Percutaneous Lapidus is a technically challenging procedure that is used in cases where a distal hallux valgus correction may not be sufficient to correct underlying midfoot instability or severe deformity. The rate of complications including nonunion and recurrence or undercorrection do appear higher, but this may be more related to the learning curve of the surgeon and the higher risk overall of the severe bunions treated with Lapidus.

References

1. Lai MC, Rikhraj IS, Woo YL, Yeo W, Ng YCS, Koo K. Clinical and radiological outcomes comparing percutaneous chevron-Akin osteotomies vs open scarf-Akin osteotomies for hallux valgus. *Foot Ankle Int.* 2018;39(3):311-317.
2. Lee M, Walsh J, Smith MM, Ling J, Wines A, Lam P. Hallux valgus correction comparing percutaneous chevron/Akin (PECA) and open scarf/Akin osteotomies. *Foot Ankle Int.* 2017;38(8):838-846.
3. Lapidus PW. A quarter of a century of experience with the operative correction of the metatarsus varus primus in hallux valgus. *Bull Hosp Joint Dis.* 1956;17(2):404-421.
4. Lapidus PW. The author's bunion operation from 1931 to 1959. *Clin Orthop.* 1960;16:119-135.
5. Do DH, Sun JJ, Wukich DK. Modified Lapidus procedure and hallux valgus. A systematic review and update on triplanar correction. *Orthop Clin N Am.* 2022;53:499-508.
6. Vernois J, Redfern D; GRECMIP soon MIFAS 3. Lapidus, a percutaneous approach. *Foot Ankle Clin.* 2020;25(3):407-412.
7. Michels F, Guillo S, de Lavigne C, Van der Bauwhede J. The arthroscopic Lapidus procedure. *Foot Ankle Surg.* 2011;17:25-28.
8. Cardoso DV, Veljkovic A, Wing K, Penner M, Gagne O, Younger A. Cohort comparison of radiographic correction and complications between minimal invasive and open Lapidus procedures for hallux valgus. *Foot Ankle Int.* 2022;43(10):1277-1284.

SECTION 2
Hallux Rigidus

6 Minimally Invasive Dorsal Cheilectomy and Moberg Osteotomy for Hallux Rigidus

Thomas L. Lewis, Robbie Ray, and Peter Lam

◆ INTRODUCTION

Hallux rigidus is a degenerative disorder of the first metatarsophalangeal joint (MTPJ) that causes substantial discomfort, as well as a decline in function and quality of life. It is common, affecting 2.5% of the population over 50 years old and disproportionately affecting females. Hallux rigidus is characterized by the formation of dorsal and peripheral osteophytes, flattening of the metatarsal head, and a reduced joint space width, giving rise to symptoms of increasing pain, dorsal tenderness, and a progressive reduction of overall mobility, especially dorsiflexion, at the first MTPJ.[1]

The operative treatment of hallux rigidus focuses on either joint-preserving interventions, such as cheilectomy or osteotomy of the metatarsal or phalanx, or joint-sacrificing surgery in the form of arthrodesis or arthroplasty.[2] Joint-preserving operations are indicated for early stages of hallux rigidus, while arthrodesis is the gold standard for advanced stages of hallux rigidus with predictable and consistent satisfactory results in 90% of cases.[3]

The most common joint preservation operations include a cheilectomy, which can be combined with a Moberg osteotomy (dorsal closing wedge osteotomy of the proximal phalanx (P1) of the hallux). One biomechanical theory based on a cadaveric study showed that a Moberg osteotomy shifted the center of pressure on the first metatarsal head in a plantar direction.[4] The plantar shift created by the Moberg osteotomy may lessen forces on the arthritic joint surfaces, especially dorsal articular chondral lesions.

The aim of this chapter is to review the indications, surgical technique, and literature outcomes following minimally invasive (MIS) dorsal cheilectomy and Moberg osteotomy for hallux rigidus.

◆ INDICATIONS AND CONTRAINDICATIONS

Clinical examination and radiographic studies are required to guide the surgical decision-making regarding whether to proceed with a joint-preserving or joint-sacrificing technique. Weight-bearing radiographs can be categorized using the Coughlin and Shurnas classification of hallux rigidus. Patients with a Coughlin and Shurnas grade less than 3 are potential candidates for joint preservation. Preoperative range of motion assessment is important, as surgery is not recommended for patients with first MTPJ dorsiflexion greater than 20°.

The aim of the cheilectomy and Moberg osteotomy are to increase range of motion by removing bony osteophytes that may be blocking dorsiflexion and effectively elevate the proximal phalanx by plantar subluxation of the first MTPJ. In the authors' experience, the combination of cheilectomy and Moberg osteotomy may increase the dorsiflexion range by at least 10° to 20°.

Patients with significant pain on applied compressive force across the joint rather than predominantly pain on dorsiflexion (Coughlin and Shurnas grade 4) are unlikely to significantly benefit from joint preservation surgery and should instead be considered for joint-sacrificing surgery.

◆ PATIENT HISTORY AND PHYSICAL EXAMINATION

When taking a history, it is important to inquire as to whether more of the pain is due to rubbing of the osteophytes on shoe wear or pain with motion at the joint. For pain due to rubbing of osteophytes, shoes with a soft upper part can be useful for reducing pain, bursitis, and ulceration. For pain with range of motion, a shoe with a stiff sole or orthotics with a Morton extension or spring steel plate can limit movement at the first MTPJ, reducing inflammation and pain. Rocker sole shoes are available that combine these two factors and can be an excellent conservative measure in the early treatment of painful first MTPJ arthritis.

Evaluation of patient history is important for identifying underlying inflammatory conditions such as gout or other inflammatory arthropathies. Although these conditions do not necessarily exclude a joint-preserving procedure, patients with continued bouts of acute inflammation and pain the patient are more likely to benefit from joint arthrodesis.

Deformity should also be assessed. If there is minor axial plane deformity, an Akin or combined Akin and Moberg osteotomy may be beneficial during surgical correction. Midrange of motion pain and, more specifically, axial compression testing in a neutral position should be performed to assess for deep intra-articular pain. Although midrange pain does not preclude joint-sparing surgery, pain on axial compression in a neutral position should push the surgeon toward joint-sacrificing surgery, as this is suggestive of central arthritic rather than dorsal impingement pain, making the patient less likely to clinically improve with joint-sparing procedures.

Range of motion should be assessed as preoperative range of movement generally dictates postoperative range of motion. In the authors' experience, although great dorsiflexion is seen intraoperatively after dorsal cheilectomy, patients generally gain only around 10° to 20° of motion after recovery from the procedure.[5]

Finally, an assessment of the hallux interphalangeal (IP) joint should be performed (Figure 6.1). If the patient has hyperdorsiflexion of the IP joint, they are more tolerant of stiffness at the MTPJ and a dorsal cheilectomy without Moberg may be sufficient to improve dorsiflexion, even in a significantly stiff first MTPJ. If the hallux interphalangeal joint does not have compensatory hyperdorsiflexion, all dorsiflexion will have to come from the first MTPJ, and it may be prudent to add a Moberg osteotomy.

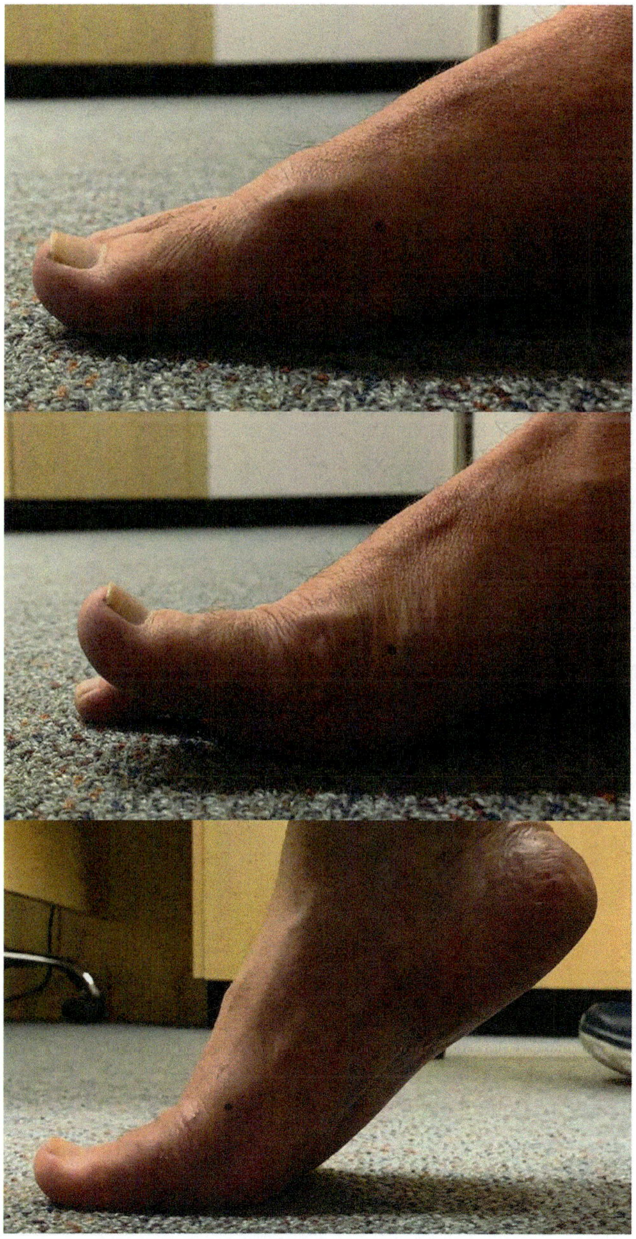

Figure 6.1 Clinical photographs demonstrating the preoperative active range of motion in a patient with hallux rigidus with loss of dorsiflexion (*top*, *middle*) and subsequent improvement following MIS dorsal cheilectomy and Moberg osteotomy (*bottom*).

◆ IMAGING STUDIES

Standard weight-bearing anterior-posterior (AP), oblique, and lateral radiographs are essential to guide decision-making with regard to performing a cheilectomy and Moberg osteotomy. The lateral view should be evaluated for dorsal osteophytes in conjunction with the AP view, which is useful in showing medial and lateral osteophytes, sclerotic changes, joint-space narrowing, and subchondral cysts (Figure 6.2).

Additional cross-sectional imaging is not usually needed, but if osteochondral abnormalities are suspected, advanced imaging may be helpful. In cases of trauma, normal radiographs, or young patients, an MRI may be recommended to evaluate for chondral injury, a loose body, or a developing osteochondral defect.

◆ PREOPERATIVE PLANNING AND PREPARATION

The setup for MIS procedures is of the utmost importance in order to improve the flow and efficiency of the procedure. The main aims of the setup are as follows:

- The surgeon should be well positioned to use the burr with their dominant hand.
- There must be adequate space and planning to use an image intensifier or mini C-arm throughout the procedure without risking sterility or the comfort of the surgeon.
- The nurse or surgical technician should be positioned so that they are available to pass instruments without impeding the surgeon or image intensifier.

The patient is positioned with the operative foot hanging from the end of the operating table by 6 in and the nonoperative leg frog-legged out of the operative field (unless the patient has an anterior total hip arthroplasty) in order to avoid obstructing the image intensifier. This allows for natural plantarflexion at the ankle and aids the surgeon in obtaining a true AP image of the first ray. It is also possible to achieve a true lateral view intraoperatively if the assistant externally rotates and flexes the knee. The authors do not recommend use a sandbag as the foot requires manipulation throughout MIS forefoot procedures, and a sandbag can impede external rotation, which is often required when taking a lateral radiographic image.

A right-handed surgeon should always position themselves to the left of the patient at the foot of the bed. This allows for full access to the first ray using medial incisions and puts their dominant hand in a relaxed position to operate. It follows that the image intensifier or mini C-arm should be brought in from the right of the patient so as not to impede access to the patient's foot.

Another important aspect of imaging positioning is that the imaging machine should be arranged so that the

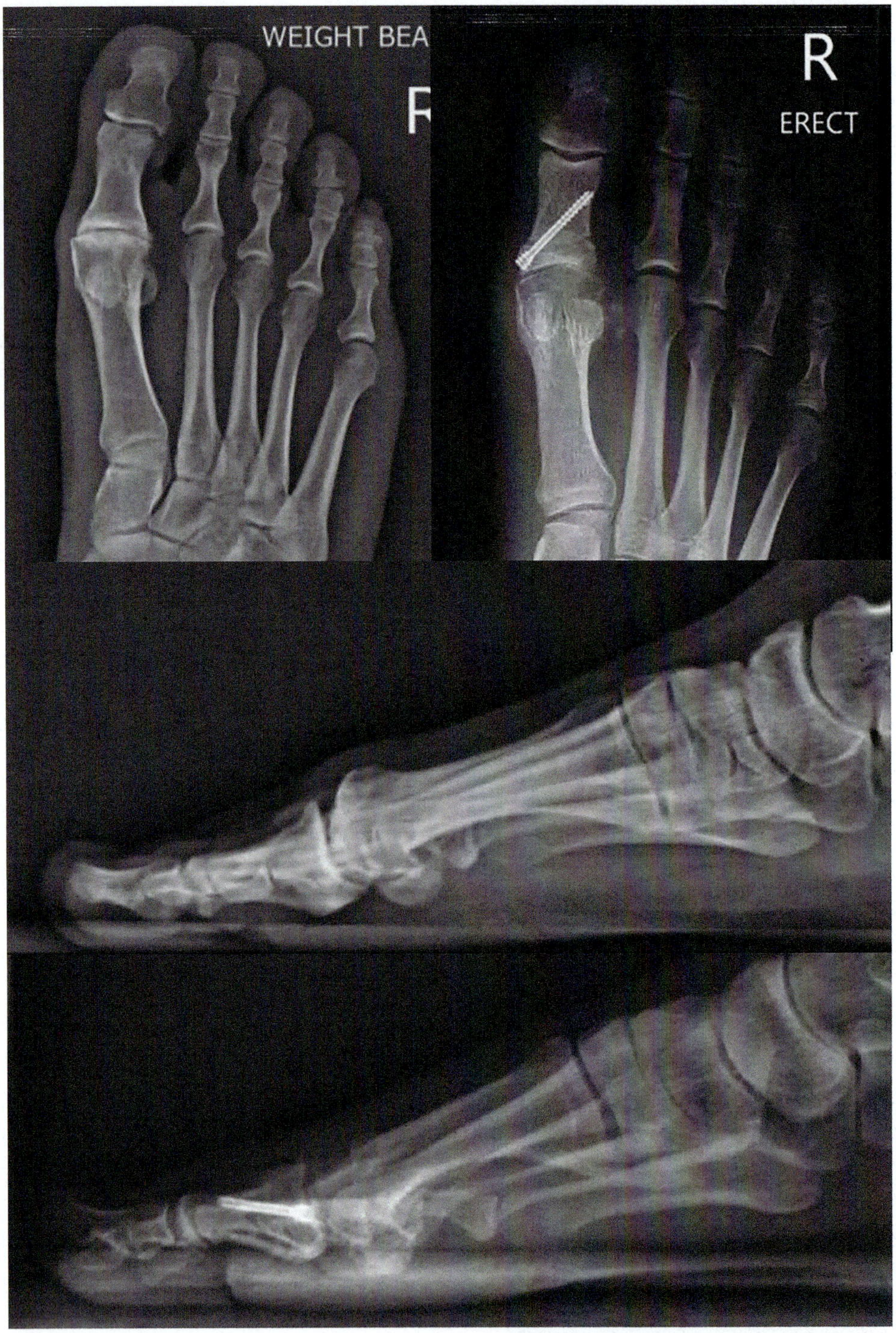

Figure 6.2 Preoperative and postoperative weight-bearing anterior-posterior and lateral radiographs demonstrating classic features of hallux rigidus including loss of joint space, large dorsal osteophytes, and subchondral sclerosis followed by MIS dorsal cheilectomy with Moberg osteotomy.

plate or drum is used as a table on which the forefoot rests. It is the authors' preference to use a mini C-arm over a large image intensifier. The other important factor to consider is that many orthopedic procedures are performed in theatres with a laminar flow Perspex box, and due to the commonly performed procedures being lower limb arthroplasty, the bed is generally positioned with the feet at the edge of this box. If this is the case, the Perspex box can impede access for the imaging machine especially if it is a larger machine, and due care must be taken to position the patient deeper into the laminar flow Perspex box prior to beginning the procedure.

The nurse or surgical technician should be positioned such that they are not in the way of the surgeon and able to assist throughout the procedure. As such, for the right-handed surgeon, the authors position the nurse to the left of the patient behind the surgeon. From this position, the assistant has ample space to open their trays and have their equipment ready. The console for the MIS system and power instruments should be set up at the patient's right hip out of the operating field.

SURGICAL TECHNIQUE

MIS DORSAL CHEILECTOMY OF FIRST MTPJ

The procedure is typically performed under total intravenous anesthesia with propofol. Once the patient is sedated, a first ray proximal digital ring block is performed using 30 mL of a combination of 1% lidocaine and 0.5% ropivacaine. A tourniquet is not used for this procedure. The skin incision for an MIS dorsal cheilectomy of the first MTPJ is made dorsomedially 2 to 3 cm proximal to the joint and adjacent to the extensor hallucis longus (EHL) tendon (Figure 6.3). This position allows for capsular release and clearance of the osteophytes from lateral to medial. The incision is made through the skin and dermis to expose the subcutaneous fat. After the dermis is cut, it is vitally important to make a safe plane down to the capsule without damaging the dorsomedial cutaneous nerve or extensor hallucis tendon.[6,7]

The MIS periosteal elevator is inserted with the blade of the periosteal elevator in line with the skin incision down to bone. This reduces the risk of iatrogenic injury to the dorsomedial cutaneous nerve. The elevator is then used to elevate the periosteum distally in order to reach the dorsomedial capsule. The proximal dorsomedial capsule is punctured with the periosteal elevator. The elevator is then directed intracapsularly toward the lateral aspect of the joint over the prominent dorsal osteophyte. The proximal dorsal capsule is then released from the lateral to the medial side. The capsular attachments are particularly adherent at the dorsomedial aspect, and if there is a combination of a dorsal osteophyte and medial exostosis, it is particularly important to focus on elevating the capsule here to make a clear path for osteophyte excision without any fragments adhering to the capsule. The complete release of the dorsal capsule from its attachment to the first metatarsal head is important to allow easier removal of the dorsal cortical fragments at the end of the cheilectomy. Once the dorsal capsular attachment to the first metatarsal head is fully released, the burr is inserted into the dorsal first MTPJ. The minimum size burr to use for dorsal cheilectomy

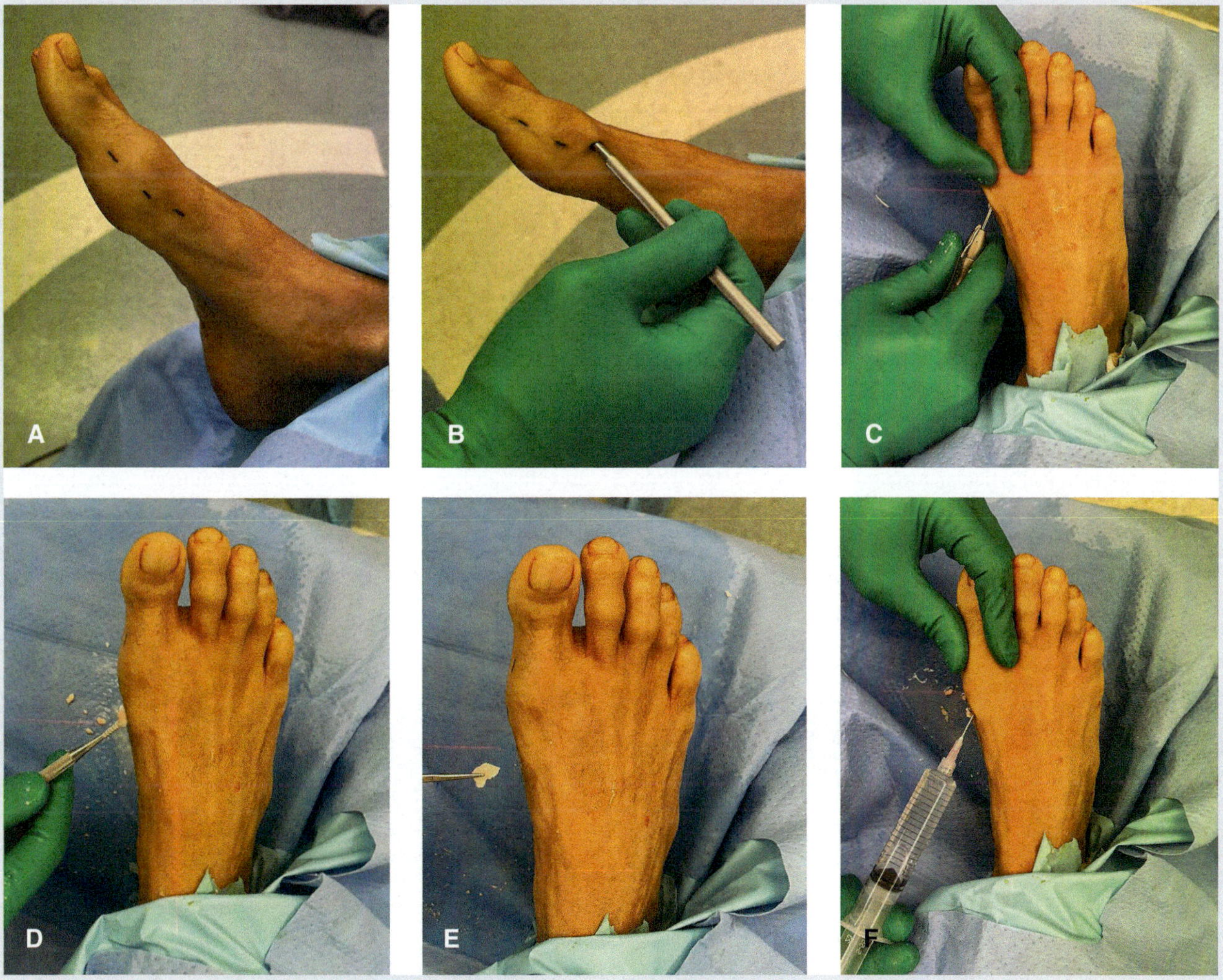

Figure 6.3 Clinical photographs demonstrating the key steps of MIS dorsal cheilectomy (*left* to *right*): **(A)** skin incision marking, **(B)** elevation of capsule off dorsal osteophytes, **(C)** excision of dorsal osteophytes with burr, **(D, E)** removal of dorsal osteophytes, and **(F)** copious irrigation to reduce bone paste.

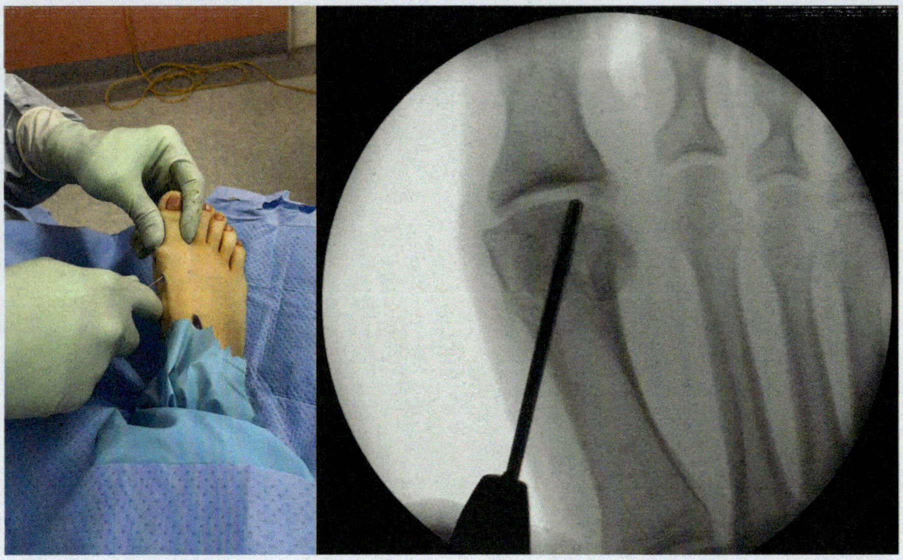

Figure 6.4 Clinical photograph and fluoroscopy image demonstrating the burr (3.1 mm × 13 mm wedge burr, Novastep, Orangeburg, New York) position for a lateral to medial bone cut for dorsal cheilectomy.

is a 2.9 or 3.1 wedge burr. The advantage of this burr is its conical shape that allows for cutting as well as grinding the bone. The primary sweep of the burr should be performed through the dorsal osteophyte, and create a plane between the osteophyte and the remaining metatarsal head. When performing a cheilectomy, the authors advocate performing a lateral to medial cut because the dorsal surface of the metatarsal is used as a guide for the burr (Figure 6.4).

For the right foot, the burr is inserted and run along the dorsal cortex of 1st metatarsal (M1) to get a feel of the line of the dorsal cortex. The tip of the burr is then directed 10° plantarly from the dorsal cortical line of M1, aiming to resect the dorsal third of the metatarsal head. The burr is used to cut the metatarsal. Once the bone cut has been initiated, a lateral radiograph is taken to confirm the trajectory of the cut (Figures 6.4 and 6.5). The first MTPJ is distracted when performing the osteotomy to protect that phalangeal articular surface (Figure 6.4). Care needs to be taken as the burr is pushed through the subchondral bone at the lateral aspect of the first metatarsal head. The burr is then directed medially while the joint is held in a neutral position with distraction of the first MTPJ. This will result in a flat cut dorsal cheilectomy and avoid leaving a small ridge of subchondral bone on the head. Once the osteotomy is complete, the index and middle fingers of the left hand are placed gently over the dorsal fragment on either side of the EHL tendon to steady the dorsal fragment while upward pressure is applied to the burr for resection of the thin the dorsal fragment. A 20-mL syringe with an 18-gauge blunt needle is used to irrigate the bony paste (Figure 6.3F). A rasp is used to help remove the bone paste. The rasp is used to pull the dorsal cortical sliver toward the portal. A straight mosquito hemostat is inserted to remove the remnant of the dorsal cortical fragment (Figure 6.3E). Further irrigation is performed to remove all remaining bone paste. A lateral radiograph is taken to confirm completion of the osteotomy and that all bone paste and any residual fragments have been removed (Figure 6.5B).

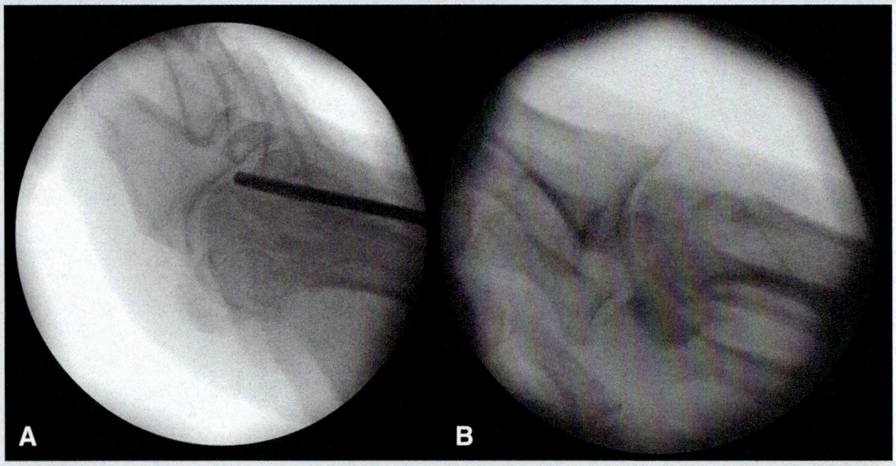

Figure 6.5 Intraoperative lateral fluoroscopy images demonstrating: **(A)** the position of the burr (3.1 mm × 13 mm wedge burr, Novastep, Orangeburg, New York) for a dorsal cheilectomy and **(B)** subsequent resection.

The authors think there is an important distinction between this described inside-out technique and the outside-in technique that involves using the burr in the plane between the dorsal osteophyte and the dorsal capsule with a gradual thinning technique. Although this technique has been described, the authors believe that it is unduly risky to the dorsal soft tissues and a significant risk factor for EHL tendon injury.

Arthroscopic Assistance

Once the cheilectomy is complete, thorough clearance of debris is recommended to reduce the risk of articular irritation from the bone paste. This can be performed with rasping and repeated syringe irrigation. Alternatively, an arthroscopic-assisted method may also be employed. Arthroscopy ensures irrigation of the joint with large volumes of saline, typically between 3 and 6 L, ensuring the maximum amount of bone paste is removed. On occasion, a small ledge of bone is left on the dorsal first metatarsal head, which could be a risk factor for future impingement. With arthroscopic assistance, the surface can be shaved smooth, and impingement-free range of movement may be visually assessed. Finally, visual assessment of the joint may be performed to evaluate for loose chondral flaps, synovitis, or osteochondral lesions that all can be addressed arthroscopically. It is important to position the camera to allow for comfortable arthroscopy without impeding the percutaneous portion of the procedure. The ideal place for the camera and arthroscopy tower is to the right of the patient just proximal to the fluoroscopy machine (Figure 6.6).

A 4-mm arthroscope is initially inserted through the dorsomedial portal, and a second portal is made at the level of the joint dorsolaterally. The capsule is punctured using blunt dissection with a straight mosquito hemostat, and a 3.5-mm shaver is inserted. Using suction, debris is cleared to allow visualization of the joint. Any loose bone is removed with the shaver, and the distal aspect of the cheilectomy is inspected (Figure 6.7). Any shelf of bone is shaved smooth, and care is taken to check the joint laterally and in the medial gutter. Finally, the portals can be switched and the camera can be used to assess the MTPJ cartilage condition.

Minimally Invasive Moberg Osteotomy (Dorsal Closing Wedge of Proximal Phalanx)

There are two 2-mm skin incisions needed to perform an MIS Moberg osteotomy. The incision for the osteotomy is made at the metaphyseal flare, and a second incision for screw fixation is made at the medial midaxial point between the dorsal and plantar aspect of the first MTPJ (Figure 6.3A).

The Moberg osteotomy is performed using a 2 mm × 12 mm Shannon burr. Care is taken to carefully resect all of the dorsal cortex followed by the plantar lateral and plantar medial corners while leaving the central plantar cortex intact (Figure 6.8).

If the plantar lateral or plantar medial cortices are not cut, closure of the Moberg osteotomy may be more difficult. A guidewire for the 2.9-mm cannulated screw is inserted from the medial base of the proximal phalanx and aimed slightly more dorsally in order to facilitate closure of the osteotomy when the screw is tightened. The guidewire is advanced through the far cortex while the osteotomy is held closed with digital pressure (Figure 6.9). Only the near cortex is overdrilled to utilize a lag screw technique to assist with closure of the osteotomy as screw is tightened. The 2.9-mm screw (Novastep, Orangeburg, New York) is inserted while the osteotomy is held closed with digital pressure. Failure to perform this step may result in gapping of the osteotomy at the dorsal cortex.

The wounds are carefully inspected for any sign of skin thermal damage in which case the skin edges are excised to reduce the risk of postoperative wound problems. The most proximal incision is closed with 4-0 Monocryl subcuticular suture. The two distal portals are closed with Steri-Strips only. The foot is wrapped with gauze, soft roll or cast padding cotton dressing, and ace wrap followed by a flat surgical shoe.

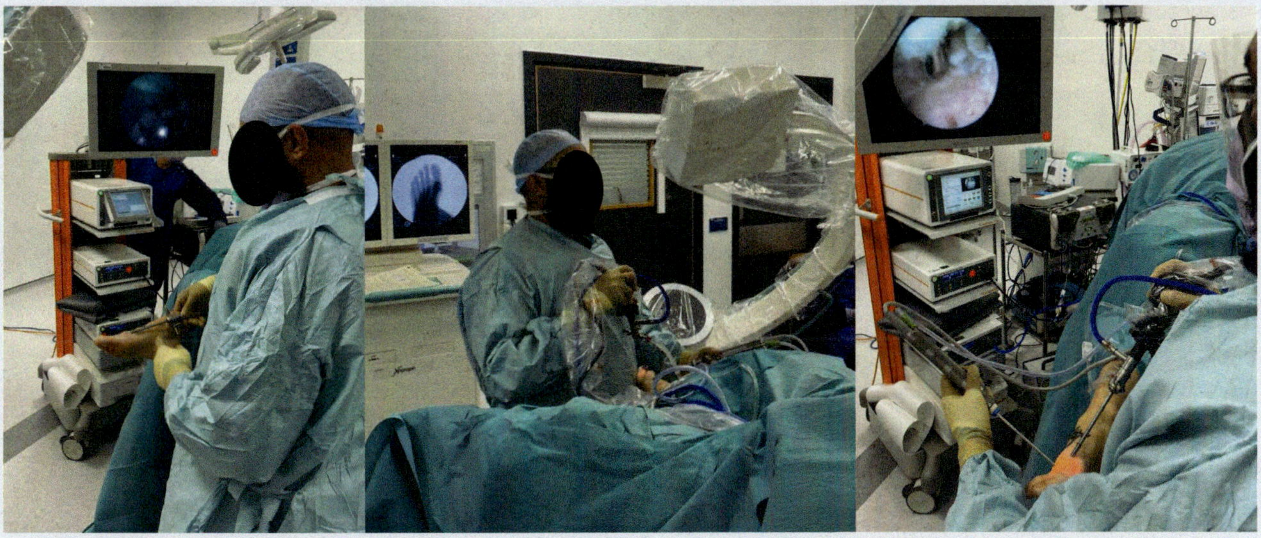

Figure 6.6 Clinical photographs demonstrating the positioning of surgeon, patient, and arthroscopy tower for first metatarsophalangeal joint arthroscopy.

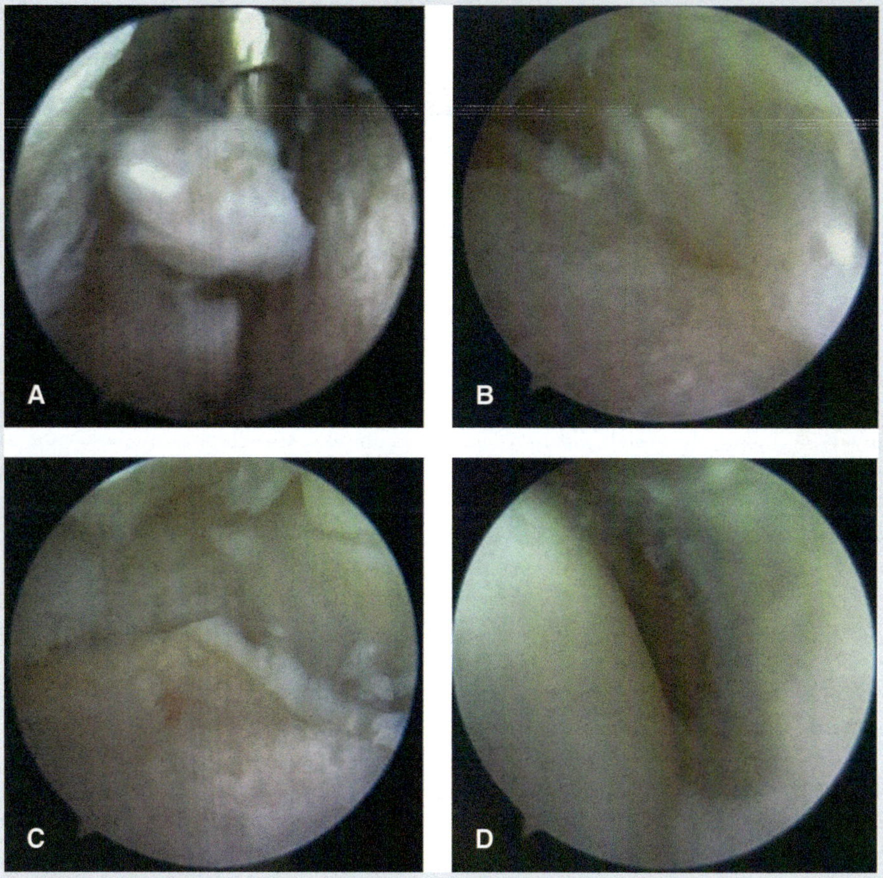

Figure 6.7 Arthroscopy pictures demonstrating (*left* to *right*): **(A)** use of a shaver to bring loose bodies into view, **(B)** unstable cartilage flap, **(C)** subsequent resection of cartilage flap, and **(D)** visual assessment of the remaining joint surface.

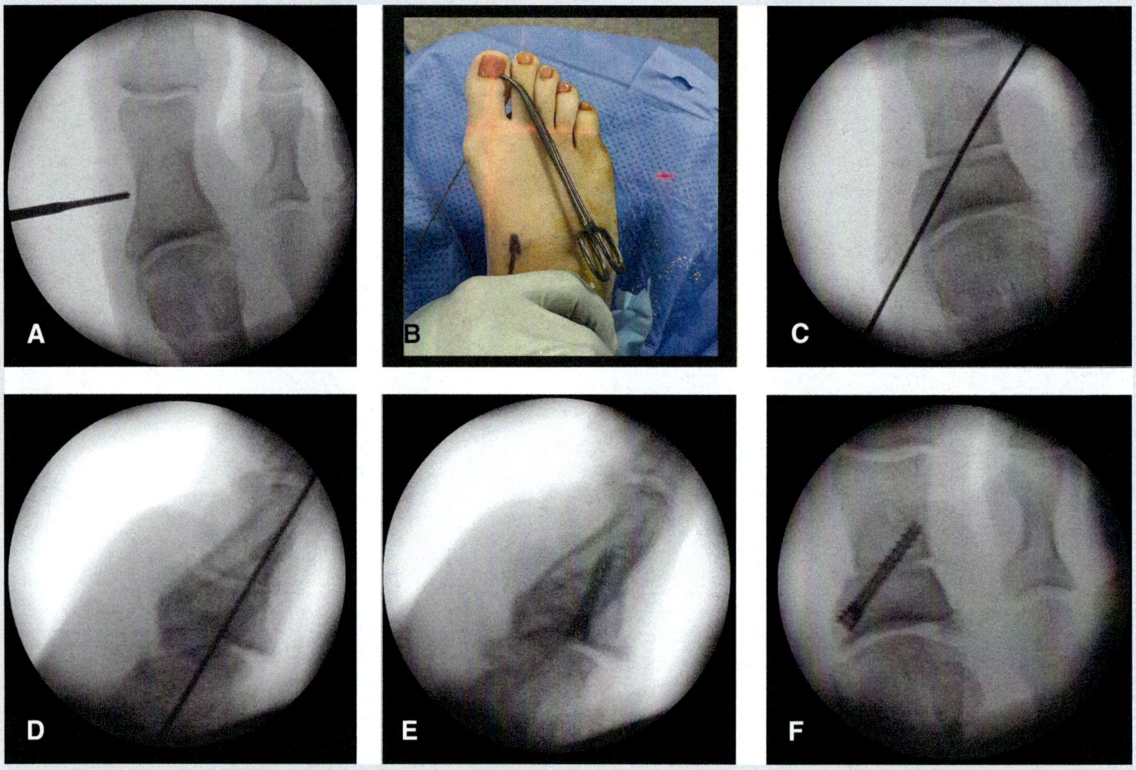

Figure 6.8 Intraoperative fluoroscopy images and clinical photograph demonstrating the steps for an MIS Moberg osteotomy (*left* to *right*): **(A)** initial burr placement (2 mm × 12 mm burr, Novastep, Orangeburg, New York) and osteotomy, **(B)** clinical picture showing wire placement, **(C)** wire placement on AP view, **(D)** wire placement on lateral view, **(E)** final screw (Nexis 2.9-mm screw, Novastep, Orangeburg, New York) placement on lateral view, **(F)** final screw placement on AP view.

◆ POSTOPERATIVE MANAGEMENT

Minimally invasive dorsal cheilectomy with Moberg osteotomy is performed on an outpatient basis with patients allowed to mobilize with full weight bearing as tolerated (with or without the aid of crutches for comfort and balance). Patients are counseled regarding the importance of elevating the foot in the first 2 weeks following surgery to reduce swelling and the risk of wound problems. Patients are advised to keep their surgical dressing dry and intact for 1 week following surgery at which point the dressing may be removed. Provided wounds are healing well, patients can commence scar massage to reduce scar sensitivity and prevent excessive scar formation at 2 weeks postoperatively. Patients are also advised to start gentle dorsiflexion and plantarflexion exercises to focus on improving the range of motion at the first MTPJ. At 2 weeks postoperative, patients are allowed to transition to mesh sneakers as swelling improves and are encouraged to gradually increase walking as tolerated. After 4 weeks postoperative, patients are allowed to participate in low-impact exercise activities including exercise bike, elliptical trainer, and swimming.

◆ OUTCOMES

There is a notable lack of literature investigating the clinical and radiological outcomes following MIS first MTPJ dorsal cheilectomy with a Moberg osteotomy. Clinical outcomes following open and MIS dorsal cheilectomy are well established with excellent improvements in both pain and function.[1,5,8-13]

Clinical Outcomes

The clinical outcomes reported in the literature following first MTPJ dorsal cheilectomy and Moberg osteotomy are limited but generally favorable as shown in Table 6.1. Further, higher-quality studies are necessary to better evaluate outcomes after this procedure.

Additional comparative studies, reported only in conference abstracts, have demonstrated positive results. One prospective study of 47 patients compared the outcome of 22 patients who underwent MIS dorsal cheilectomy to a matched group of 25 patients who underwent open dorsal cheilectomy. Both groups demonstrated significant improvement in Manchester-Oxford Foot Questionnaire (MOXFQ) score; however, there was no statistically significant difference in outcomes between the two groups.[16] Other studies have demonstrated improvements in American Orthopedic Foot and Ankle Society Score (AOFAS) and satisfaction following MIS dorsal cheilectomy.[17]

Complications

Complications following MIS cheilectomy and Moberg osteotomy can be categorized into general MIS-related

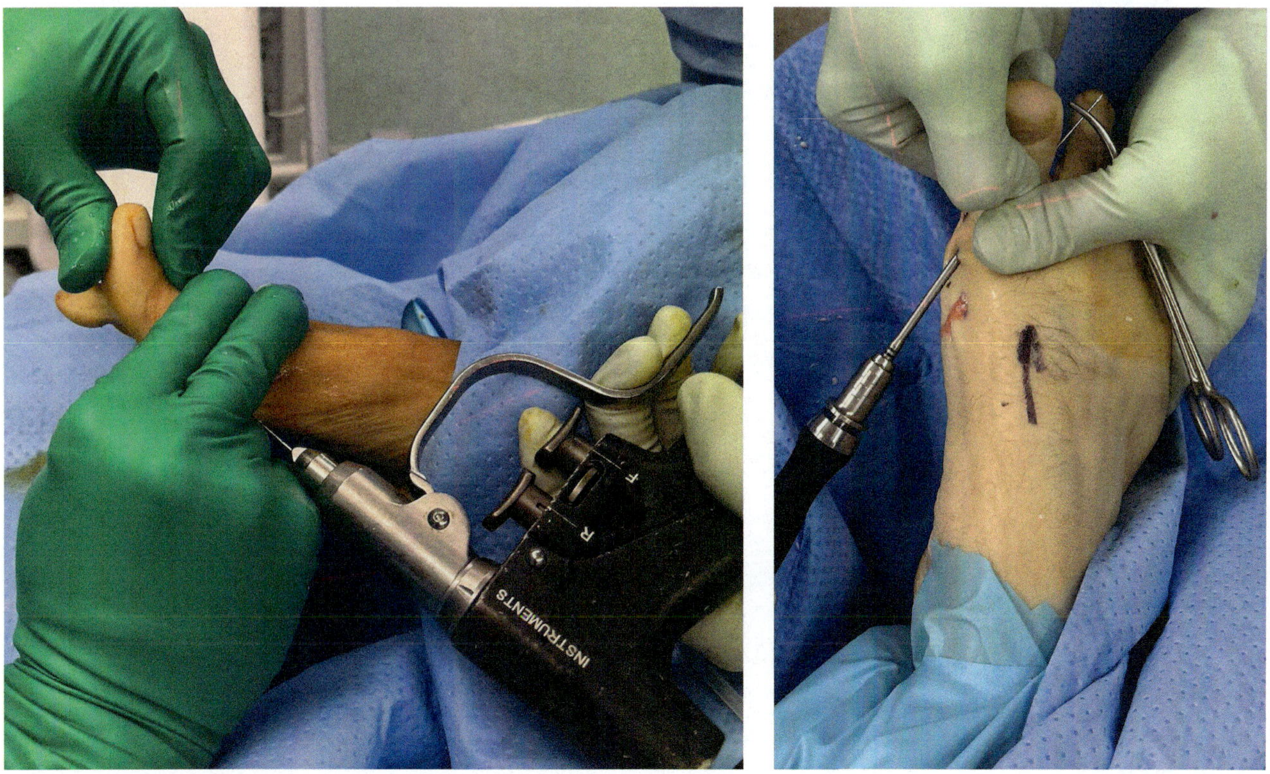

Figure 6.9 Wire placement for the Moberg osteotomy (*left*) and subsequent closure of the Moberg osteotomy as the hallux proximal phalanx screw is inserted (*right*).

Table 6.1

Clinical Studies of Minimally Invasive Cheilectomy and/or Moberg Osteotomy

Study	Design	Operative Technique	No. of Cases	Follow Up (Months)	Clinical Outcomes	Complication Rate
De Prado and Cuervas-Mons (2022)[10]	Retrospective case series	Minimally invasive technique combining cheilectomy, Moberg P1 base osteotomy, and distal dorsal closing M1 descending osteotomy	42	27	Mean AOFAS score was 44 preoperatively and 82 at the end of follow-up, and outcomes were classified as good or excellent in 86% of patients	2 transfer metatarsalgia, 1 delayed union, 1 postoperative stiffness, 1 postoperative hematoma
Glenn et al. (2021)[11]	Retrospective case series	Isolated minimally invasive dorsal cheilectomy with arthroscopy	20	16.5	Average VAS score improved from 7.05 preoperatively to 0.75 postoperatively ($P < .05$). Average ROM in dorsiflexion increased from 32° to 48° ($P < .05$) and plantarflexion increased from 15° to 19° plantarflexion ($P < .05$)	1 patient converted to arthrodesis 3 y following index procedure. No nerve injuries, damage to the EHL, wound infections, or wound complications
Stevens et al. (2020)[12]	Retrospective comparative study	Isolated minimally invasive dorsal cheilectomy compared with open technique	133 MIS 38 Open	36 MIS 34 Open	Complication and reoperation rates	MIS reoperation rate 12.8% compared to 2.6% Complications 11.3% in MIS group vs 2.6%
Hickey et al. (2020)[5]	Retrospective case series	Isolated minimally invasive dorsal cheilectomy with arthroscopy	36	56	83% of patients reported they would recommend the procedure. At follow-up, mean postoperative improvement in pain was 69% (range 0-100). A total of 84% of patients reported either no pain (28%) or mild pain (56%)	1 EHL rupture, 3 postoperative numbness, 1 repeat cheilectomy, 3 postoperative stiffness → MUA and steroid injection

(Continued)

Table 6.1

Clinical Studies of Minimally Invasive Cheilectomy and/or Moberg Osteotomy *(Continued)*

Study	Design	Operative Technique	No. of Cases	Follow Up (Months)	Clinical Outcomes	Complication Rate
Teoh et al. (2019)[13]	Retrospective case series	Isolated minimally invasive dorsal cheilectomy	98	50	Average VAS score improved from 8.0 preoperatively to 3 postoperatively. The mean MOXFQ summary index score decreased from 58.6 preoperatively to 30.5 postoperatively with a corresponding improvement in all 3 MOXFQ domains also improved	2 wound infections 2 delayed wound healing 2 transient postoperative numbness 2 permanent postoperative numbness 12 patients (12%) underwent reoperation, of which 7 had a first metatarsophalangeal joint arthrodesis for ongoing pain, 4 had repeat cheilectomy for residual impingement, and 1 had an open removal of loose bone
Mesa-Ramos et al. (2008)[14]	Prospective case series	Minimally invasive dorsal cheilectomy +/– Weil osteotomy	26	18	Pain relief was noted in all cases, with mean pain scores falling from 7.44 before surgery to 1.69. Quality of life also improved, while AOFAS scores rose from 58.45 to 92.36	2 postoperative numbness
de Arruda and Baptista (2019)[15]	Prospective case series	Minimally invasive dorsal cheilectomy + Watermann osteotomy + Moberg osteotomy	7	8	Increased ROM in both plantarflexion and dorsiflexion. Improvement in AOFAS score and VAS pain score	None

AOFAS, American Orthopedic Foot and Ankle Society Score; EHL, extensor hallucis longus; M1, 1st metatarsal, MOXFQ, Manchester-Oxford Foot Questionnaire; MUA, manipulation under anesthesia; P1, proximal phalanx; ROM, range of motion; VAS, visual analog scale.

complications and procedure-specific complications.[18] Studies utilizing an open Moberg osteotomy technique have reported complication rates of approximately 10.6% and 14.3% of all cases needing some form of reoperation.

General MIS complications include thermal skin damage leading to wound problems and dehiscence. Procedure-specific complications reported in the literature include EHL injury/rupture, hematoma formation, superficial/deep infection, osteotomy nonunion/malunion, and recurrence of pain.

There are also reports of increased rates of complication and reoperation when compared to the open technique secondary to learning curve–associated technical errors, incomplete resection, retained bone fragments within the MTPJ, and other associated MTPJ pathology. Further studies are necessary to determine if arthroscopy-assisted MIS first MTPJ dorsal cheilectomy is superior to MIS first MTPJ dorsal cheilectomy alone with regard to complications and reoperation.

References

1. Coughlin MJ, Shurnas PS. Hallux rigidus. Grading and long-term results of operative treatment. *J Bone Joint Surg Am.* 2003;85(11):2072-2088.
2. Lam A, Chan JJ, Surace MF, Vulcano E. Hallux rigidus: how do I approach it? *World J Orthop.* 2017;8(5):364-371.
3. Stone OD, Ray R, Thomson CE, Gibson JNA. Long-term follow-up of arthrodesis vs total joint arthroplasty for hallux rigidus. *Foot Ankle Int.* 2017;38(4):375-380.
4. Kim PHU, Chen X, Hillstrom H, Ellis SJ, Baxter JR, Deland JT. Moberg osteotomy shifts contact pressure plantarly in the first metatarsophalangeal joint in a biomechanical model. *Foot Ankle Int.* 2016;37(1):96-101.
5. Hickey BA, Siew D, Nambiar M, Bedi HS. Intermediate-term results of isolated minimally invasive arthroscopic cheilectomy in the treatment of hallux rigidus. *Eur J Orthop Surg Traumatol.* 2020;30(7):1277-1283.
6. Dalmau-Pastor M, Vega J, Malagelada F, Peña F, Manzanares-Céspedes MC. An anatomical study of nerves at risk during minimally invasive hallux valgus surgery. *J Vis Exp.* 2018;(132):56232.
7. Teoh KH, Haanaes EK, Alshalawi S, Tanaka H, Hariharan K. Minimally invasive dorsal cheilectomy of the first metatarsal: a cadaveric study. *Foot Ankle Int.* 2018;39(12):1497-1501.
8. Easley ME, Hodges Davis W, Anderson RB. Intermediate to long-term follow-up of medial-approach dorsal cheilectomy for hallux rigidus. *Foot Ankle Int.* 1999;20:147-152.
9. Roukis TS. Outcomes after cheilectomy with phalangeal dorsiflexory osteotomy for hallux rigidus: a systematic review. *J Foot Ankle Surg.* 2010;49(5):479-487.
10. De Prado M, Cuervas-Mons M. Minimal incision surgery in hallux rigidus. *J Foot Ankle.* 2022;16(1):9-11.
11. Glenn RL, Gonzalez TA, Peterson AB, Kaplan J. Minimally invasive dorsal cheilectomy and hallux metatarsal phalangeal joint arthroscopy for the treatment of hallux rigidus. *Foot Ankle Orthop.* 2021;6(1):2473011421993103.
12. Stevens R, Bursnall M, Chadwick C, et al. Comparison of complication and reoperation rates for minimally invasive versus open cheilectomy of the first metatarsophalangeal joint. *Foot Ankle Int.* 2019;41(1):31-36.
13. Teoh KH, Tan WT, Atiyah Z, Ahmad A, Tanaka H, Hariharan K. Clinical outcomes following minimally invasive dorsal cheilectomy for hallux rigidus. *Foot Ankle Int.* 2018;40(2):195-201.
14. Mesa-Ramos M, Mesa-Ramos F, Carpintero P. Evaluation of the treatment of hallux rigidus by percutaneous surgery. *Acta Orthop Belg.* 2008;74(2):222-226.
15. de Arruda JF, Baptista AD. Percutaneous cheilectomy combined with Watermann and Moberg osteotomies for the treatment of hallux rigidus. *Sci J Foot Ankle.* 2019;13(2):135-139.
16. Morgan S, Jones C, Palmer S. Minimally invasive cheilectomy: functional outcome and comparison with open cheilectomy. *Orthopaedic Proceedings.* The British Editorial Society of Bone & Joint Surgery; 2012:14.
17. Dawe ECJ, Ball T, Annamalai S, Davis J. Early results of minimally invasive cheilectomy for painful hallux rigidus. *Orthopaedic Proceedings.* The British Editorial Society of Bone & Joint Surgery; 2012:33.
18. Lewis TL, Mason L, Ray R. The Clavien-Dindo complication classification modified for foot and ankle orthopaedic surgery. *Foot Ankle Surg.* 2022;28(6):800-802. https://www.sciencedirect.com/science/article/pii/S1268773122000534.

7 Minimally Invasive First Metatarsophalangeal Fusion

Christopher P. Miller and Philip B. Kaiser

◆ INTRODUCTION

Hallux rigidus is a common condition encountered by foot and ankle surgeons. It was originally described in 1887 as condition affecting the great toe causing stiffness and pain.[1] The first metatarsophalangeal (MTP) joint is one of the most common joints affected by degenerative changes with almost 8% of adults reporting symptomatic hallux rigidus in their lifetime and radiographic evidence of arthritis present in at least 27% of adults over 50 years.[2-4]

Drs. Coughlin and Shurnas described their classification system of hallux rigidus and recommended that, when nonoperative treatment fails, mild grade 1 and 2 cases can be treated with cheilectomy and arthrodesis considered for higher grades.[5] However, recently, there has been realization that the radiographic imaging and classification grades do not necessarily correlate with patient's symptoms and treatment options.[6,7]

In general, patients with severe arthritis of the joint with limited motion and pain in the mid arc of motion typically correlate to grades 3 and 4 on the Coughlin classification.[5] Open arthrodesis has been the traditional gold standard treatment for these patients with excellent long-term reported outcomes and function.[8-10] Minimally invasive (MIS) surgical techniques offer a new approach to treat forefoot pathologies with the potential to limit postoperative wound complications and pain.[11] The first reported minimal incision first MTP joint fusion was in 1999 as case report of a successful arthroscopic-assisted MTP joint fusion.[12] Since then, the role of arthroscopy in foot and ankle conditions as well as the authors' understanding of the anatomy, safe zone, and portal placement has expanded, and the first MTP joint arthroscopy and minimally invasive forefoot surgery have become much more common.[12-23]

As foot and ankle surgeons gain MIS experience with bunion correction, cheilectomy, and metatarsal osteotomies, these skills are readily applicable to joint fusions. Hallux rigidus, one the most commonly treated degenerative foot and ankle conditions, coupled with the relatively simple anatomy of the first MTP joint allow the benefits of MIS to be applied to one of the most commonly performed foot surgeries. This chapter will describe the technique of MIS fusion of the hallux MTP joint. Results from early case series demonstrate 93% to 97% fusion rates with low complications, indicating that this is a promising surgery that could benefit many pati ents.[12,14,16,22,24-26]

◆ INDICATIONS AND CONTRAINDICATIONS

Arthrodesis remains the gold standard for the treatment of advanced arthritis of the first MTP joint. Additionally, certain patient factors including poor bone quality, soft-tissue compromise, concomitant coronal or sagittal plane deformities, bony erosions, or in the setting of neuromuscular disorders make fusion of the hallux MTP joint a good option when nonoperative care does not relieve pain.[8]

Patients, regardless of initial symptoms or radiographs, should be offered nonoperative treatments such as shoe modifications, carbon fiber inserts, rocker bottom shoes, and possible steroid injections. However, if this fails, surgery may be considered. As described in the prior chapter, MIS cheilectomy may work well when the pain from hallux rigidus is primarily with toe dorsiflexion or shoe wear impinging on the arthritic spur.[5] However, if there is pain at the mid arc of motion or a positive grind test on examination, then a cheilectomy is less likely to achieve adequate long-term pain relief, and therefore, a fusion may be preferred.

The indications for an MIS or open first MTP fusion are largely equivalent. Beyond surgeon preference and experience, an MIS approach may be favored in certain conditions such as in the presence of significant scar tissue or adherent skin that could lead to poor wound healing if approached with a traditional open technique. With the percutaneous technique, a plate and screw construct is not possible; however, screw-only constructs have been shown to allow for early, protected, weight bearing without increased risk of nonunion.[27]

Relative contraindications of MIS fusion compared to open include severe angular deformity requiring open ligament releases to achieve reduction and/or poor bone quality as in the setting of severe osteoporosis or rheumatoid arthritis. In these cases, the surgeon should give consideration to an open approach since a dorsal plate with lag screw has been shown to be the strongest construct biomechanically.[28]

Contraindications to MIS procedures would include revision fusion for nonunion, cases with significant bone loss requiring bone block arthrodesis, conversion of arthroplasty or other implant to fusion, as well as cases with active infection or vascular compromise sufficient to preclude healing of the wounds.

Dorsal spurring is not a contraindication as this can be treated with an MIS cheilectomy at the time of fusion. In the authors' practice, the MIS first MTP fusion has become the workhorse procedure for more than 90% of cases.

◆ PATIENT HISTORY AND PHYSICAL EXAMINATION

Patients often present with pain and stiffness at the first MTP joint with or without deformity. There may be a history of trauma, but typically, there is no inciting event that the patient recalls. Usually, the pain is worse with actions involving toe dorsiflexion and loading across the MTP joint, such as the push-off phase of gait. Similarly, stairs, running, and plank position during activities such as yoga or push-ups may cause discomfort.[8,10,29]

When there is a large dorsal osteophyte, there may be tenderness due to impingement in shoes. The dorsal medial cutaneous nerve will course over the spur and may be a source of additional pain if stretched over the spur with plantarflexion of the toe, and there is often evidence of neuritis with a positive Tinel sign at the site.[30] The patient may also report lateral foot discomfort due to abnormal gait patterns in an effort to off-load the painful hallux MTP joint. Finally, evaluating the pain with range of motion is one of the most important deciding factors. If the patient has pain at the mid arc of motion or with axial loading of the joint in the mid position, this likely indicates a loss of cartilage in the central joint, and in those cases, a fusion as opposed to a cheilectomy will be more beneficial as discussed above.

◆ IMAGING STUDIES

At a minimum, initial imaging of hallux rigidus should include standard three-view weight-bearing radiographs of the foot to include AP, lateral, and oblique views. In the presence of any other clinical deformities, weight-bearing ankle radiographs should be obtained as well, and sometimes, imaging of the contralateral foot can assist with preoperative planning.

The hallmarks of hallux rigidus include joint space narrowing, sclerosis of the joint, and flattening of the metatarsal head with dorsal osteophyte formation at the metatarsal head (Figure 7.1). Sometimes, there may be osteophytes at the proximal phalanx as well or loose bodies within the joint. Typically, these are noted on the lateral view.

Evidence of prior surgery should be noted; particularly prior bunion correction as this may alter the trajectory of screws needed for fixation or require removal of prior hardware. In addition, attention must be given to any angular deformities and bone erosion as this may require conversion to open procedure.

◆ PREOPERATIVE PLANNING AND PREPARATION

The setup for an MIS hallux MTP joint fusion begins with the patient positioned supine with the operative foot overhanging the end of the bed. The foot may be elevated on a rolled blanket or patient positioner taped to the end of the bed. The entire foot should be off the table and the table or position should contact the leg at the midportion of the Achilles tendon (Figure 7.2B). This permits passive plantarflexion of the ankle and will make intraoperative fluoroscopy easier, particularly for AP views.

Some surgeons will place a bump under the hip on the operative side. This can be helpful if there is significant external rotation of the leg when the patient is sedated; however, this may also be left out and the surgeon can utilize external rotation of the foot to more easily obtain lateral imaging with the mini C-arm (Figure 7.2B).

The nonoperative leg should be padded and draped out of the field. It can be helpful to frog-leg the nonoperative leg to avoid impeding the mini C-arm.

The mini C-arm may be carefully positioned during the case similar to what is described for the MIS bunion procedure. Surgeons may have individual preference for C-arm position, but in general, for right-handed surgeons, the mini C-arm should come in from the patient's right side (Figure 7.2B). If performing surgery on the left foot, the surgeon will stand on the patient's left facing the dorsal foot. If

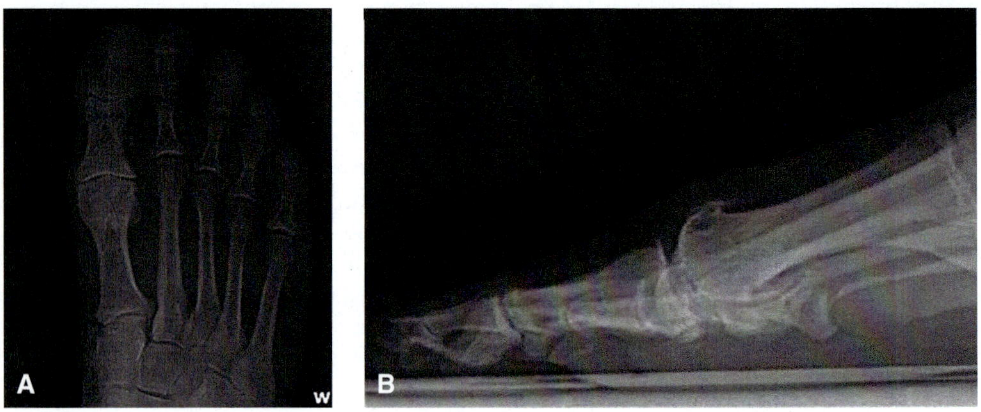

Figure 7.1 Radiographs of the foot demonstrating joint space narrowing on the AP **(A)** and dorsal metatarsal head osteophyte formation on the lateral view **(B)**. (With permission from Christopher P. Miller MD, MHS © 2022.)

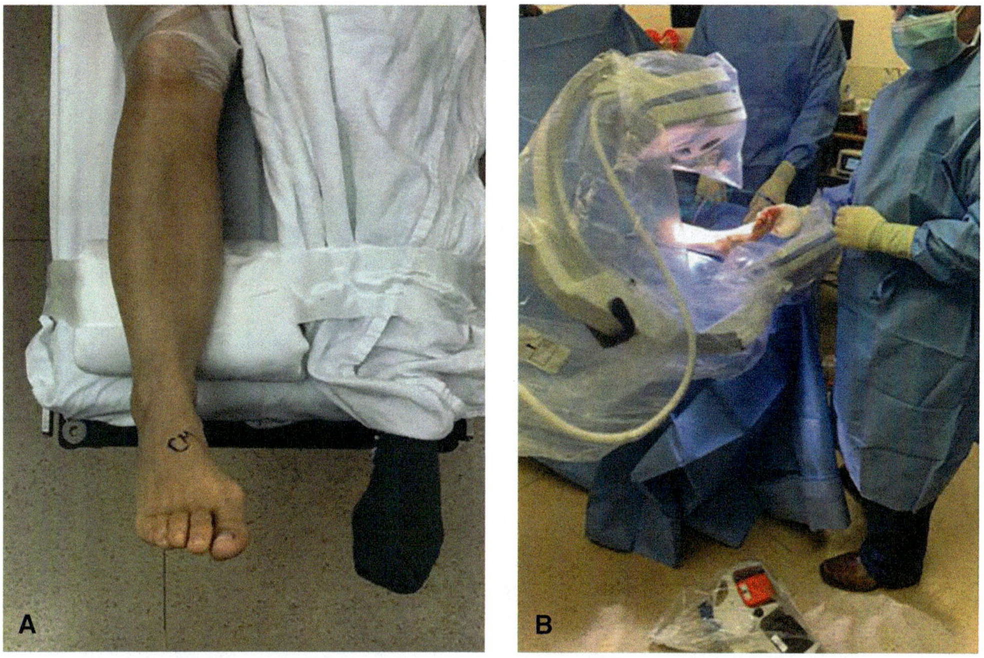

Figure 7.2 **A.** Foot position hanging off end of the bed. **B.** The mini C-arm is used as part of the table to support the forefoot and provide imaging throughout the surgery. (With permission from Christopher P. Miller MD, MHS © 2022.)

operating on the right foot, the surgeon will stand at the bottom of the bed facing the plantar aspect of the foot. In either case, the mini C-arm will be entering the sterile field from the patient's right side.

If the surgeon is left handed, then the mini C-arm and surgeon positioning will be opposite of what is described above.

It is often useful, particularly early in the MIS learning curve, to give the fluoroscopy control pedal to an assistant. When using a pedal for both the burr and the mini C-arm, the surgeon may inadvertently press the wrong pedal, which may cause unnecessary radiation to the patient and surgeon, or contaminate the surgical field if the burr is accidentally activated.

SURGICAL TECHNIQUE

A standard surgical preparation and draping is performed. Tourniquet is not recommended in an effort to prevent thermal injury during the surgery.

1. Commonly a popliteal/saphenous nerve block, ankle block, or first ray field block is performed, and monitored anesthesia care is sufficient anesthesia for the case. Alternatively, the surgical team can perform a local forefoot block, but in this case, the patient may require general anesthesia to maintain comfort during the case.
2. The anatomy is marked with attention paid to the course of the extensor hallucis longus (EHL) tendon and the dorsal medial cutaneous nerve, which is sometimes palpable. When imagining the metatarsal head in the transverse plane as a clock with the EHL at the 12 o'clock position, the dorsomedial and dorsolateral cutaneous nerves are reliably found at the 10 and 2 o'clock positions.[19] This can be useful to avoid iatrogenic injury.
3. The joint line is then identified fluoroscopically, and a direct medial portal is developed. The portal is typically about 5 mm in length (Figure 7.3A).
4. A secondary dorsolateral portal may be developed as well. If a percutaneous lateral release is required, it may be performed via this same portal with a Beaver blade (Figure 7.3B).
5. A small blunt hemostat can be used to dissect through the capsule and enter the joint through both portals.
6. A freer or MIS elevator is then used to help define the joint and release the dorsal capsule off the spur. This will allow easier access when performing the cheilectomy as well. The instrument is rotated first dorsal and then plantar to the sesamoids (Figure 7.4).
   - Pearl: Take time to palpate the joint surfaces. Areas of cartilage will feel smooth, while areas of eburnation have granular feel. At the end of the joint preparation, this should be repeated and the surgeon will now feel the rough subchondral and cancellous bone that has been exposed. This will help ensure that the entire joint is adequately prepared. The surgeon can also gain tactile feel of the contour of the joint, which will assist with accurate burr preparation.
7. Joint preparation should occur in two stages. A 2 × 12 mm Shannon burr, similar to what is utilized for an Akin osteotomy, is utilized to first remove any residual cartilage in the joint (Figure 7.5A and B).
   - Pitfall: Irrigation must be contacting the burr and skin at the portal site to avoid iatrogenic thermal burns. Additionally, the burr should not be activated for more than 20 seconds before resting it to allow cooling.[31]

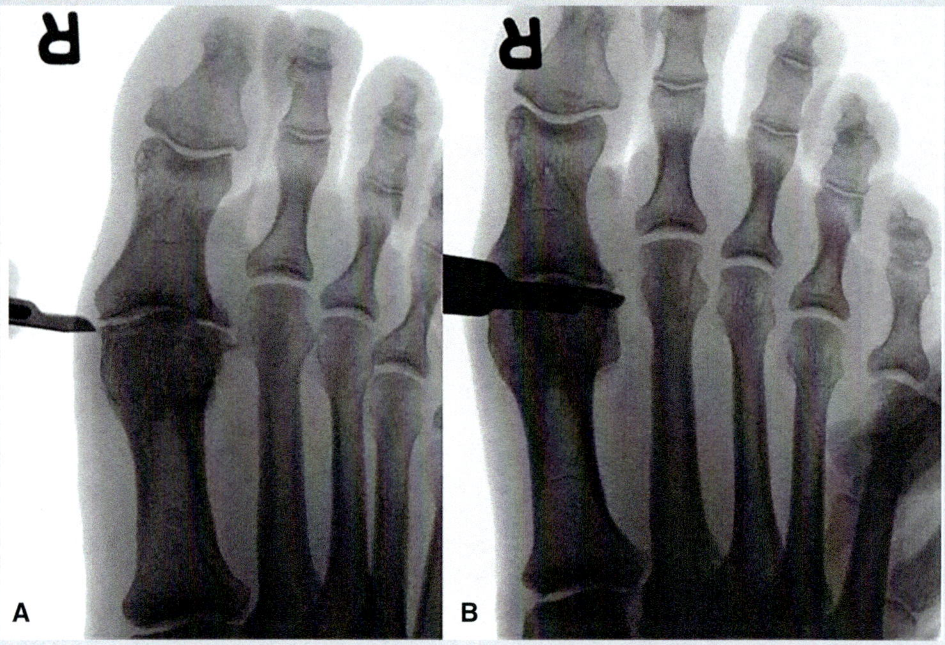

Figure 7.3 **A.** The medial portal. **B.** Dorsolateral portal. (With permission from Christopher P. Miller MD, MHS © 2022.)

8. Joint preparation is performed under fluoroscopic guidance. Begin by removing bone and cartilage from the medial portion of the joint.
9. Débridement should be performed in a systematic fashion. First, begin at the medial metatarsal head. Attempt to follow the natural curvature of the joint to allow congruent compression at the end.
10. Once the medial portion of the metatarsal head is prepared, perform the same débridement on the proximal phalanx. This relies on tactile feedback and intermittent fluoroscopy to ensure that the burr remains in the proper plane.
11. Next, the lateral joint is prepared in a similar fashion using the dorsolateral portal (Figure 7.5C).
    - Pitfall: It is possible to asymmetrically prepare the joint by débriding too much dorsal bone. To avoid this, the surgeon should take regular lateral fluoroscopy views.
12. Once the initial débridement is completed, the site should be irrigated thoroughly to remove the cartilaginous slurry.
13. A freer may be used to palpate the joint surfaces for any unprepared areas.

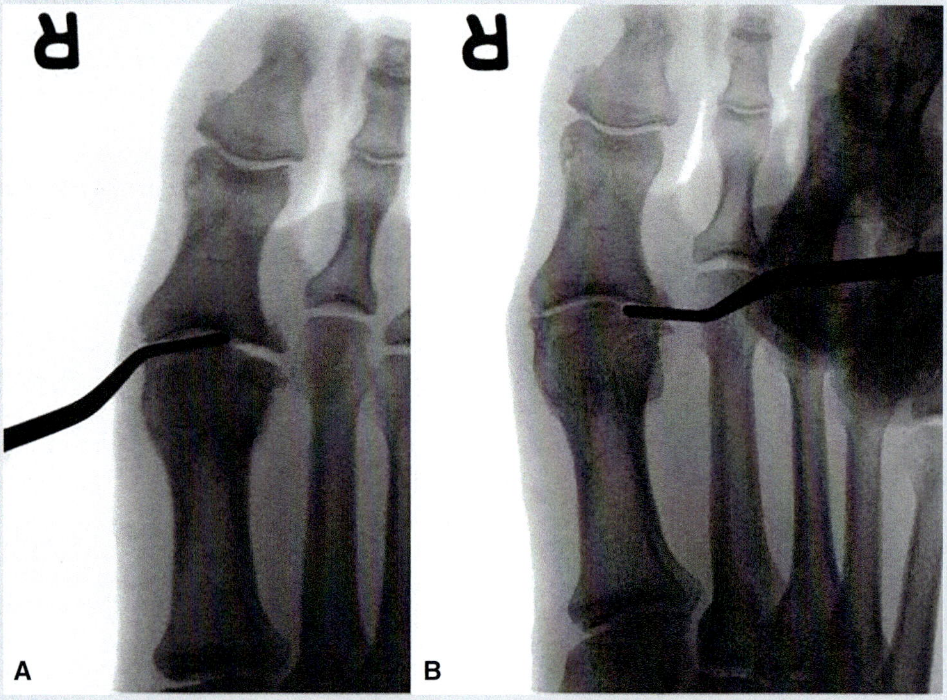

Figure 7.4 Blunt dissection into joint and capsular release from medial **(A)** and dorsolateral portals **(B)**. (With permission from Christopher P. Miller MD, MHS © 2022.)

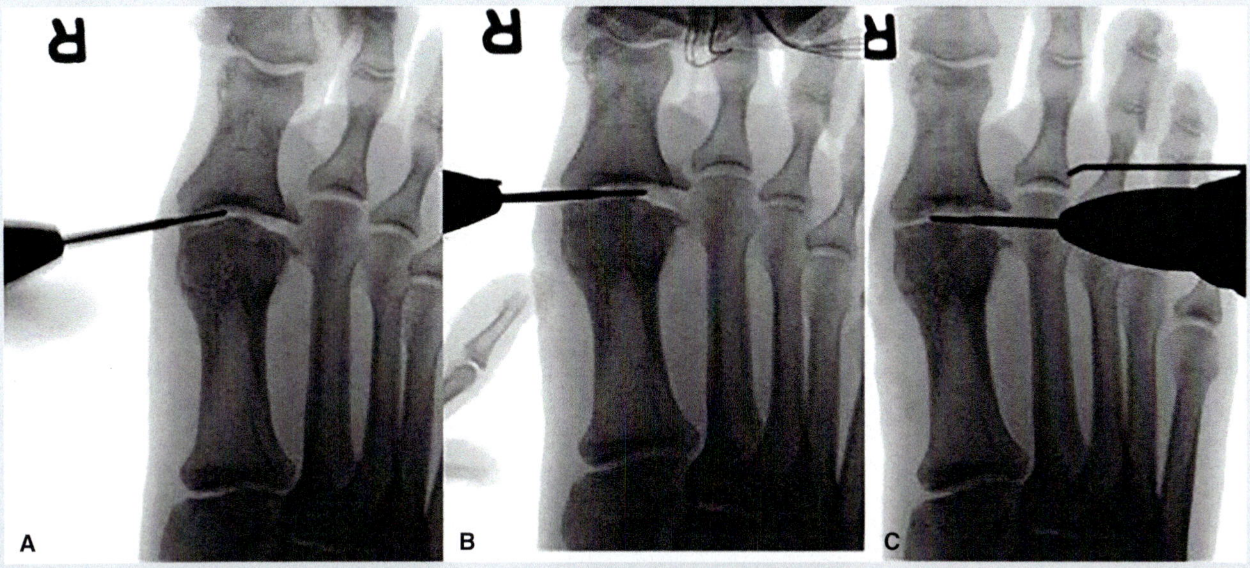

Figure 7.5 A 2 × 12 Shannon burr working from medial portal **(A, B)** and dorsolateral portal **(C)** to prepare joint for fusion. (With permission from Christopher P. Miller MD, MHS © 2022.)

14. If desired, a small joint arthroscope may be inserted to check preparation as well; however, with practice, it is possible to achieve joint preparation that is similar in quality to open (Figure 7.6).[32]
15. Reducing the joint manually and checking that there is no residual joint space on fluoroscopy can also confirm joint preparation.
16. A secondary débridement is then performed with either the 2 × 12 mm burr or a 3-mm wedge burr to resect the residual subchondral bone and generate local bone slurry to facilitate fusion.
17. The 2-mm Shannon burr or a small drill can be used through the portals to fenestrate the joint surfaces and further expose subchondral bone (Figure 7.7).
18. If there is a large bone spur, a cheilectomy may now be performed as well. For full details on the MIS cheilectomy, see the previous chapter. Any large fragments are removed.
19. If a cheilectomy is performed, the morselized bone slurry may be left in place as additional bone graft for fusion. The cheilectomy may either be performed through the medial and dorsolateral portals,

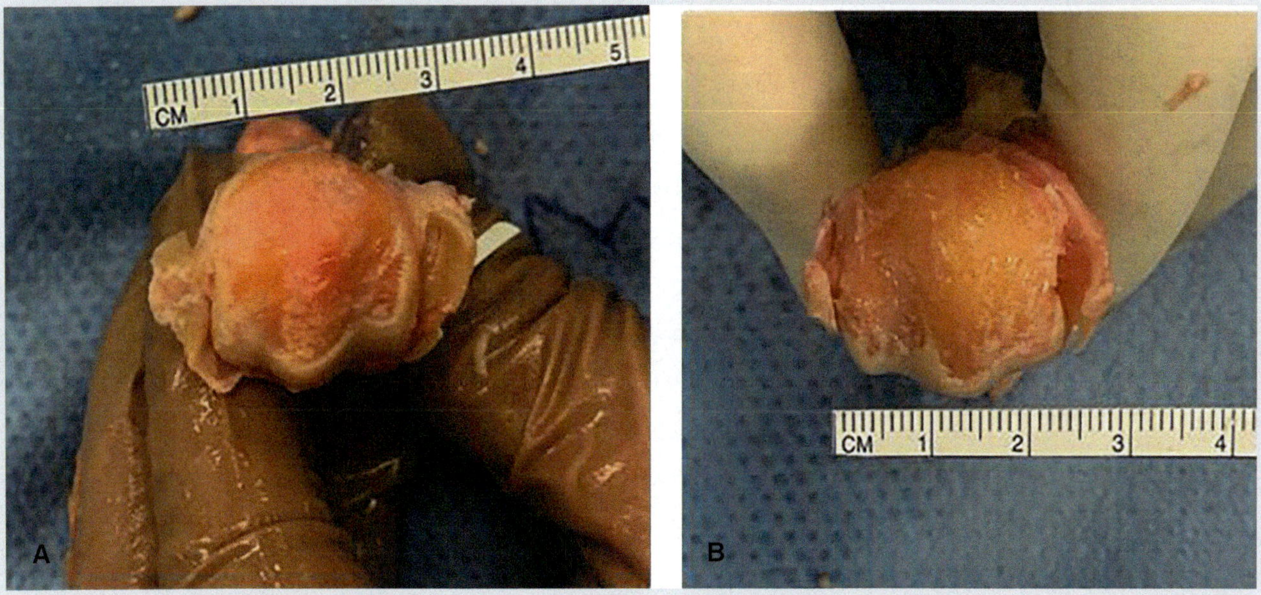

Figure 7.6 Cadaveric dissection following MIS burr for joint preparation **(A)** as compared to traditional open surgery **(B)**. Equivalent joint preparation quality is noted. (With permission from Christopher P. Miller MD, MHS © 2022.)

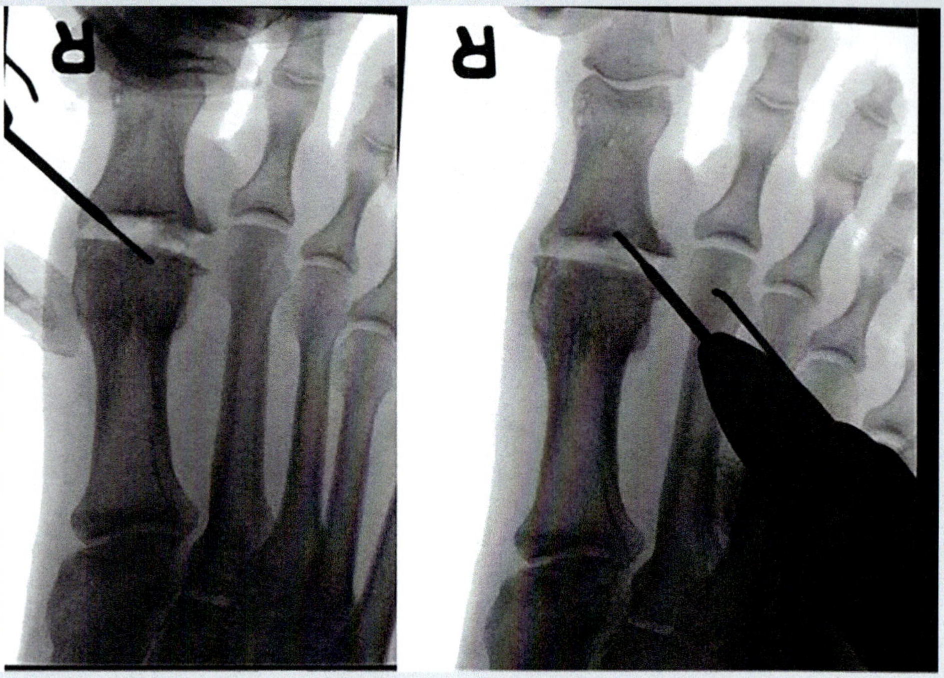

Figure 7.7 The Shannon burr is used to fenestrate the subchondral bone surface for fusion. (With permission from Christopher P. Miller MD, MHS © 2022.)

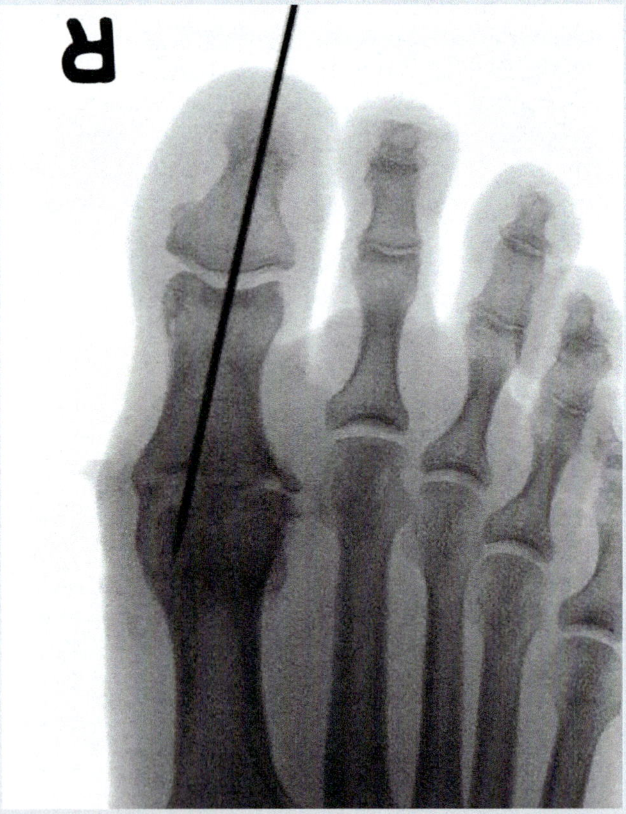

Figure 7.8 With manual compression, the joint space is obliterated, indicating adequate joint débridement. The toe is positioned for fusion and held temporarily with an axial K-wire until definitive fixation is placed. (With permission from Christopher P. Miller MD, MHS © 2022.)

or a proximal incision may be utilized and the spur taken down from proximal to distal. This incision may also be used for screw placement if planned appropriately.

20. If additional bone graft or bone graft substitute is desired, it may be injected into the joint at this point.
21. The access portals are now closed prior to compression in order to keep the graft in place.
22. Positioning of the toe should be in neutral rotation, 5° to 15° of valgus, and 10° to 15° dorsiflexion relative to a simulated weight-bearing surface. The hallux should be parallel to the second toe in the coronal plane, and the pad should not only rest on the simulated floor but also be able to dorsiflex through the interphalangeal joint (IP) about 5 to 10 mm passively to permit a forefoot rocker during the toe off phase of gait (Figure 7.8).[5,8,33]
23. Finally, K-wires are positioned across the joint. These are most typically crossed K-wires but can also be parallel or intramedullary if needed depending on the bony geometry and surgeon preference.[14,24,25,28,29]
24. The K-wires are over drilled and replaced with the appropriate partially or fully threaded compression screws. Typically, these are 3.5-, 4.0-, or 5.0-mm cannulated screws (Figure 7.9).
25. Closure is performed with 3-0 nylon sutures (Figure 7.10).
26. A wet spica gauze dressing is applied to the great toe for compression and edema control followed by dry gauze wrap and compression wrap.

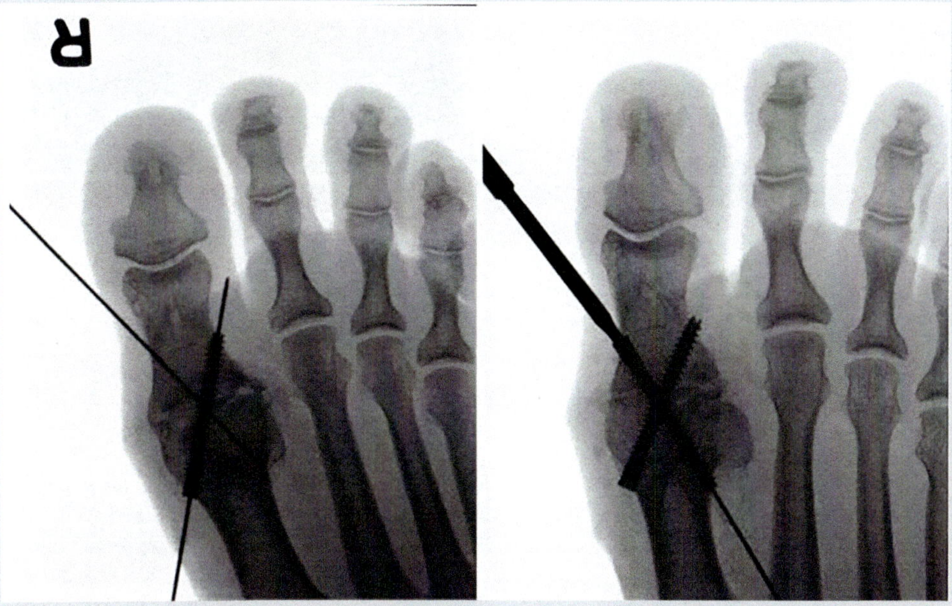

Figure 7.9 Crossed K-wires over drilled and then replaced with cannulated compression screws. (With permission from Christopher P. Miller MD, MHS © 2022.)

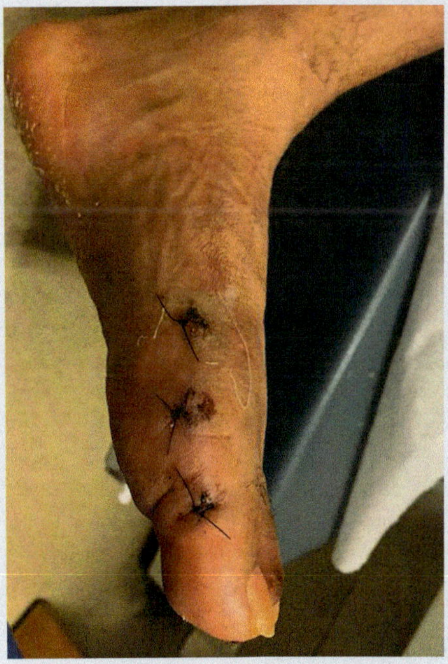

Figure 7.10 Clinical photo of incisions at 2-week follow-up visit after surgery. (With permission from Christopher P. Miller MD, MHS © 2022.)

◆ POSTOPERATIVE MANAGEMENT

The patient is seen at 10 to 14 days, 6 weeks, 3 months, and 6 months for routine postoperative visits. Weight bearing may be permitted once the surgical block has worn off. The authors generally permit heel weight bearing in a postoperative stiff-soled shoe or short boot for 4 weeks. After 4 weeks, the patient can transition to weight bearing as tolerated (WBAT) in the shoe or boot and wean to regular shoes at 6 to 8 weeks if there is no pain and radiographs show signs of healing. Light exercise is permitted at 6 weeks. Impact exercise may begin at 3 months postoperatively (Figure 7.11).

Sutures are removed at the first visit after surgery and Steri-Strips applied. The wet spica dressing may be reapplied if there is substantial swelling at this time and removed in 1 to 2 weeks by the patient at home.

◆ OUTCOMES

There are limited reports on the postoperative outcomes of MIS the first MTP joint fusion compared to open procedures. However, the existing literature demonstrates favorable outcomes and safety of the procedure.

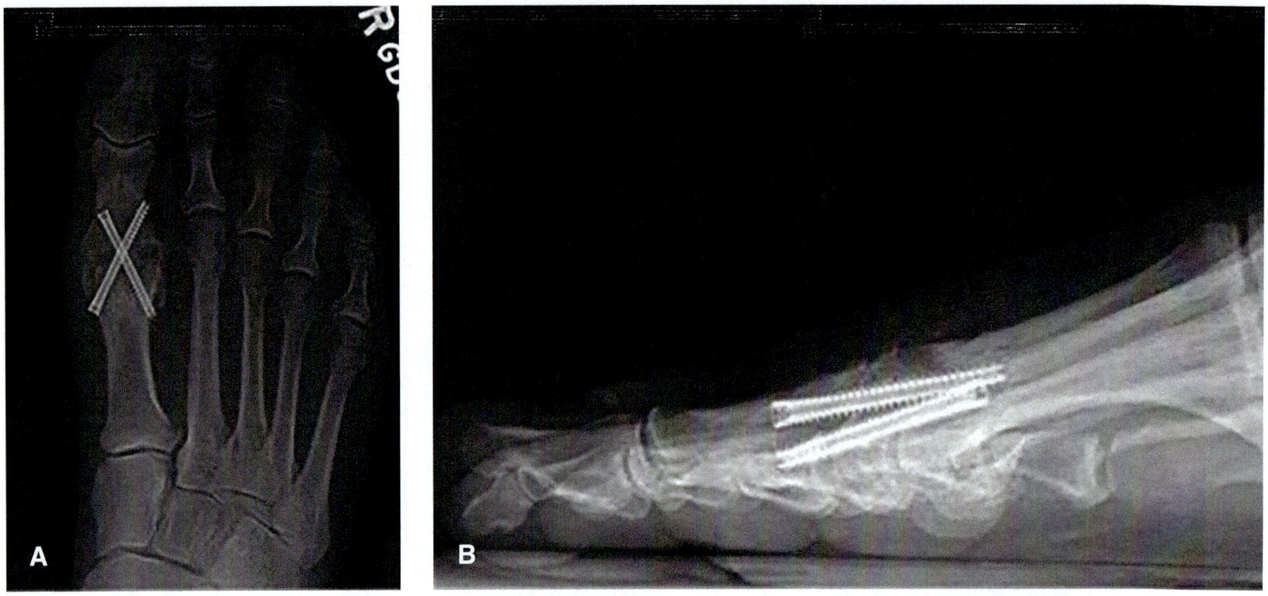

Figure 7.11 Final postoperative weight-bearing radiographs demonstrating healing on AP **(A)** and lateral **(B)** views with resection of the dorsal osteophyte. (With permission from Christopher P. Miller MD, MHS © 2022.)

The first and largest reported case series to date by Bauer et al.[24] in 2010 reported a fusion rate of 97% (31 of 32 cases). There was significant improvement in AOFAS scores from 36 preoperatively to 80 at final follow-up. Patients reported that they were satisfied or very satisfied with their final outcome in 30 of 32 cases (94%). Of those who were satisfied, the mean return to walking in regular shoes was 50 days. There was one case requiring screw removal. There was one deep infection requiring antibiotics, which then progressed to subsequent pseudoarthrosis.

In 2014, Fanous et al. reported a 93% fusion rate (24 of 26 cases) in their case series. The study showed a significant improvement in MOxFQ from 42 to 18 at final follow-up.[25] The authors specifically discussed the need for advanced training in MIS prior to considering these procedures as well as the need to be thoughtful regarding radiation exposure to the surgeon's hands during the case. Sott reported 16 out of 18 patients successfully fused by 6 weeks with 91% patient satisfaction with the procedure and no postoperative infections.[22]

Carlucci et al.[14] reported the results of an intramedullary screw (5.5 mm fully threaded compression screw) with an additional crossed screw for rotational stability. They demonstrated fusion in 14 of 15 cases (93.3%) at 18 months. There was one case of superficial infection that was managed medically and one asymptomatic pseudoarthrosis. The patients were allowed to WBAT in a rigid sole shoe immediately and had weekly dressing changes. They transitioned to a regular shoe at 1 month. AOFAS scores improved from a mean of 49 to 90 at final follow-up.

The results of arthroscopic-assisted first MTP fusion have also been reported by Carro et al.[34] and Kaufmann[26] These two studies combined report on 30 cases with 28 radiographic fusions (93%) and 2 asymptomatic nonunions, which did not require revision. They utilized a combination of parallel, crossed, and single fully threaded compression screws (Figure 7.12).

In summary, the outcomes with modern techniques for MIS first MTP joint fusion are similar to those found in open procedures.[16] The fusion rate is reported to be 93% to 97%, and many of the cases with radiographic nonunion were asymptomatic or minimally symptomatic. Patient-reported outcomes improved significantly in all studies, and patient satisfaction was high, with low complication rates.

In the authors' experience, postoperative pain is substantially less than with open procedures with many patients requiring no opiate pain medications and the vast majority weaning off narcotics within 2 to 3 days postoperatively. It should be noted that there are no studies specifically evaluating pain medication usage for the first MTP fusion. However, the average 5-mg oxycodone pill usage after MIS bunion correction is 2.2 pills indicating a substantial decrease in pain compared to traditional open procedures.[11]

Full union may take 3 to 6 months, although the majority (>90%) show evidence of bone healing by 6 to 8 weeks. In the rare case that a patient does not show healing by 8 weeks, the authors will still progress activities per protocol as long as there is no pain at the operative site and reimage every 3 to 4 months until healed.

With appropriate training and experience, MIS first MTP joint fusion is a safe and effective procedure that is reproducible and often takes less time than open as the approach and closure are much faster as well. The benefit to the patients may include less pain, easier recovery with less scarring, and fewer wound complications.

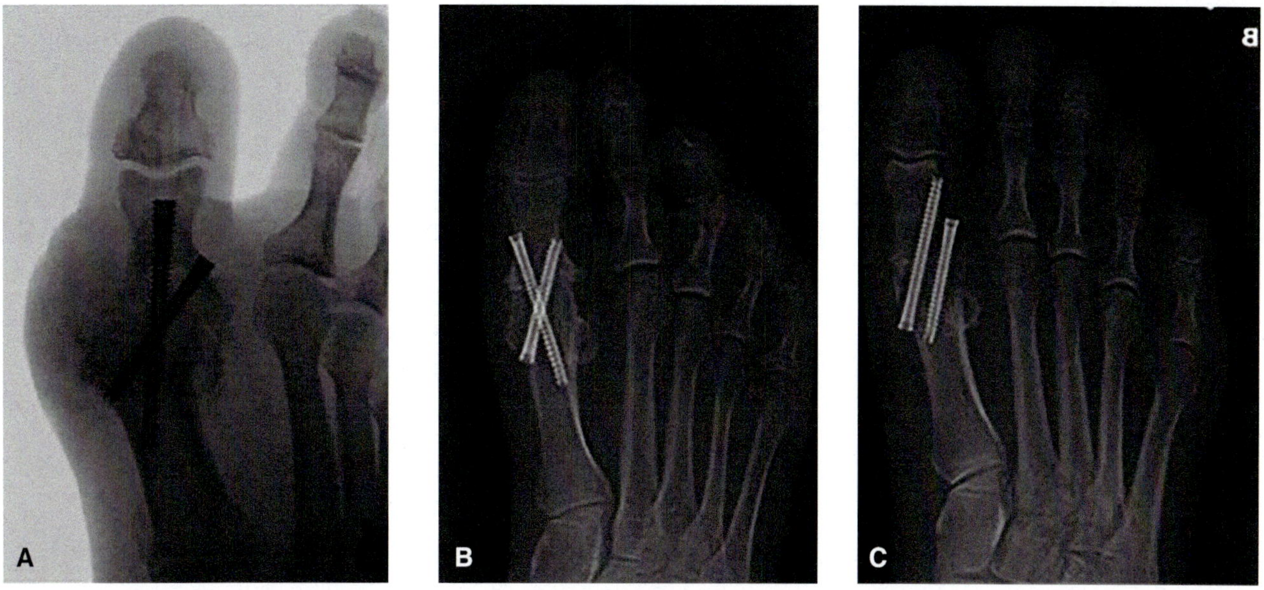

Figure 7.12 Alternative screw constructs. **A.** An axial intramedullary screw with crossed screw was placed to avoid a large gouty tophus medially. **B.** Standard crossed screw fixation. **C.** Parallel screws construct used due to screw interference with attempted crossed fixation. All cases went on to fusion by 8 weeks. (With permission from Christopher P. Miller MD, MHS © 2022.)

References

1. Cotterill JM. Stiffness of the great toe in adolescents. *Br Med J*. 1887;1:1158.
2. Roddy E, Thomas MJ, Marshall M, et al. The population prevalence of symptomatic radiographic foot osteoarthritis in community-dwelling older adults: cross-sectional findings from the clinical assessment study of the foot. *Ann Rheum Dis*. 2015;74:156-163.
3. Senga Y, Nishimura A, Ito N, Kitaura Y, Sudo A. Prevalence of and risk factors for hallux rigidus: a cross-sectional study in Japan. *BMC Musculoskelet Disord*. 2021;22:786.
4. Wilder FV, Barrett JP, Farina EJ. The association of radiographic foot osteoarthritis and radiographic osteoarthritis at other sites. *Osteoarthritis Cartilage*. 2005;13:211-215.
5. Coughlin MJ, Shurnas PS, Hallux rigidus. Grading and long-term results of operative treatment. *J Bone Joint Surg Am*. 2003;85:2072-2088.
6. Baumhauer JF, Singh D, Glazebrook M, et al. Correlation of hallux rigidus grade with motion, VAS pain, intraoperative cartilage loss, and treatment success for first MTP joint arthrodesis and synthetic cartilage implant. *Foot Ankle Int*. 2017;38:1175-1182.
7. Nixon DC, Lorbeer KF, McCormick JJ, Klein SE, Johnson JE. Hallux rigidus grade does not correlate with foot and ankle ability measure score. *J Am Acad Orthop Surg*. 2017;25:648-653.
8. Anderson MR, Ho BS, Baumhauer JF. Current concepts review: hallux rigidus. *Foot Ankle Orthop*. 2018;3:11.
9. Curran MG, Murphy EP, Murphy FM, Fenelon CG, Kearns SR. Functional capabilities after first metatarsal phalangeal joint arthrodesis using a locking plate and compression screw construct. *J Foot Ankle Surg*. 2022;61:79-83.
10. Da Cunha RJ, MacMahon A, Jones MT, et al. Return to sports and physical activities after first metatarsophalangeal joint arthrodesis in young patients. *Foot Ankle Int*. 2019;40:745-752.
11. Mikhail CM, Markowitz J, Di Lenarda L, Guzman J, Vulcano E. Clinical and radiographic outcomes of percutaneous chevron-akin osteotomies for the correction of hallux valgus deformity. *Foot Ankle Int*. 2022;43:32-41.
12. Carro LP, Vallina BB. Arthroscopic-assisted first metatarsophalangeal joint arthrodesis. *Arthroscopy*. 1999;15:215-217.
13. Angthong C, Rajbhandari P, Handoyo HR. Minimally invasive surgery versus an arthroscopic procedure for the first metatarsophalangeal arthrodesis: a comparative study of the effectiveness and safety profile. *Eur J Orthop Surg Traumatol*. 2021;31:497-501.
14. Carlucci S, Parise AC, Santini-Araujo MG, et al. Minimally-invasive hallux arthrodesis with endomedullary and a crossed screw fixation. *Foot Ankle Surg*. 2020;26:744-749.
15. Carreira DS. Arthroscopy of the hallux. *Foot Ankle Clin*. 2009;14:105-114.
16. Hodel S, Viehofer A, Wirth S. Minimally invasive arthrodesis of the first metatarsophalangeal joint: a systematic literature review. *Foot Ankle Surg*. 2020;26:601-606.
17. Hunt KJ. Hallux metatarsophalangeal (MTP) joint arthroscopy for hallux rigidus. *Foot Ankle Int*. 2015;36:113-119.
18. Kaplan DJ, Chen JS, Colasanti CA, et al. Needle arthroscopy cheilectomy for hallux rigidus in the office setting. *Arthrosc Tech*. 2022;11:e385-e390.
19. Malagelada F, Dalmau-Pastor M, Fargues B, Manzanares-Cespedes MC, Pena F, Vega J. Increasing the safety of minimally invasive hallux surgery—an anatomical study introducing the clock method. *Foot Ankle Surg*. 2018;24:40-44.
20. Schipper ON, Day J, Ray GS, Johnson AH. Percutaneous techniques in orthopedic foot and ankle surgery. *Orthop Clin North Am*. 2020;51:403-422.
21. Siclari A, Piras M. Hallux metatarsophalangeal arthroscopy: indications and techniques. *Foot Ankle Clin*. 2015;20:109-122.
22. Sott AH. Minimally invasive arthrodesis of 1st metatarsophalangeal joint for hallux rigidus. *Foot Ankle Clin*. 2016;21:567-576.
23. Walter R, Perera A. Open, arthroscopic, and percutaneous cheilectomy for hallux rigidus. *Foot Ankle Clin*. 2015;20:421-431.
24. Bauer T, Lortat-Jacob A, Hardy P. First metatarsophalangeal joint percutaneous arthrodesis. *Orthop Traumatol Surg Res*. 2010;96:567-573.
25. Fanous RN, Ridgers S, Sott AH. Minimally invasive arthrodesis of the first metatarsophalangeal joint for hallux rigidus. *Foot Ankle Surg*. 2014;20:170-173.
26. Kaufmann G. Minimally invasive arthroscopic-assisted arthrodesis of the first metatarsophalangeal joint. *Oper Orthop Traumatol*. 2021;33:465-470.
27. Crowell A, Van JC, Meyr AJ. Early weight-bearing after arthrodesis of the first metatarsal-phalangeal joint: a systematic review of the incidence of non-union. *J Foot Ankle Surg*. 2018;57:1200-1203.
28. Politi J, John H, Njus G, Bennett GL, Kay DB. First metatarsal-phalangeal joint arthrodesis: a biomechanical assessment of stability. *Foot Ankle Int*. 2003;24:332-337.
29. Brodsky JW, Passmore RN, Pollo FE, Shabat S. Functional outcome of arthrodesis of the first metatarsophalangeal joint using parallel screw fixation. *Foot Ankle Int*. 2005;26:140-146.

30. Keiserman LS, Sammarco VJ, Sammarco GJ. Surgical treatment of the hallux rigidus. *Foot Ankle Clin.* 2005;10:75-96.
31. Robinson D, Heller E, Yassin M. Comparing the temperature effect of dedicated minimally invasive motor system to the discontinuous use of rotatory burrs in the correction of hallux valgus. *Foot Ankle Spec.* 2020;13:478-487.
32. Zhao JZ, Kaiser PB, DeGruccio C, Farina EM, Miller CP. Quality of MIS vs open joint preparations of the foot and ankle. *Foot Ankle Int.* 2022;47(7):948-956.
33. Strony JT, Rascoe AS, Marcus RE. Validation of the artificial floor technique in first metatarsophalangeal joint arthrodesis. *Clin Orthop Relat Res.* 2022;480(10):2002-2009.
34. Carro L, Golano P, Escajadillo N, Vallejo MR, de Diego V, Biazzio A. Hallux rigidus: arthroscopic-assisted first metatarsophalangeal joint arthrodesis. *Tech Foot Ankle Surg.* 2013;12:5.

SECTION 3
Metatarsalgia

8 Distal Minimally Invasive Metatarsal Osteotomy

Olivier Laffenêtre

◆ INTRODUCTION

Lesser ray osteotomies are an effective treatment for metatarsalgia when conservative management fails. They potentially allow three-dimensional displacement of the distal capital fragment, thus modifying the weight bearing on the metatarsal head. Stephen Isham, DPM, designed this distal, extra-articular, and unfixed osteotomy in the 1980s. It was subsequently introduced to European surgeons by Mariano De Prado in Spain in 1994 who established, along with anatomist Pau Golanó, the surgical and anatomical bases essential for a safe and reproducible practice.[2] This technique was further developed in France from 2002, under the aegis of the Research Group and Study in Minimally Invasive Surgery of the Foot (GRECMIP),[3] now MIFAS *by Grecmip*.

A thorough understanding of forefoot anatomy and proper osteotomy technique depending on the deformity is mandatory as each osteotomy may have a functional impact on the adjacent metatarsals. When performing one or more lateral metatarsal osteotomies, the surgeon must aim to obtain sufficient stability to maintain the desired correction and to respect the anterior arch of the metatarsal heads in the coronal and sagittal planes. In general, the more proximal a procedure is, the less stable it is. In addition, osteotomies oriented from dorsal-distal to plantar-proximal are more stable than those that are vertical or perpendicular to the metatarsal axis or those oriented from plantar-proximal to dorsal-distal. Many surgeons have adopted percutaneous techniques to treat lesser metatarsal pathology even with a relative lack of literature on the subject. With lesser ray osteotomies, the main challenge remains the ability to sufficiently balance the correction of the plantar hyperpressure while at the same time preserving a harmonious metatarsal arch in the anteroposterior and frontal planes, by avoiding a transfer metatarsalgia.[1]

Principles

This technique is performed through a working 1- to 3-mm incision, guided by intraoperative fluoroscopy. The absence of osteosynthesis is the main asset of this procedure, providing the ability to allow "self-adjustment" of the metatarsal heads according to ground reaction forces. However, this does require some control, and the osteotomies are maintained first by a postoperative dressing, which is removed generally after 2 weeks and replaced by cohesive strips for a few more weeks. During this time, walking and thus loading of the metatarsal heads is encouraged as this facilitates normalization of the pressure under the metatarsal heads. The developments of this technique discussed later also demonstrate the importance of the direction of the cut line to orient the displacement.

◆ INDICATIONS AND CONTRAINDICATIONS

Indications

De Prado and separately members of GRECMIP have described this procedure to treat metatarsalgia.[4,5] A nonpropulsive or static metatarsalgia, which appears during the second rocker of gait, when the entire foot contacts the ground under the gastrocnemius eccentric contraction control, is the best indication for 2/3/4 distal metatarsal metaphyseal osteotomies (DMMOs). However, when the second metatarsal (M2) and the third metatarsal (M3) are long relative to first metatarsal, it is possible to perform only two DMMOs even if other associated lesser ray deformities and/or a bunion are present (Figure 8.1).

Furthermore, another excellent indication is a propulsive metatarsalgia, which appears during the third rocker, the last part of the stance phase, when only the forefoot contacts the ground just before the swing phase. In this case, the metatarsalgia is considered secondary to excessive of lesser metatarsal length.

DMMO and variations of percutaneous metatarsal osteotomies are useful for recurrence of metatarsalgia after classical open surgery (Figure 8.2).

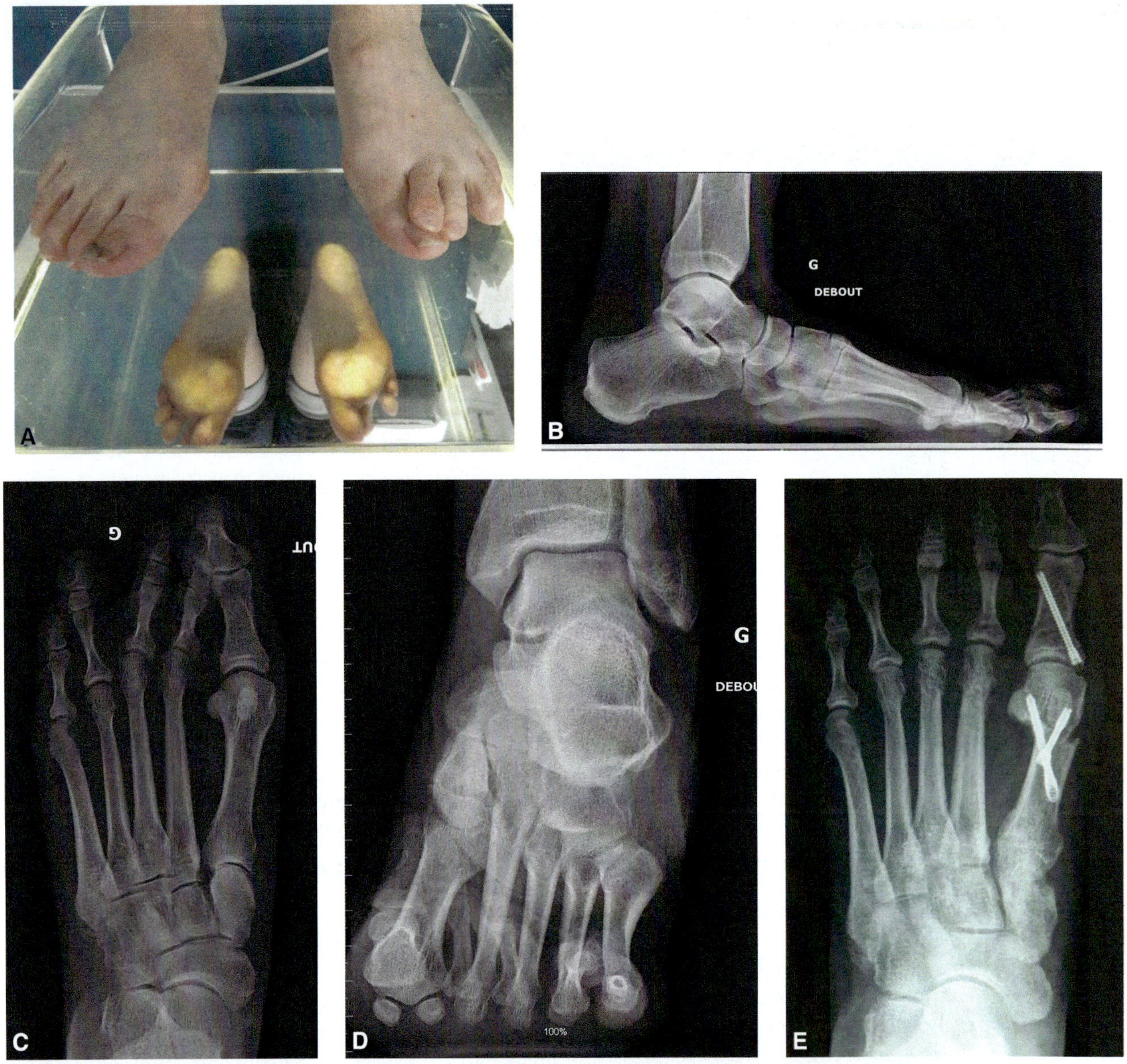

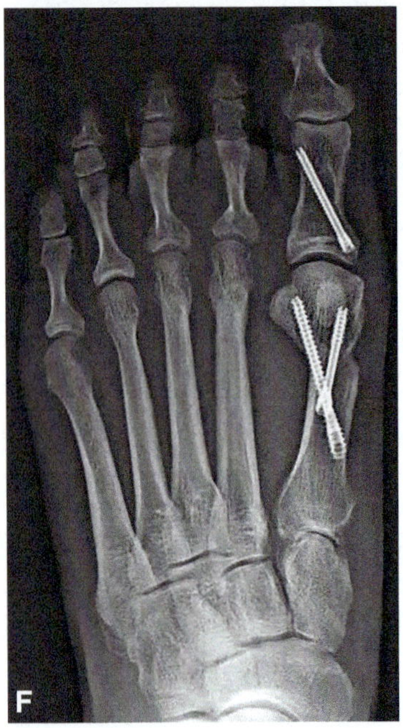

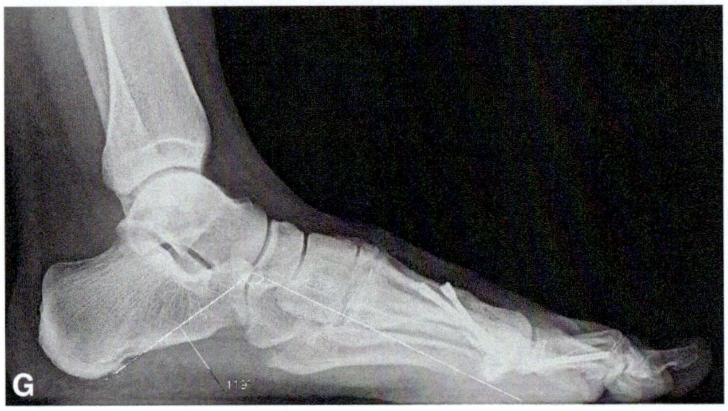

Figure 8.1 A 45-year-old female suffering from a bunion associated to static metatarsalgia and crossover toes. **A-D.** Preoperative aspect and AP, lateral, and sesamoid Guntz incidence radiographs. **E.** AP view after 6 weeks (percutaneous chevron, distal metatarsal metaphyseal osteotomy M2-M3, percutaneous lesser toes M2-M3 procedures). **F-I.** Postoperative aspect and radiographs at 6 months.

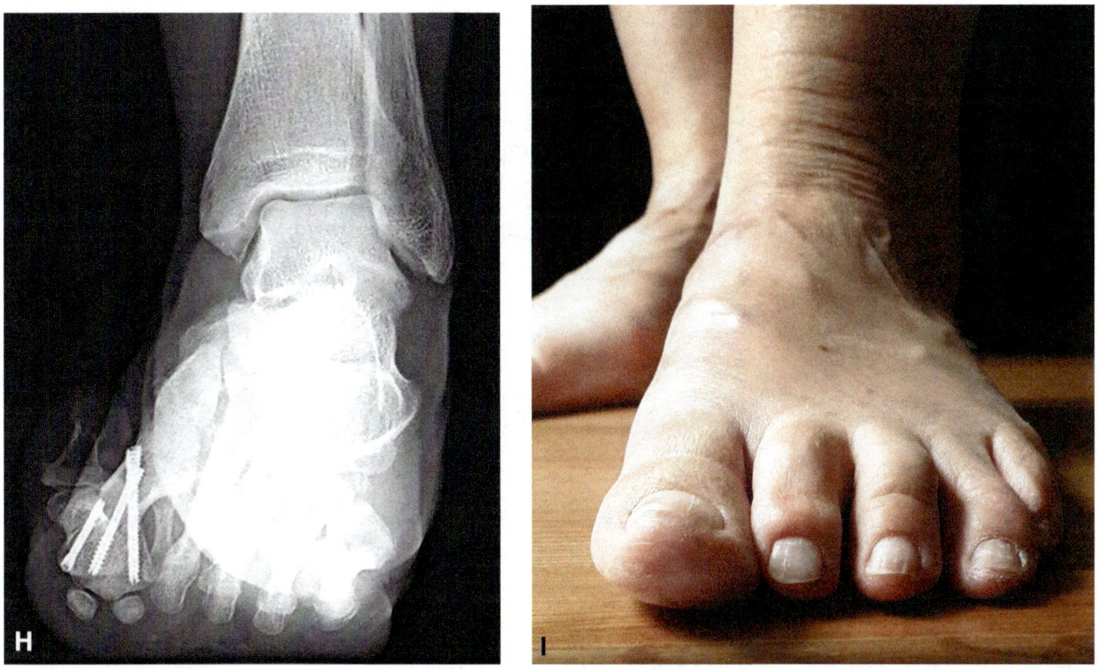

Figure 8.1 *(Continued)*

Contraindications

Because of the anatomical connection of the metatarsal heads by the intermetatarsal transverse ligaments, they tend to move together. Thus, an isolated osteotomy will not move back very much but may on the contrary significantly elevate the head and cause a load transfer. The main rule is never to perform an isolated DMMO and to be very careful by performing only two. Transfer metatarsalgia is a great risk after a single metatarsal shortening, and transfer pain to the fourth metatarsal may be experienced after M2 and M3 DMMOs performed in isolation. The DMMO allows a maximum shortening of only 5 mm; therefore, if the toe is subluxated or dislocated completely, sufficient shortening and/or joint reduction may not be possible.

◆ PREOPERATIVE PLANNING AND PREPARATION

Planning for DMMO requires careful understanding of the concepts and power of each osteotomy. Generally, it is necessary to perform osteotomies on the M2, M3, and fourth metatarsal (M4), even if the M4 is less overloaded and thus usually asymptomatic. The addition of the M4 osteotomy does appear to permit a more harmonious alignment of the metatarsal heads in relation to one another.

The patient is in supine position, with the surgeon facing the end of the table (Figure 8.3).

The use of a tourniquet is not recommended for an exclusive percutaneous procedure as natural blood flow helps to cool the bone during the osteotomy.

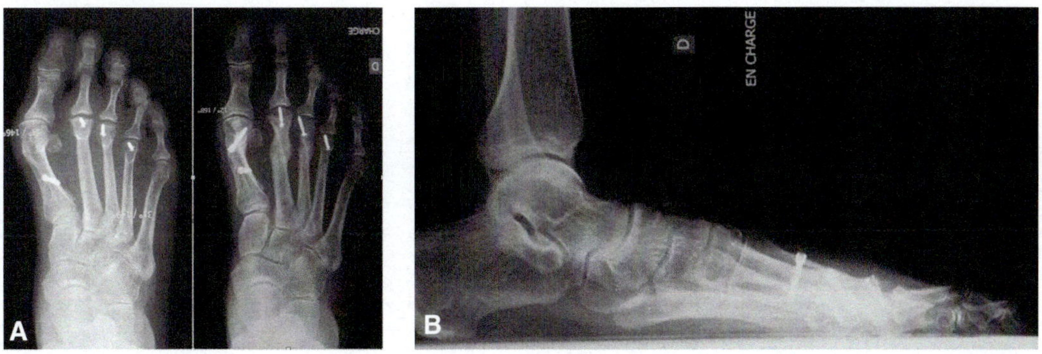

Figure 8.2 Weil revision using distal metatarsal metaphyseal osteotomy M2-M4; **(A)** pre- and postoperative (3 years) and **(B)** AP views.

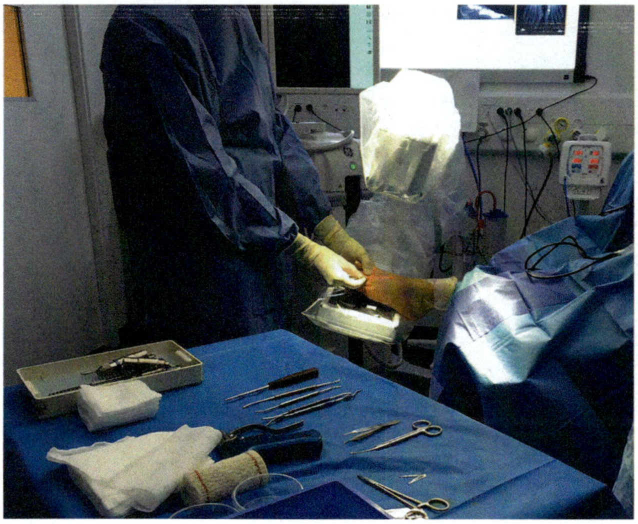

Figure 8.3 Setup.

SURGICAL TECHNIQUE

Note: Described for DMMO surgery on the left foot by a right-handed surgeon.

This is an extra-articular osteotomy where the correction occurs slightly more proximally than the Weil osteotomy and begins 2 to 3 mm from the articular surface at the metatarsal neck.

The use of dedicated instrumentation, and particularly of a high torque low-speed drill, lower than 8,000 rpm, is fundamental. A 2 × 12 mm Shannon burr is required for the osteotomy. For surgery on a left foot by a right-handed operator, the precise top of the metatarsal head must first be palpated with the left thumb (Figure 8.4). Then, at this level in the interspace, on the right side from top of the head (ie, lateral side for the left foot), the surgeon makes a 2-mm incision, parallel to the extensor tendons, preparing a path for the burr using a periosteal elevator to move along the flare on the proximal part of the head onto the neck. A thin curved mosquito clamp may also be used to create space for the burr (Figure 8.5). The burr is positioned obliquely at a 45° angle to the metatarsal axis, against the neck.

A 1-cm area at the osteotomy site is carefully dissected, peeling, and therefore preserving, the integrity of the soft tissue. This allows a precise location of the distal point on the neck corresponding to the beginning of the head. Once the surgeon reaches it, they angle the burr 45° to the metatarsal axis.

Before cutting, the head is held firmly between the left thumb and the forefinger.

The correct positioning of the burr may be checked with a C-arm at the beginning, but with experience, this will

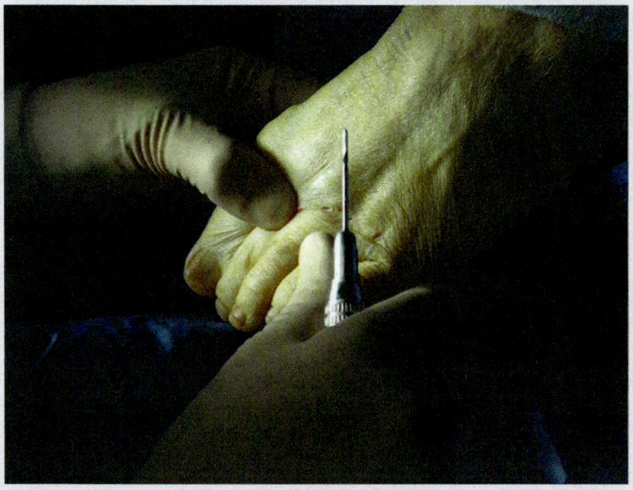

Figure 8.4 High torque low-speed drill and Shannon 2 × 12 burr.

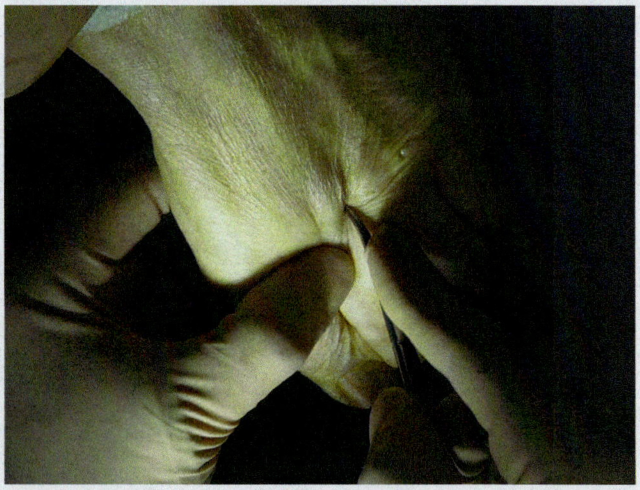

Figure 8.5 Mosquito clamp preparing the path for the burr.

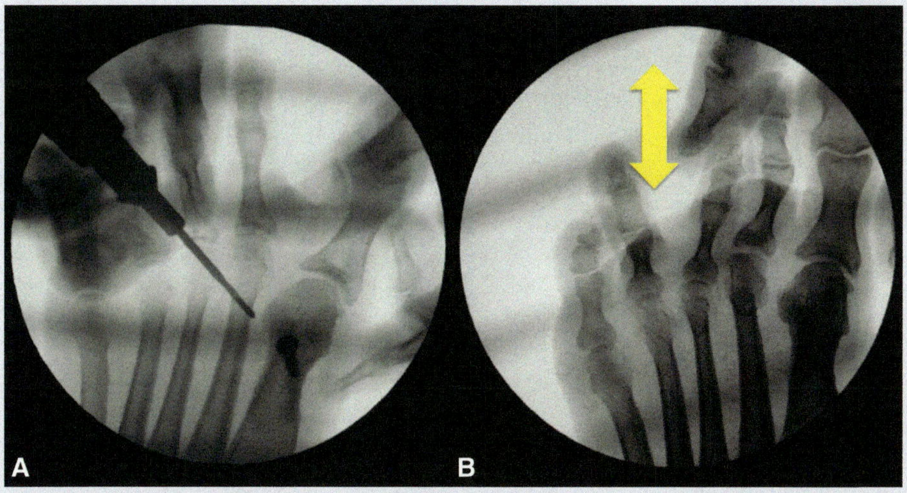

Figure 8.6 Distal metatarsal metaphyseal osteotomy M2-M3. **A.** Location of the burr in the neck area under preoperative fluoroscopic control. **B.** Axial mobilization allowing the expected postoperative displacement.

not be necessary (Figure 8.6A). Identification of the transition from the flare of the head to the narrower neck may be achieved by feel alone.

The osteotomy begins at the lateral cortex, and the burr is moved plantar and medial, completing the cut at the dorsal cortex. This is done by pivoting the hand with the burr in a rotational movement from the point of skin entry, supinating the wrist through a 90° arc. The burr thus comes to almost lie flat on the foot at 90° to the metatarsal axis in the AP plane (Figure 8.7).

To avoid a lateral translation, it is necessary, depending on the side, right or left of the foot, to finish the cut with an angle of 135° or 45°, respectively, with respect to the metatarsal axis, again for a right-handed operator (Figure 8.8). By producing a somewhat oblique cut in the dorsoplantar projection, the lateral cortex is slightly longer than the medial cortex, thus producing a buttress to lateral displacement as this is the natural direction for drift.

It is very important to mobilize the toe in the metatarsal axis to make sure that the metatarsal heads can move together with full weight bearing by mobilizing periosteal adhesions that could prevent the shortening and elevation of the distal fragment (Figure 8.6B). This is performed using the straight elevator through the incision to release the soft tissues.

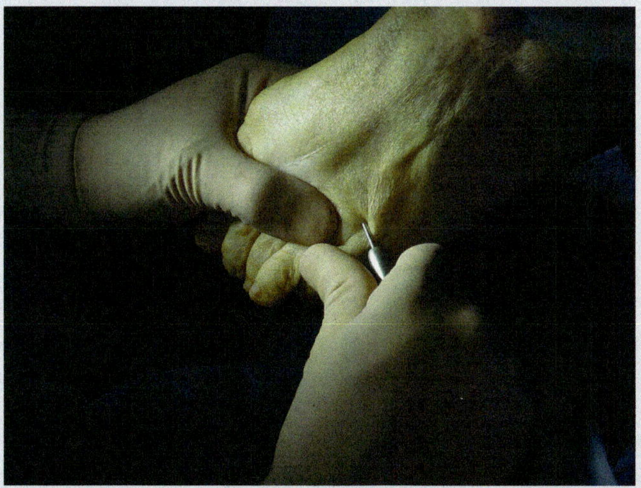

Figure 8.7 Distal metatarsal metaphyseal osteotomy M4: Position of the burr at a 90° angle from the metatarsal axis at the end of the cut.

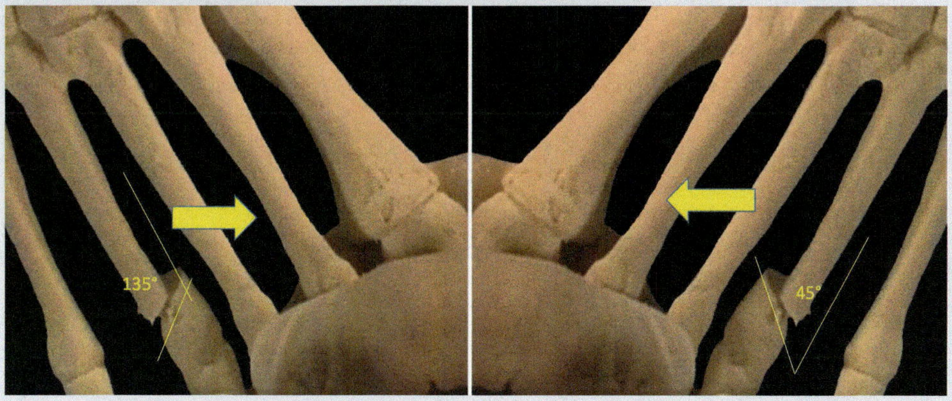

Figure 8.8 Direction of the final cut by 135° (right foot) and 45° (left foot) to avoid a lateral displacement.

◆ POSTOPERATIVE MANAGEMENT

DMMOs are not often done in isolation and are often associated with a bunion and lesser toe deformities, which are also usually into valgus. Postoperative dressings therefore must help to control this drift into valgus but can also help to control the metatarsal heads, which may drift into valgus if multiple DMMOs have been performed. It can be difficult when the second to fourth or fifth are done together. The natural drift is lateral, and therefore, dressing gauze and crepe are used to hold the toe in a straight alignment while permitting natural motion of metatarsophalangeal (MTP) and proximal interphalangeal joints (Figure 8.9A). Fluoroscopy should be used to check the appropriate positioning of the osteotomies after the dressing is placed in the operating room. The dressing is changed only after 2 weeks or more and replaced with small self-gripping strips directing the toes. Patients can remove them for the shower and replace them afterward (Figure 8.9B).

Immediate and full weight bearing allows forefoot self-adjustment, with the metatarsal heads aligning with one another and the ground reaction force. It is preferable for this to be done in a more physiologic postoperative flat shoe. The shoe needs to be worn for 3 weeks until the swelling reduces sufficiently for normal but comfortable footwear. Range of motion of the MTP joints is encouraged immediately after surgery.

Physiotherapy is very helpful after the 3rd week to limit edema and to restore mobility and gait. The patient needs to be aware that the foot will be swollen and sore, with symptoms decreasing slowly over the course of 3 months. DMMOs result in a longer recovery compared with a percutaneous hallux valgus done in isolation.

◆ OUTCOMES

Though many osteotomies have been advocated for the treatment of metatarsalgia, the Weil osteotomy[6] has been established as the procedure of choice around the world.

The ability to correct the metatarsal parabola to accepted norms[7] and furthermore the ability to control this correction with fixation is seen as key to the success of this operation. The DMMO, as a nonfixed osteotomy, had been unfavorably compared to the Helal osteotomy[8] and its very poor results.[9] The Helal osteotomy is performed open and is angled in the opposite direction, plantar to dorsal. As a result, uncontrolled elevation often resulted in transfer metatarsalgia. In addition to the metatarsal head destabilization, the open operation creates significantly more scar tissue postoperatively at the incision site.

As experience with the Weil osteotomy has increased, there has been a growing awareness of its failings. While it effectively shortens the metatarsal, it does not allow sufficient elevation. In fact, studies have shown that there is a risk of plantarizing the head instead, often causing a floating toe deformity. Other complications include stiffness and arthrofibrosis,[10,11] likely influenced by the significant soft-tissue dissection and the intra-articular nature of the osteotomy. Interest has therefore grown in finding alternatives to the Weil osteotomy, such as the unfixed Weil osteotomy.[12] The DMMO, as an extra-articular osteotomy performed percutaneously with minimal soft-tissue dissection, permits elevation as well as shortening. The direction of the osteotomy and the soft-tissue preservation allow better control of excessive dorsiflexion.

Though the lack of fixation is key to the mode of action of a DMMO, there has been concern that this may result in uncontrolled displacement. However, a comparative study[13] of 39 patients treated with DMMO and 33 patients treated with the Weil osteotomy, the head being placed at a predetermined position, showed that the postoperative correction was similar. In this study, the overall outcomes as scored by the AOFAS score were similar and the incidence of recurrent metatarsalgia was similar. The key difference was that the incidence stiffness was less for DMMO (normal movement or slight stiffness was 62% vs 43%). Notably, there was more swelling in DMMO patients at 3 months postoperatively. All the DMMOs went on to unite, but the incidence of delayed union was higher compared to the fixed Weil osteotomy.

Similar results have been shown in other papers with comparison to the Weil osteotomy[14-16] and case series.[17] In Magnan's series,[18] 88% of patients had excellent outcomes with excellent range of motion and a low complication rate. There was a 1.4% incidence of skin necrosis, a frequent complication during the learning curve.[19]

In another study[20] of 30 patients assessed by MOXFQ, visual analog scale and radiological measures showed excellent

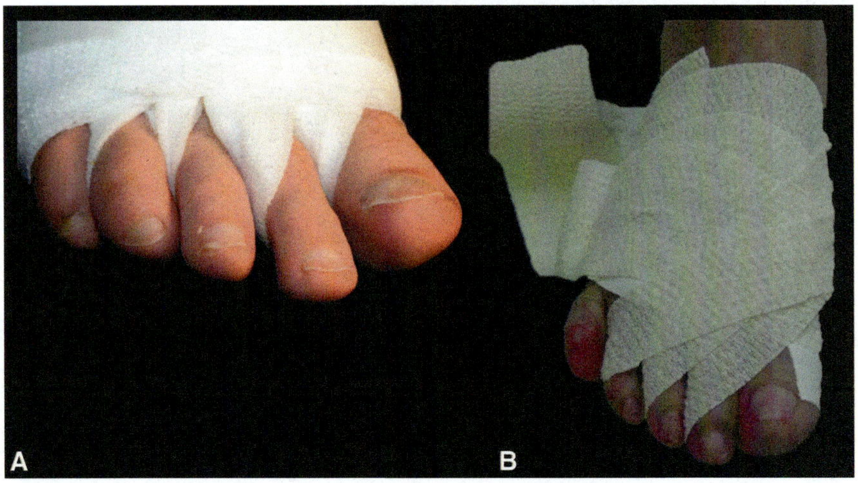

Figure 8.9 **A.** Postoperative dressing. **B.** After its removal at 2 weeks, cohesive elastic strips can be used to maintain the direction of the operated toes.

results with a low risk of infection. One was one nonunion and one patient who had a second and third DMMO who went on to develop transfer metatarsalgia to the M4 and which then required shortening. This confirms the concept that DMMOs M2-M4 are usually required, and an isolated DMMO is formally contraindicated due to the risk of iatrogenic load transfer.

Postoperative edema is the most frequent complaint due to the osteotomy self-adjustment, which leads to micromotion for a few weeks until bone healing occurs. Continued swelling is noted in 59% of cases at 3 months[13] or 22% after 4 months,[21] but reliably resolves once complete bony healing has occurred.

Malunion rates up to 14% have been reported in one study[13] leading to transfer metatarsalgia in one case of an elevation, recurrence in case of an excess of plantarflexion, or poor positioning leading to deformity lesser toes. Positional control of the osteotomies is essential after cuts are made, maintained initially by intraoperative dressing, and later during the first 3 to 6 weeks of the postoperative course.

Despite the absence of fixation, pseudarthrosis is rare, reported in 1 of 693 (0.14%) osteotomies in Darcel's study[21] and in 1.4%[20] to 3.3%[18] in other studies but may remain asymptomatic. Nonunion can be blamed by a technical error where the osteotomy performed too proximally in the shaft rather than the metaphysis or performed using the burr at too high speed, which burns the bone. This may result in overshortening or excessive dorsiflexion of the metatarsal head. If orthotic treatment fails, revision surgery may be needed. In revision cases for nonunion, De Prado suggested performing new DMMOs around the pseudoarthrosis site.[1] In such cases, postoperative care is the same as in an initial surgery. In cases where a lack of immobilization is considered the cause of nonunion, the osteotomy can be stabilized on either side by placing K-wires in the adjacent metatarsals for 6 weeks, with weight bearing allowed in a postoperative flat shoe. This procedure was described by Diebold before the arrival of percutaneous surgery[22] and has always led a complete healing in the author's hands (Figure 8.10).

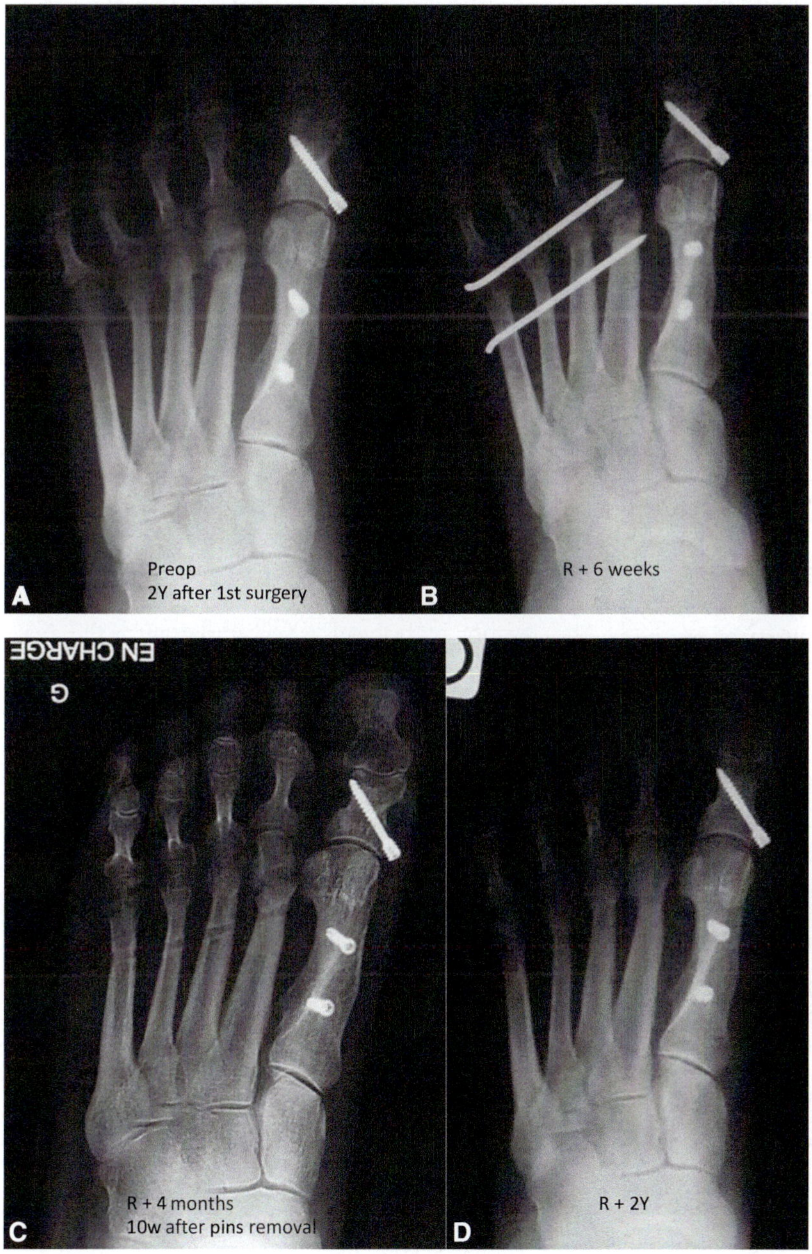

Figure 8.10 Nonunion of the distal metatarsal metaphyseal osteotomy M2 after a 2-year follow-up **(A)** treated according the Diebold's method **(B)**. Aspect 10 weeks after the removal of both wires **(C)** and 2 years after the revision **(D)**.

Evolutions

As simple and beneficial as this technique may seem, it should not be applied to every case of metatarsalgia, and it is not exempt from complications.

The evolution of different DMMOs was designed to address these shortcomings.

Distal Intra-capsular Minimally Invasive Osteotomy (DICMO)

While DMMO has the potential for significant displacement through self-adjustment via weight bearing, due to the instability of the osteotomy, this technique can be associated with more edema that resolves only when bone healing is complete.[13,21,23] To address this lack of stability, an intra-articular osteotomy, a "DICMO" may be performed instead of a DMMO. Unlike the DMMO, the DICMO may be performed in isolation, especially in case of a painful instability of the M2 or M3. The cut is more stable, allowing controlled elevation, 2 mm (the width of the 2-mm burr) and shortening of 0 to 1 mm. This is performed through a medial or lateral approach with a Beaver blade, respecting the extensor system laterally. The capsule is penetrated, and the 2 × 12 mm Shannon burr is placed at the dorsal aspect of the articular surface. Following a 45° angle cross the plantar cortex proximal to the joint, the burr penetrates the head ideally at the level of the notch that notes the end of the articular cartilage. A scan of the burr then makes it possible to cut the bone while remaining within the capsular limits, avoiding any major displacement, particularly laterally or medially (Figure 8.11).

The advantage of the DICMO is that single or double osteotomies may be made, with less edema in the postoperative period due to the inherent stability of the osteotomy being intracapsular. However, the surgeon must be careful at the beginning of the learning curve to check the position of the burr during the cut so as not to be too proximal, creating a DMMO that will be too mobile, or too distal, causing damage to the articular surface or devascularization of the metatarsal head.

The best indication for DICMO is an isolated case of MTP joint instability, and it may be combined with other types of metatarsal osteotomies.

Distal Oblique Metatarsal Minimally Invasive Osteotomy (DOMMO)

In case of a nonreducible dislocation, Weil osteotomies or equivalent are considered better at correcting MTP deformity as they allow the most amount of shortening with control of the joint.

Compared with the DMMO, the DOMMO allows more significant shortening.

The direction of the burr may be convergent (Figure 8.12) or divergent toward the first ray. This allows the surgeon to guide the displacement with shortening or displacement often exceeding 1 cm. The direction of the approach, either medial or lateral, depending on the desired effect, is metaphyseal from dorsal-distal to plantar-proximal. No osteosynthesis is required, and the longer the cut is, the higher the expected shortening is.

This osteotomy can be combined with an open Weil on an adjacent metatarsal for a dislocated ray (ie, when major shortening is needed). This hybrid technique avoids an extensive scarring Weil procedures can cause when performed on multiple lesser rays, leading to much better functional results (Figure 8.13).

Reverse or Converse DMMO

Lastly, this osteotomy variant is an "upside-down" DMMO. Its approach is much more proximal, and the direction of the cut is almost vertical from dorsal-proximal to distal-plantar. It is still an extra-articular osteotomy in the metatarsal neck area, but this cut is strictly transverse without seeking supination of the DMMO (Figure 8.14). The goal is to elevate the metatarsal heads without significant shortening. Indications are limited but include recurrence of operated metatarsalgia with soft-tissue retractions, particularly in cavus foot, and chronic plantar ulcers in diabetic patients with high risks for delayed skin and bone healing. The ergonomics are different, and the surgeon must position themselves in a manner that enables them to hold the metatarsal in order to feel the elevation of the metatarsal head.

The elevation of the heads is very important as the shortening is limited to the width of the cutting portion of the burr. Consider operating on M2 to M5 to avoid a load transfer.[24]

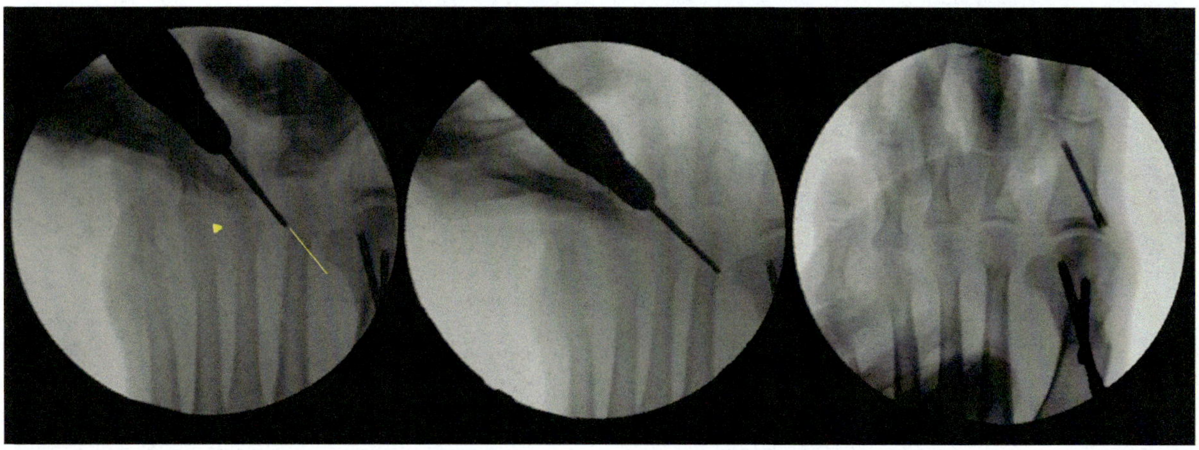

Figure 8.11 Distal intracapsular minimally invasive osteotomy procedure under fluoroscopy.

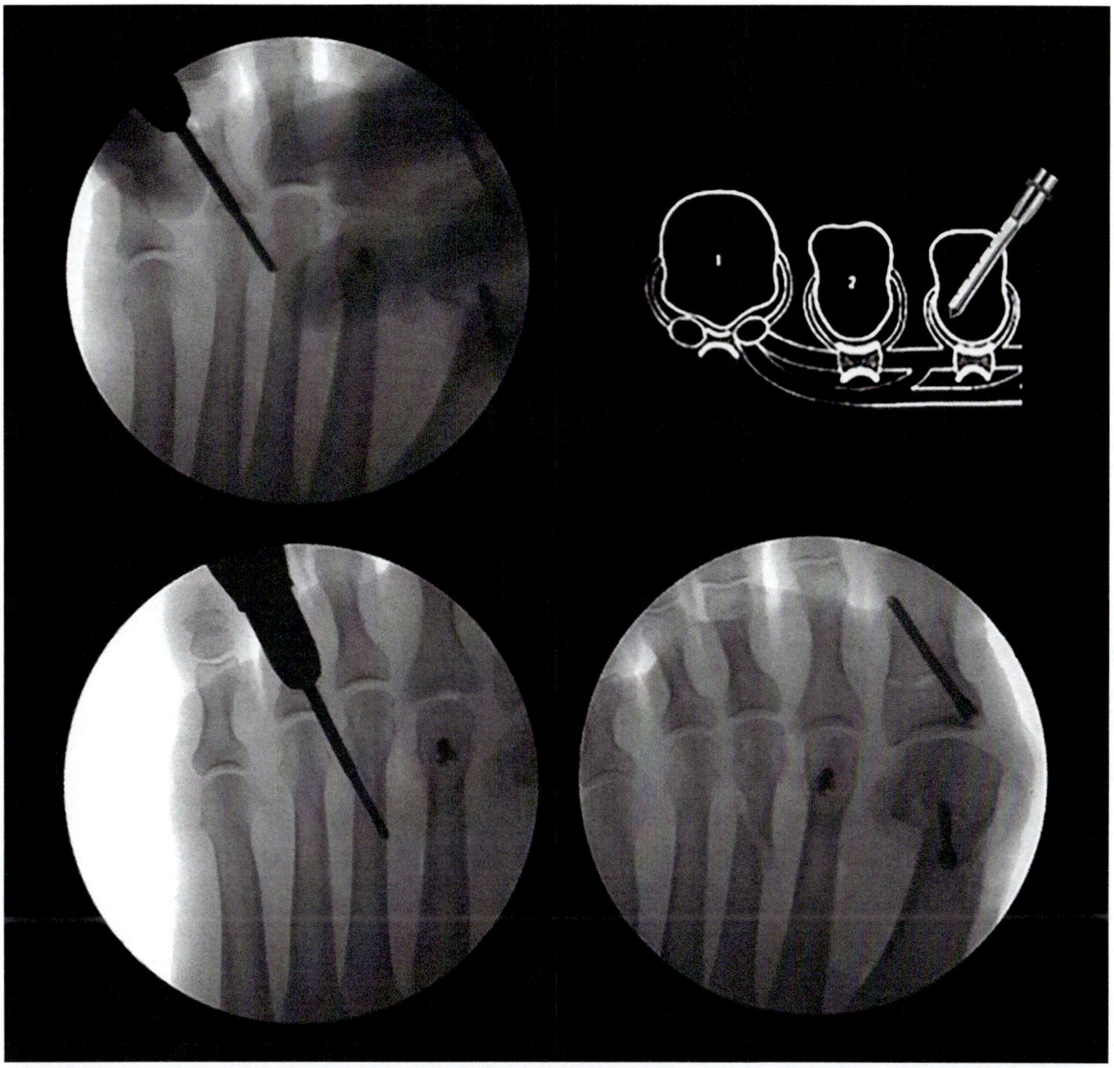

Figure 8.12 Convergent distal oblique metatarsal minimally invasive osteotomy procedure under fluoroscopy.

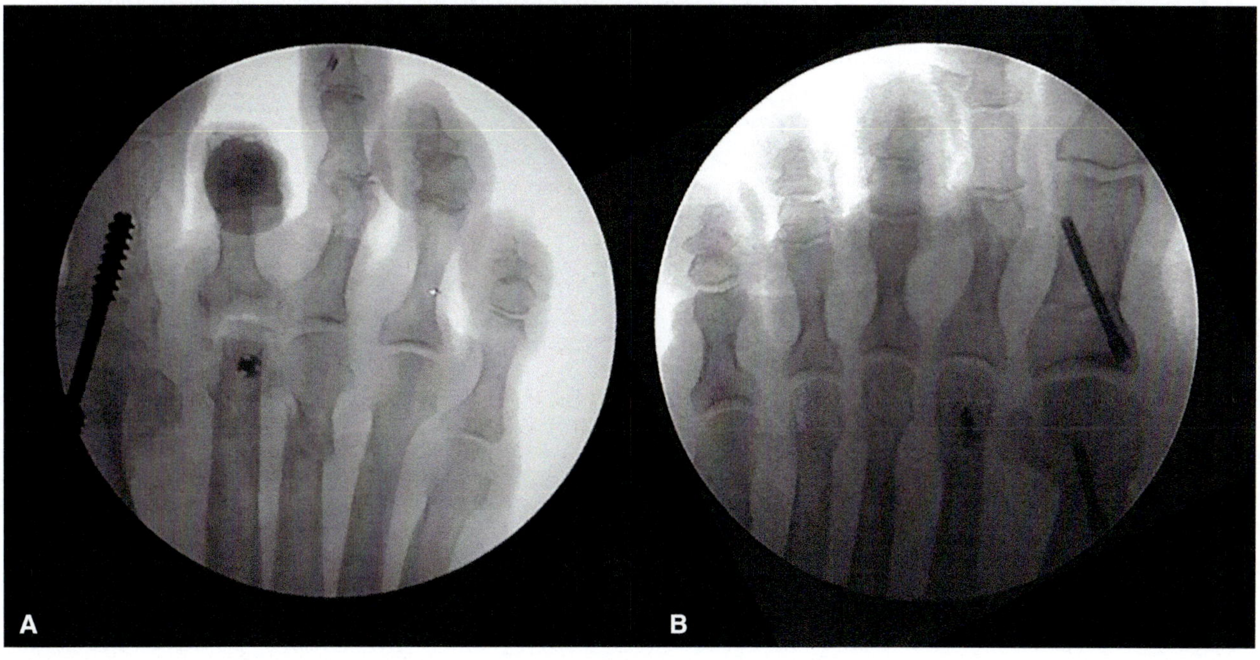

Figure 8.13 **A.** Hybrid surgeries mixing Weil 2 and divergent distal oblique metatarsal minimally invasive osteotomy (DOMMO) M3 and **(B)** Weil 2 and convergent DOMMO M3 and distal metatarsal metaphyseal osteotomy M4.

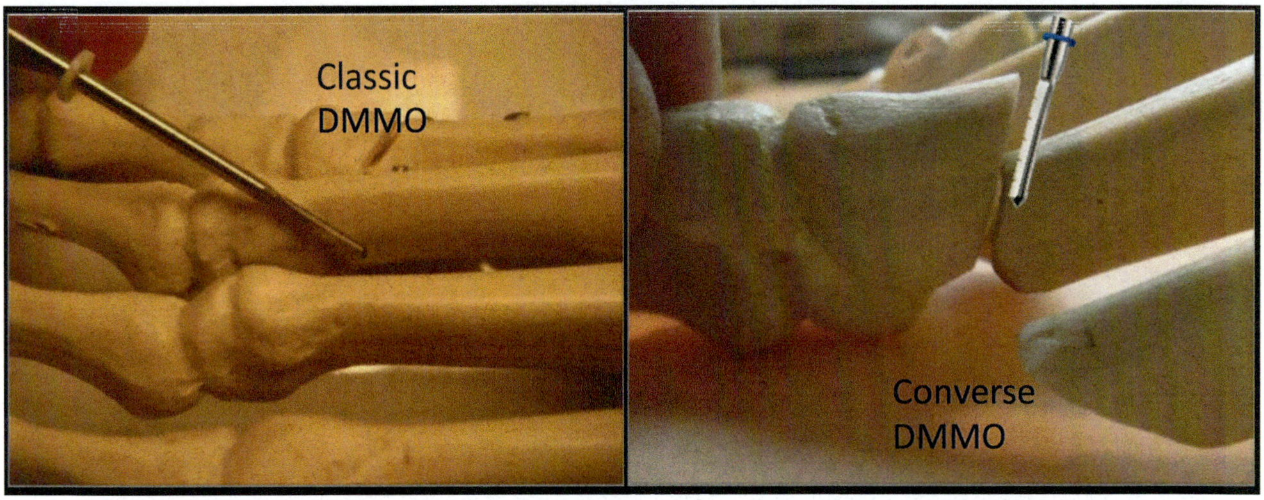

Figure 8.14 Converse distal metatarsal metaphyseal osteotomy (DMMO); place of the cut compared to DMMO.

◆ CONCLUSION

Understanding the multiple types of metatarsal osteotomies available provides the surgeon with flexibility to determine the ideal indication for each clinical situation in order to obtain the most reliable result.

For the treatment of metatarsalgia, percutaneous distal metatarsal osteotomies provide results comparable to those obtained by the open Weil osteotomy with the benefit of fewer complications like stiffness and wound healing problems due to the absence of extensive dissection.

DMMO, DICMO, and DOMMO can be mixed with each other and even with a classic open Weil osteotomy when reduction of a MTP dislocation is required.

The percutaneous tool is an alternative that offers immediate weight bearing, less scarring and stiffness, and fewer soft-tissue complications for lesser rays based the concept of self-adjustment. More prospective research needs to be published in order to determine exact indications, surgical techniques, and long-term results.

References

1. De Prado M, Ripoll PL, Golanó P. *Cirugia Percutanea del pie. Tecnicas quirurgicas, indicaciones, bases anatomicas*. Masson; 2003.
2. Laffenêtre O, Golanó P; GRECMIP. Introduction à la chirurgie mini-invasive du pied et de la cheville: pourquoi, quand, comment? *e-Mém Acad Chir*. 2010;9(1):52-60.
3. Feibel JB, Tisdel CL, Donley BD. Lesser metatarsal osteotomies. A biomechanichal approach to metatarsalgia. *Foot Ankle Clin*. 2001;6:473-489.
4. De Prado M, Ripoll PL, Golanó P. Metatarsalgias. *Cirurgia percutanea del pie*. Masson SA; 2003:167-182.
5. Coillard JY, Laffenêtre O, Cermolacce C, et al. Traitement chirurgical des métatarsalgies statiques par technique percutanée. *Chirurgie de l'avant-pied*. 2nd ed. Cahiers d'enseignement de la SOFCOT Elsevier; 2005:153-157.
6. Leemrijse T. Ostéotomie de weil. *Chirurgie de l'avant-pied*. 2nd ed. Cahiers d'enseignement de la SOFCOT Elsevier; 2005:126-141.
7. Mastro M, Besse JL, Ragusa M, Berthonnaud E. Forefoot morphotype study and planning method for forefoot osteotomies. *Foot Ankle Clin N Am*. 2003;8:695-710.
8. Helal B. Metatarsal osteotomy for metatarsalgia. *J Bone Joint Surg (Br)*. 1975;57:187-192.
9. Trnka H-J, Kabon B, Kaider A, Salzer M, Ritschi P. Helal metatarsal osteotomy for the treatment of metatarsalgia: a critical analysis of results. *Orthopedics*. 1996;19(5):457-461.
10. Trnka H-J, Nyska M, Parks B, Myerson M. Dorsiflexion contracture after the Weil osteotomy: results of cadaver study and three-dimensional analysis. *Foot Ankle Int*. 2001;22(1):47-50.
11. Highlander P, VonHerbulis E, Gonzalez A, Britt J, Buchman J. Complications of the Weil osteotomy. *Foot Ankle Spec*. 2011;4(3):165-170.
12. Garcıa-Fernandez D, Gil-Garay E, Lora-Pablos D, De-la-Cruz-Bertolo J, Llanos-Alcazar LF. Comparative study of the Weil osteotomy with and without fixation. *J Foot Ankle Surg*. 2011;17(3):103-107.
13. Henry J, Besse JL, Fessy MH; AFCP. Distal osteotomy of the lateral metatarsals: a series of 72 cases comparing the Weil osteotomy and the DMMO percutaneous osteotomy. *Orthop Traumatol Surg Res*. 2011;97:S57-S65.
14. Johansen JK, Jordan M, Thomas M. Clinical and radiological outcomes after Weil osteotomy compared to distal metatarsal metaphyseal osteotomy in the treatment of metatarsalgia—a prospective study. *Foot Ankle Surg*. 2019;25(4):488-494.
15. Yeo NEM, Loh B, Chen JYQ, Yew AKS, Ng SY. Comparison of early outcome of Weil osteotomy and distal metatarsal mini-invasive osteotomy for lesser toe metatarsalgia. *J Orthop Surg*. 2016;24:350-353.
16. Thomas M, Jordan M. Minimally invasive correction of lesser toe deformities and treatment of metatarsalgia. *Oper Orthop Traumatol*. 2018;30(3):171-183.
17. Wong T-C, Kong S-W. Minimally invasive distal metatarsal osteotomy in the treatment of primary metatarsalgia. *J Orthop Trauma Rehab*. 2013;17(1):17-21.
18. Magnan B, Bonetti I, Negri S, Maluta T, Dall'Oca C, Samaila E. Percutaneous distal osteotomy of lesser metatarsals (DMMO) for treatment of metatarsalgia with metatarsophalangeal instability. *Foot Ankle Surg*. 2018;24(5):400-405.
19. Krenn S, Albers S, Bock P, Mansfield C, Chraim M, Trnka HJ. Minimally invasive distal metatarsal metaphyseal osteotomy of the lesser toes: learning curve. *Foot Ankle Spec*. 2018;11(3):263-268.
20. Haque S, Kakwani R, Chadwick C, Davies MB, Blundell CM. Outcome of minimally invasive distal metatarsal metaphyseal osteotomy (DMMO) for lesser toe metatarsalgia. *Foot Ankle Int*. 2016;37(1):58-63.
21. Darcel V, Villet L, Chauveaux D, Laffenêtre O. Prise en charge de métatarsalgies statiques par ostéotomies distales percutanées: suivi prospectif de 222 pieds. *Monographie AFCP*. Vol. 5. Sauramps Ed; 2009:229-242.
22. Diebold P-F, Daum B. *Le Pied Post Traumatique*. Masson Ed; 1991:8-15.
23. Salinas Gilabert JE, Lajara Marco F, Ruiz Herrera M. Distal percutaneous osteotomy in the treatment of lesser ray metatarsalgia. *Rev Esp Cic Ortop Traumatol*. 2009;53(3):192-197.
24. Coillard J-Y, Lalevée M, Tourné Y. Distal metatarsal minimally invasive osteotomy (DMMO): surgical technique, variants, indications, and treatment decision-tree. *Foot (Edinb)*. 2021;47:101801.

9 Bunionette

Paulo Carvalho

◆ INTRODUCTION

Bunionette or tailor's bunion is a forefoot deformity characterized by a bony prominence in the lateral aspect of the fifth metatarsal (M5) head, accompanied, in most cases, by varus deviation of the fifth toe (Figure 9.1).

The bunionette was first described by Davies in 1949.[1] The name "tailor's bunion" derives from the pressure and callous over the lateral aspect of the M5 head tailors would experience after spending long periods in a cross-legged sitting position.

The main classifications commonly accepted are those described by Fallat and Buckholz,[2] DuVries,[3] and Coughlin.[4] These classifications are based on the anatomical characterization of M5. There are three anatomical variants that define three types of bunionette: M5 in normal position with hypertrophic metatarsal head and prominent lateral condyle (type 1); M5 with lateral bowing, often called saber deformity (type 2); and M5 in valgus alignment where a wider intermetatarsal angle (IMA) exists between the fourth metatarsal (M4) and M5 (type 3) (Figure 9.2). The latter is the more frequent type, varying between authors (50% to 74%).[2,5] Combinations of the three types are often observed,[2,5,6] defined as type 4 by some authors.[2]

Bunionette deformity is much more frequent in women than in men. There are few demographic studies with a large series of patients. In two studies with more than 100 cases, very different female-male ratios were found.[2,6] Fallat and Buckholz found a ratio of 2:1,[2] and Shimobayashi et al. found a ratio of 21:1.[6] Based on the average of seven studies frequently cited in the literature, the author found a 5:1 female to male ratio.[2,5-10]

◆ PATHOGENESIS

There are intrinsic and extrinsic causes of bunionette deformity. In intrinsic causes, the three anatomical variants previously described play an important role in the pathogenesis of the bunionette causing an increased pressure over the lateral aspect of M5, resulting in local hyperkeratosis and inflammation with swelling and bursitis. In extrinsic causes, footwear, especially women's narrow toe box footwear, may promote or exacerbate symptoms through constant rubbing and pressure over the head of M5.

◆ CLINICAL PRESENTATION

Patients present with pain over the lateral and/or plantar aspect of the M5 head that worsens with footwear and activity. On physical examination, callous and local inflammation such as swelling and erythema are typically present. Bursitis or even ulceration may be noted as well. In addition, very often, there is an associated varus of the fifth toe, which can present a supradductus or infradductus component as well as a claw deformity (Figure 9.3).

◆ IMAGING STUDIES

Standard weight-bearing radiographs (lateral, anteroposterior, and oblique views) are recommended and typically the only imaging required. In the anteroposterior plane, the fourth-fifth IMA, the fifth metatarsophalangeal angle (MPA), lateral deviation angle, as well as the width of the M5 head should be assessed (Figure 9.2).

The IMA is formed by the lines of the longitudinal axis of the fourth and fifth metatarsals. The normal IMA is proposed to be less than 8°.[10] In normal feet, the average IMA is 6.5°, whereas it is greater than 9.6° in feet with symptomatic bunionette.[2,10-12]

The MPA is the angle between the axis of the M5 and the axis of the proximal phalanx of the fifth toe. A normal angle is considered to be 14° or less.[10,13]

The lateral deviation angle is formed between a line connecting the midpoint of the width of the head and the midpoint of the neck of the M5 and a line along the proximal one-half of the medial cortex of the M5's shaft. Normally, this measures less than 3°, but it is considered normal up to 7°.[2] However, according to some studies, there is no difference in the lateral deviation angle between patients with and without bunionette complaints.[6,10] The width of the M5 head is considered normal up to 13 mm.[10]

Spreading between the first metatarsal (M1) and the second metatarsal (M2), spreading between M4 and M5, or spreading between all the metatarsals ("splayfoot") is frequently present in patients with a bunionette[5,6,10,14]

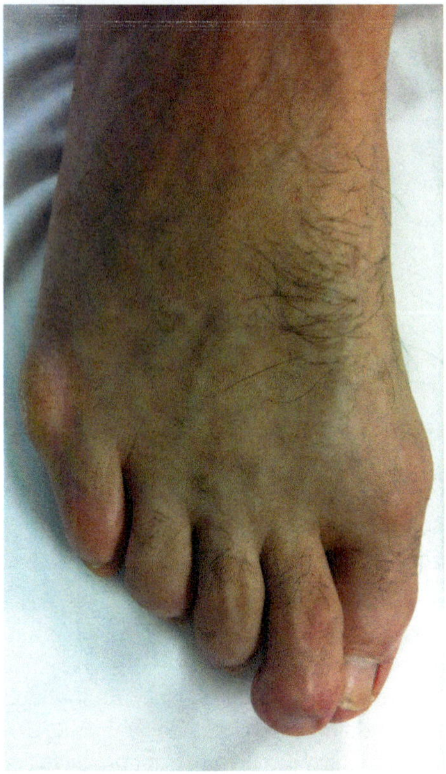

Figure 9.1 Bunionette with varus of the fifth toe.

(Figure 9.4). A splayfoot may also be present with a normal M4-M5 IMA. Therefore, it is possible to encounter patients with a symptomatic bunionette in the setting of a normal IMA, lateral deviation angle, and M5 head width, due to a large width between the M1 and M5.

◆ TREATMENT

Conservative treatment is the recommended initial approach. This includes adapted shoes (with a wide toe box or with cutouts or stretching) that can accommodate the prominent M5 head, padding the inflamed area, hyperkeratosis débridement, and the use of anti-inflammatory drugs or corticosteroids to treat the inflammation, pain, and bursitis.

Surgical treatment is indicated when conservative measures fail to control the symptoms or in patients with special demands, such as high-performing athletes.

The aim of surgery is to decrease the width of the forefoot and the prominent M5 lateral condyle. Anatomical characteristics such as IMA, MPA, lateral deviation angle, and width of the M5 head should be evaluated as it may influence the correct surgical technique. In the author's opinion, the angle between M1 and M5 should also be evaluated, as there may be a bunionette in a splayfoot with a normal IMA.

Several open surgical procedures have been described in the literature such as condylectomy, osteotomy, phalanx or metatarsal head resection, and amputation. Phalanx or metatarsal head resection and amputation should be reserved for salvage procedures.[15,16]

Lateral condylar resection was described by Davies. The lateral condylectomy of the M5 head does not change the IMA, and therefore, it is only indicated for type 1 deformities without splayfoot. It is also not effective for bunionette with associated plantar keratosis. The presence of pes planus or forefoot pronation can also be a relative contraindication as the pressure will continue due to position of the hindfoot and forefoot. Other disadvantages to simple condylectomy

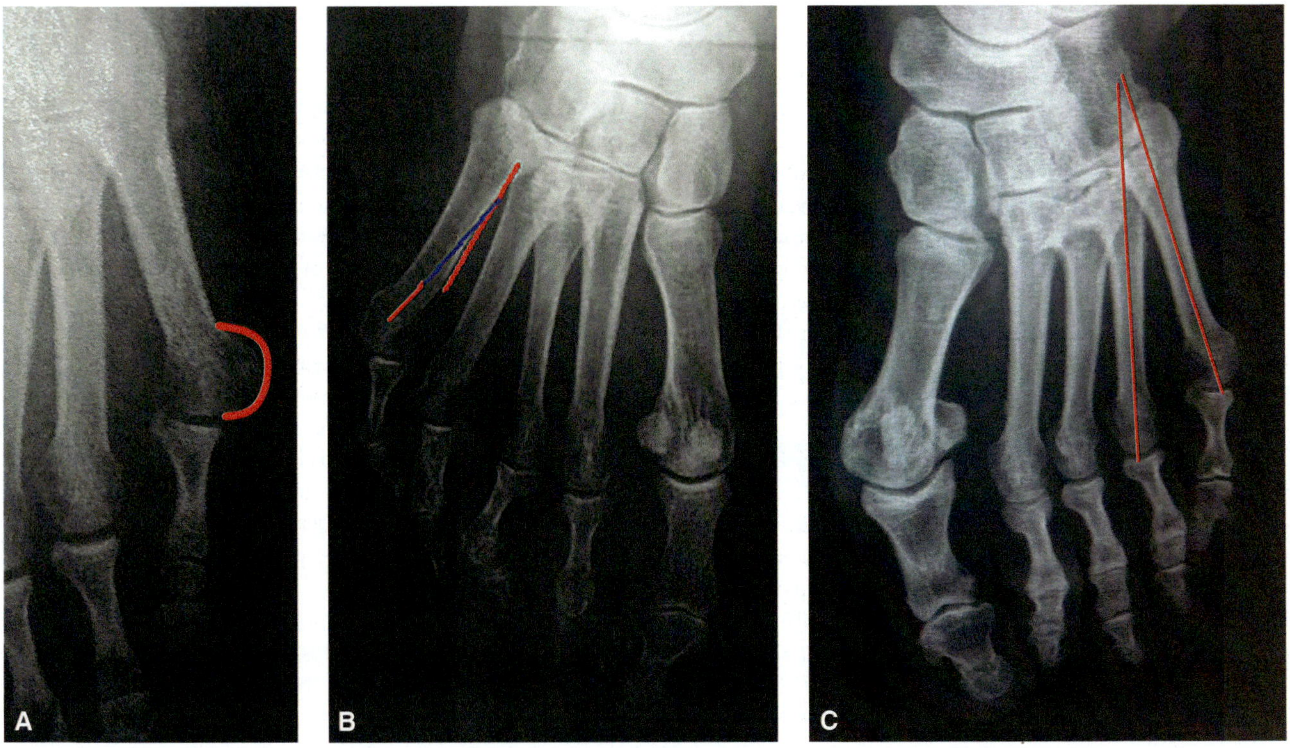

Figure 9.2 Types of bunionette, **(A)** type 1, large head; **(B)** type 2, saber deformity; **(C)** type 3 increased intermetatarsal angle.

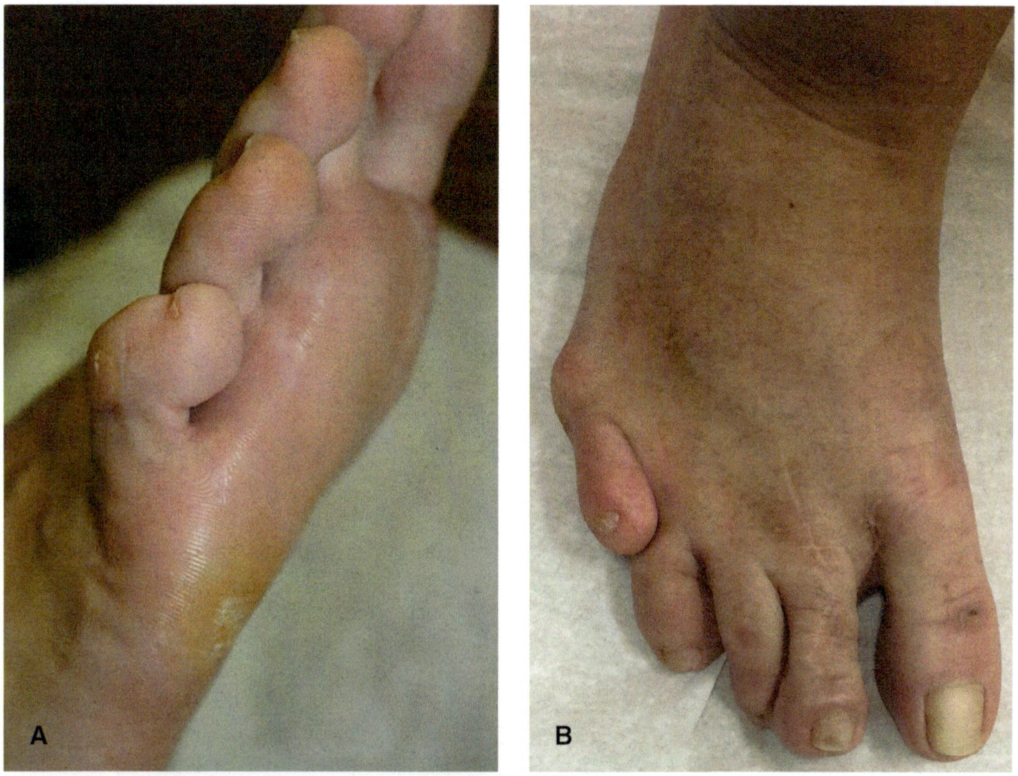

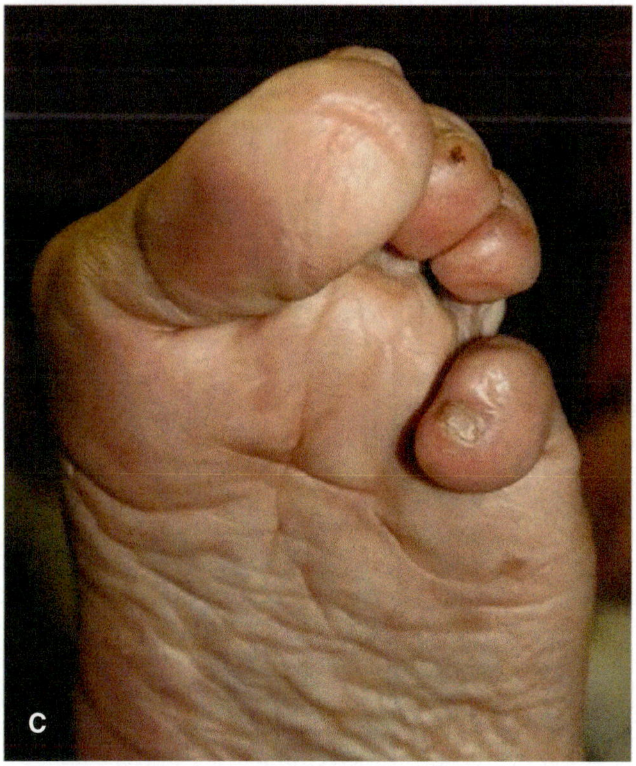

Figure 9.3 Different presentations of the fifth toe, **(A)** claw toe, **(B)** supradductus, **(C)** infradductus.

that have been reported include recurrence of deformity, joint instability with incongruous joint (Figure 9.5), and residual pain.[17]

Recurrence may be seen as the IMA is not decreased with isolated exostectomy, and a type 3 deformity or a splayfoot may develop. Weakening of the lateral capsular structures might also play a role in postoperative instability.

Metatarsal osteotomies are used to decrease the width of the forefoot and M5 head prominence. Several open M5 osteotomies have been described (oblique, transverse, chevron, crescentic, peg-in-hole, etc.), which can be grouped into proximal, diaphyseal, or distal. Although prospective, randomized, and comparative studies are lacking,[18] the existing literature reveals that the outcome of metatarsal

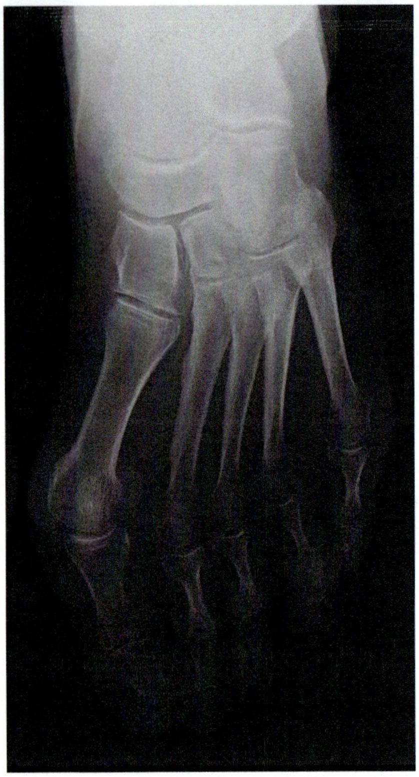

Figure 9.4 Splayfoot.

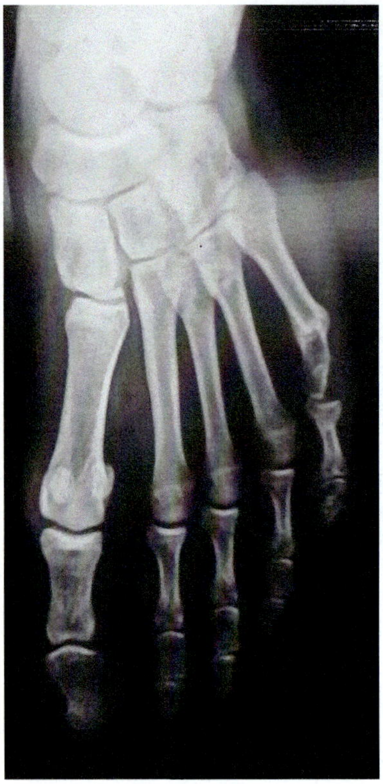

Figure 9.5 Condylectomy with metatarsophalangeal joint instability with production of an incongruous joint with possible lateral dislocation of the fifth joint.

osteotomies seems to be satisfactory. However, according to the only published meta-analysis of the M5 osteotomies,[19] a relatively high degree of complications has been reported. An overall complication rate of 14% was found, 6% of them being major. Proximal and diaphyseal osteotomies have higher complication rate, respectively, 22% and 21%. Distal osteotomies have a complication rate of 11%.[19] In this meta-analysis, percutaneous osteotomies were included as distal osteotomies.

Regarding proximal osteotomies, the literature often reports delayed union or nonunion,[19-22] which seems to be due to a poor blood supply to the metatarsal at this level that is interrupted either by the osteotomy itself or the approach.[23]

While a high rate of delayed union was reported in non-fixated diaphyseal osteotomies,[24] this complication was not reported in fixated cases.[5,25-27] However, a high rate of complications has been reported with diaphyseal osteotomies, mainly recurrence of the plantar hyperkeratosis with necessity of revision surgery.[19,28,29] Another disadvantage of this osteotomies includes a more extensive dissection leading to longer recovery.

Distal osteotomies have the advantage of being technically easier and more stable. As a disadvantage, they are limited in the amount of correction they can offer.[19,30] Several studies concluded that fixation is needed to reduce the risk of dorsal displacement, transfer metatarsalgia, and delayed union and nonunion.[5,24,31,32] However, a high rate of complications related to hardware are reported in the literature, including loosening, breakage, wound healing problems, infection, and residual pain.[5,19,27,29,30] According to Martijn et al. meta-analysis,[19] more than 50% of the complications were related to hardware.

Percutaneous Osteotomy

Minimally invasive distal metatarsal osteotomies stabilized with a K-wire have been described and studied. Although good results were obtained, some soft-tissues complications related to K-wires were reported.[33-35]

The percutaneous treatment was first described by De Prado et al.[36] It is performed trough 3-mm incisions, under fluoroscopy, without direct visualization of the anatomical structures, and hardware is not used. Several clinical studies have been published about the percutaneous approach, reporting excellent results.[8,9,37,38] An anatomical study concluded that percutaneous M5 osteotomy to be a reproducible and safe technique with a short learning curve.[39] A review study[40] compared two different groups of minimally invasive surgery: a group of six studies using a mini-open technique fixated with K-wire and a group of three studies using the percutaneous technique without fixation.[8,9,38] A high satisfaction rate was found in both groups, but more complications were found, particularly soft tissues related, in the group with K-wire fixation. The most commonly reported complication in the percutaneous treatment was delayed union, which often resulted in a hypertrophic callus (Figure 9.6).[8,9,37]

Ferreira et al.[41] reported a 5% nonunion rate on a percutaneous distal osteotomy, which is oblique in the horizontal plane with shortening and medialization of the M5.

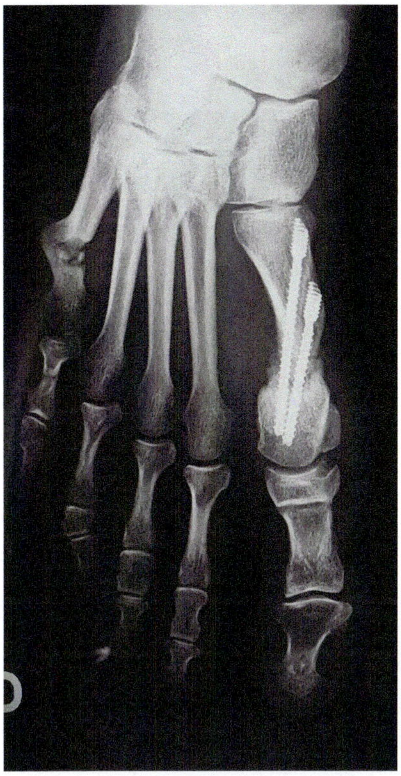

Figure 9.6 Delayed union with a hypertrophic callus.

◆ INDICATIONS

The M5 condylectomy is rarely indicated, and only for type 1 deformity without splayfoot. In the author's opinion, it should almost never be performed, corroborated by recently published literature.[37,41,42] The M5 osteotomy itself medializes the metatarsal head thereby removing the lateral condyle prominence, rendering exostectomy unnecessary. Furthermore, the percutaneous condylectomy is not easy to perform and several complications often occur, such as joint instability and residual pain. However, very rarely an exception to this rule may be found. The author only had one case in which a patient presented bilateral dorsolateral complaints with normal IMA and M5 divergence angle, without a significant splayfoot (Figure 9.7).

The metatarsal osteotomy is the fundamental procedure to correct the bunionette. The precise level of the osteotomy, and whether it is complete or incomplete, depends on the type of deformity and on the surgeon's experience. The level of the osteotomy is usually between the distal and the middle third of the diaphysis. It can be completed with medialization of the distal fragment, or via an incomplete medial closing wedge osteotomy, as described by De Prado et al.[36] By preserving the lateral cortex and stability of the metatarsal osteotomy site, a faster consolidation with less pain may result compared with a complete osteotomy. An oblique orientation in the sagittal plane minimizes the risk of dorsal displacement (Figure 9.8A and B).

Normally, the higher the IMA, the greater the need to complete the osteotomy or to perform it more proximally. As the incomplete osteotomy has less capacity for correction, it should be performed more proximally than a complete osteotomy (Figure 9.9A).

The author usually performs a complete osteotomy at the distal third of the diaphysis (Figure 9.9B). In saber

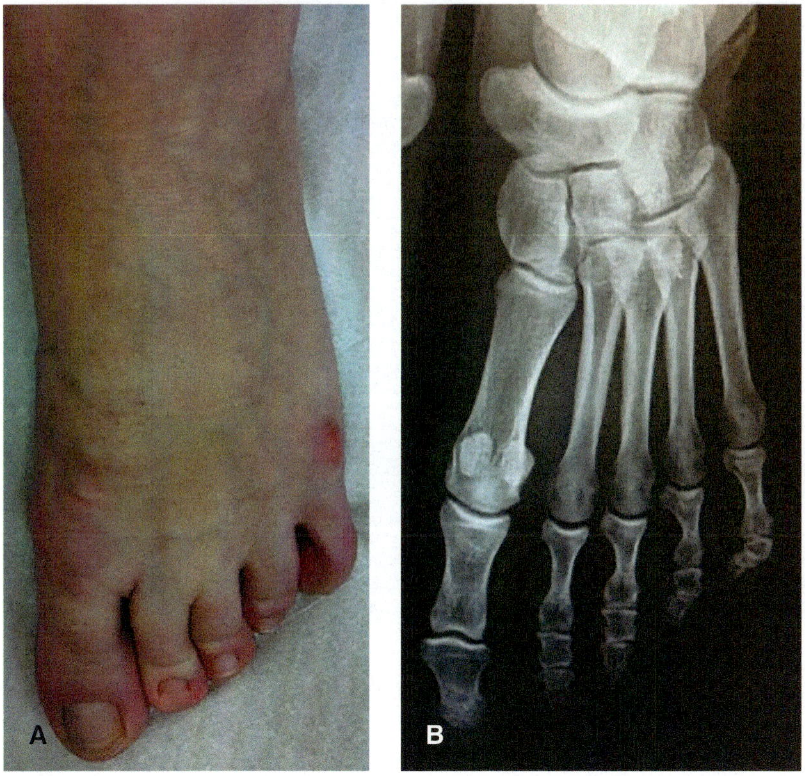

Figure 9.7 Very rare case with indication for condylectomy. **A, B.** Preoperative. **C, D.** Postoperative.

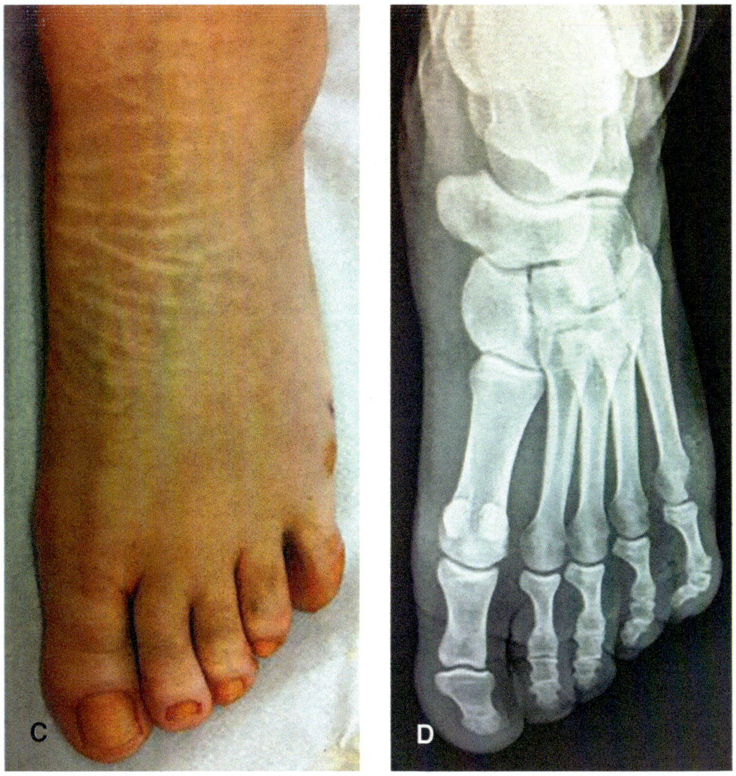

Figure 9.7 *(Continued)*

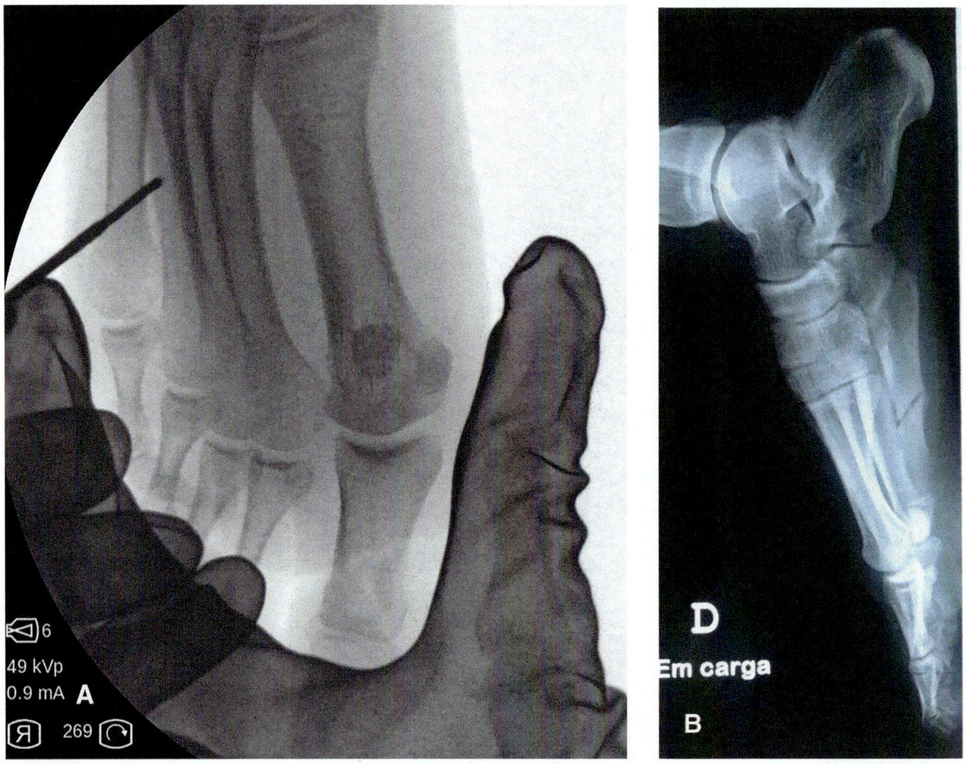

Figure 9.8 **A.** Osteotomy at the distal third of the diaphysis with a 2 × 12 mm Shannon burr. 45° oblique in the sagittal plane, with a plantar-proximal to dorsal-distal orientation. **B.** The obliquity of the osteotomy minimizes the risk of dorsal displacement.

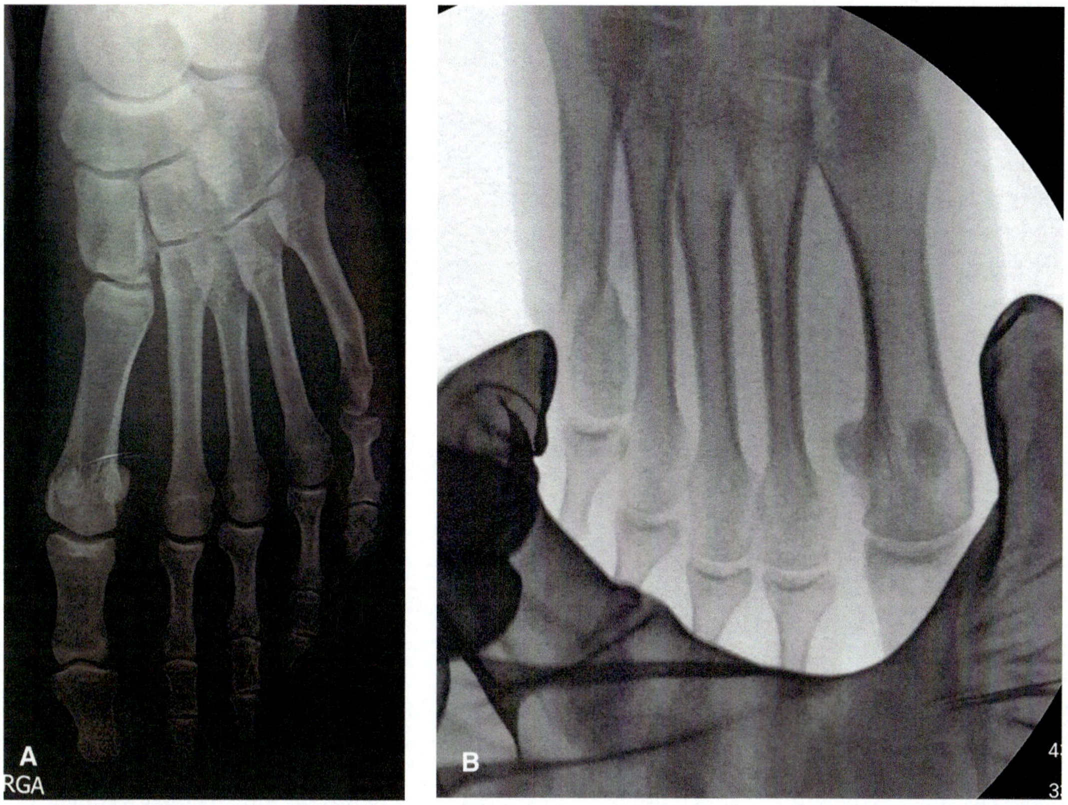

Figure 9.9 **A.** Incomplete middiaphysis osteotomy. **B.** Complete distal third osteotomy. Pushing to medialize fifth metatarsal's head.

deformities, it is advised to make the osteotomy at the apex of the deformity.

Careful consideration must be taken in pes cavovarus supinated with forefoot varus where there is often overload with plantar-lateral hyperkeratosis on the M5 head. In these cases, the varus and its cause must be treated, without indication for an M5 osteotomy in isolation.

Frequently, there is an associated varus of the fifth toe. In this scenario, a medial capsulotomy with a proximal phalanx (P1) osteotomy is needed. With a supradductus or extension of the MP5 joint, an extensor tenotomy must be performed and a dorsal capsulotomy might also be needed. In cases with flexion of the interphalangeal joint, a flexor tenotomy must be performed (Figure 9.10).

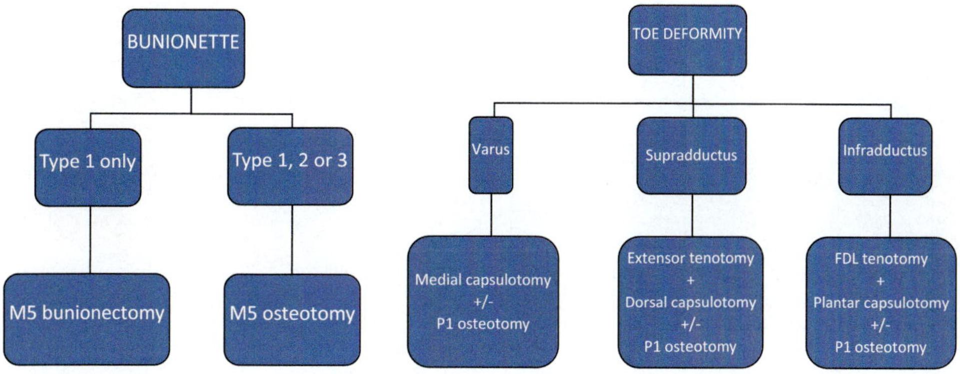

Figure 9.10 Algorithm for the treatment of the fifth ray pathologies.

SURGICAL TECHNIQUE

As in all percutaneous forefoot surgeries, the patient is in supine position with the feet over the end of the table. The image intensifier is placed with the C-arm under the patient's foot. The author usually prefers to be positioned on the left side of the patient (Figure 9.11). No tourniquet should be used as the blood arising from the osteotomy helps to cool down the burr. A foot-operated electrical microdrill with high torque and low speed, less than 7,000 rpm, should be used. A 64-Beaver mini blade is used for skin incisions. A rasp, a periosteal elevator, and specific Shannon and wedge burrs should be available. The author prefers an ankle block regional anesthesia as it provides adequate analgesia while allowing weight bearing. Patients are operated on in the ambulatory setting.

Condylectomy

The 64-Beaver blade is used to perform a 2- to 3-mm vertical incision on the lateral or plantar-lateral aspect of the M5 just proximal to the head (Figure 9.12). The Beaver blade can be used to detach the soft tissues from the bone and to create a working space. The condylectomy is performed using a 3.1 mm × 13 mm wedge burr, using a "windshield wiper" back and forth movement. Cool the burr with saline irrigation. Cleaning the burr may also be necessary. The bone resection is checked with the image intensifier. Bone paste should be removed by compression of the skin, using a rasp, and washing out area copiously with saline through an angiocatheter or a syringe.

Osteotomy

A 2- to 3-mm longitudinal incision is done lateral to the extensor tendon, immediately proximal to the metatarsal head or few millimeters distal to the middiaphysis in cases where a more proximal osteotomy is needed (Figure 9.13). A rasp or a periosteal elevator can be used to remove the periosteum. Then, a 2 × 12 mm Shannon burr is introduced and placed against the medial cortex of M5, 45° oblique in the sagittal plane, with a plantar-proximal to dorsal-distal orientation (Figures 9.8 **and** 9.14). Confirm fluoroscopically the orientation of the burr and that the cutting part of the burr is on the bone (Figure 9.8A). For a left foot and a right-handed surgeon positioned on the left side of the patient, the osteotomy is performed by making a supination movement. In this case, the osteotomy may also be performed with the surgeon positioned at the foot of the patient, similar to the position for completing a distal metatarsal metaphyseal osteotomy. For the right foot, a pronation movement is performed. For the left-handed surgeon, the positioning and gestures are inverted. Saline irrigation should be used to cool the skin and bone during the osteotomy. At the end of this procedure, the surgeon pushes on the lateral side of the metatarsal head to close the incomplete osteotomy or to medialize the distal fragment (Figure 9.9B). Correction is confirmed under fluoroscopy.

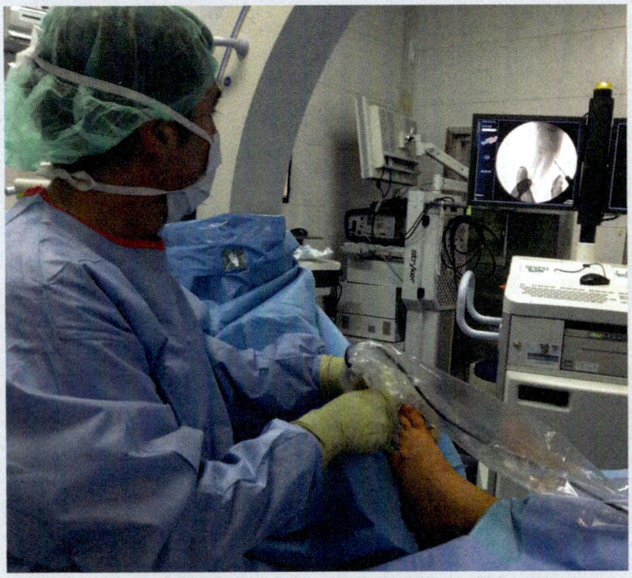

Figure 9.11 Positioning.

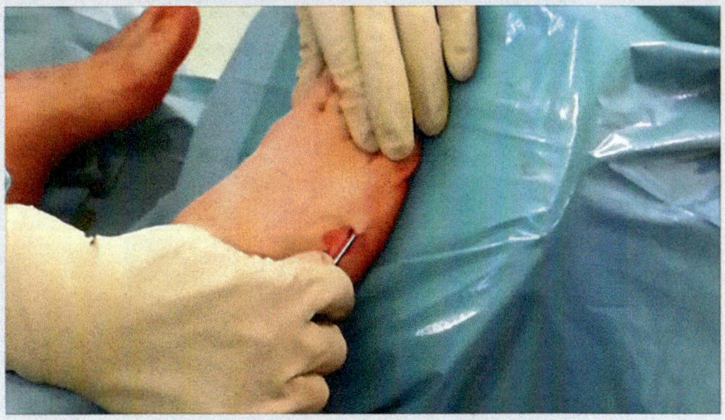

Figure 9.12 Lateral condylectomy.

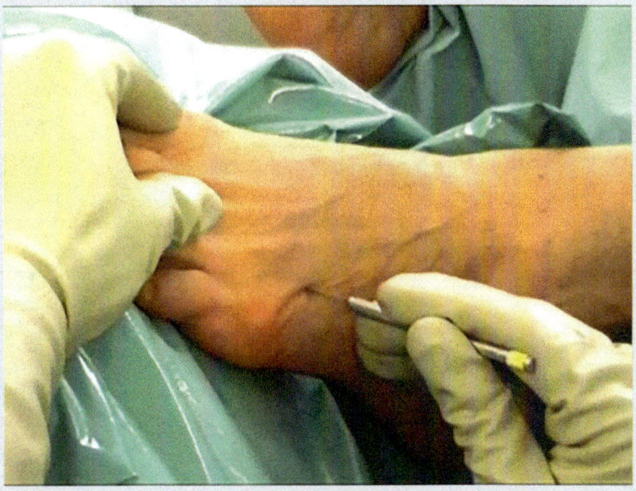

Figure 9.13 Incision for the fifth metatarsal osteotomy.

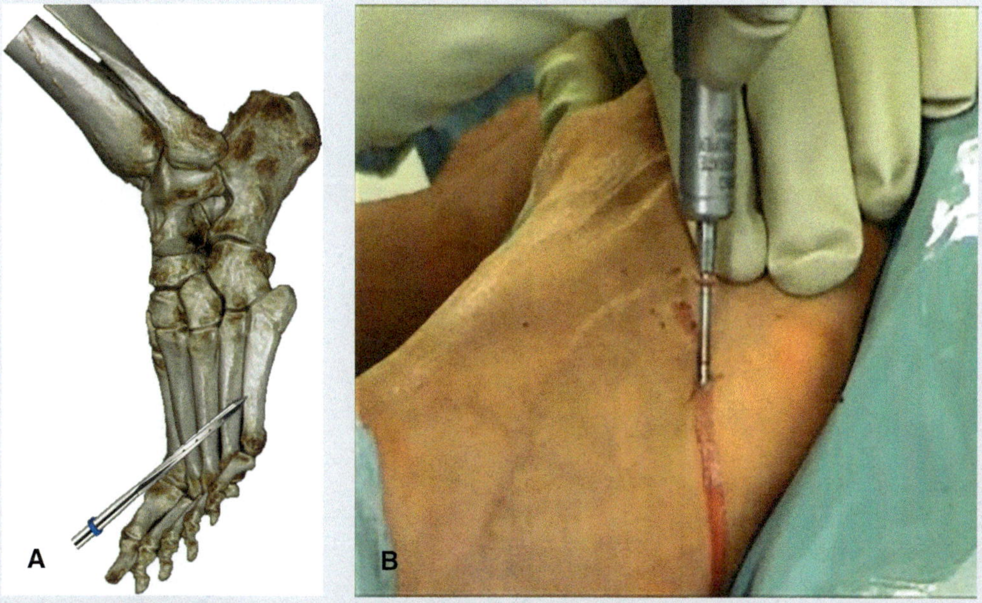

Figure 9.14 Burr orientation –45° oblique in the sagittal plane, plantar-proximal to dorsal-distal, **(A)** schematic and **(B)** intraoperative views.

Varus of the Fifth Toe

For the medial capsulotomy, a dorsal incision is performed on the medial side of the metatarsophalangeal joint (MPJ). A 64-Beaver blade is introduced into the medial joint space, perpendicular to the long axis of M5 and the medial capsule, and the collateral ligament is cut (Figure 9.15). For the extensor tenotomy, a transversal dorsal skin incision at the level of the MPJ is done. Then, the extensor tendon is cut at this level. When necessary, the dorsal capsulotomy is performed by advancing the blade deep to the tendon and making a lateral incision at the capsule. If needed, a flexor tenotomy is performed through a plantar incision at the level of the proximal phalanx, introducing the Beaver blade until it reaches the bone (Figure 9.16). With tension on the toe in extension, the blade is placed against the flexor and the tendon is sharply released.

For the phalanx osteotomy, the author makes a lateral incision at the base of P1 and performs the osteotomy at the metaphyseal-diaphyseal junction using a 2 × 12 mm or 2 × 8 mm Shannon burr (Figure 9.17).

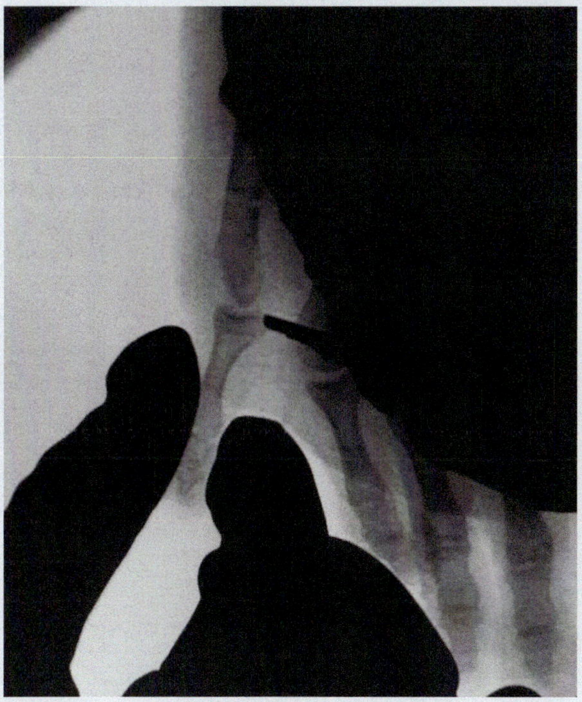

Figure 9.15 Medial capsulotomy.

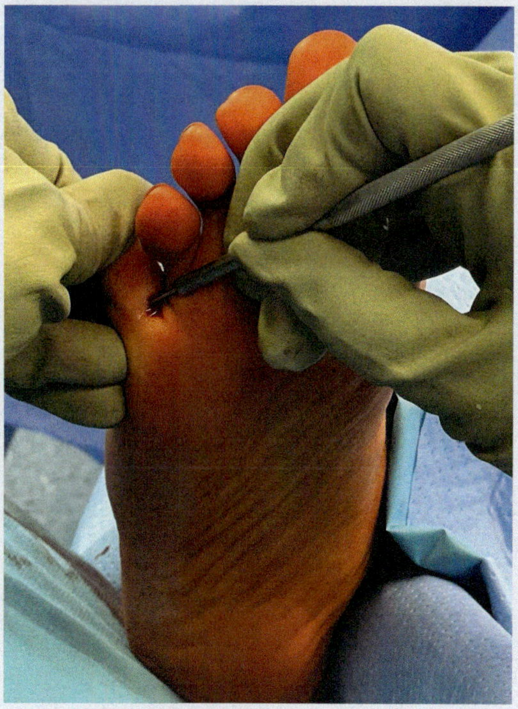

Figure 9.16 Flexor tenotomy.

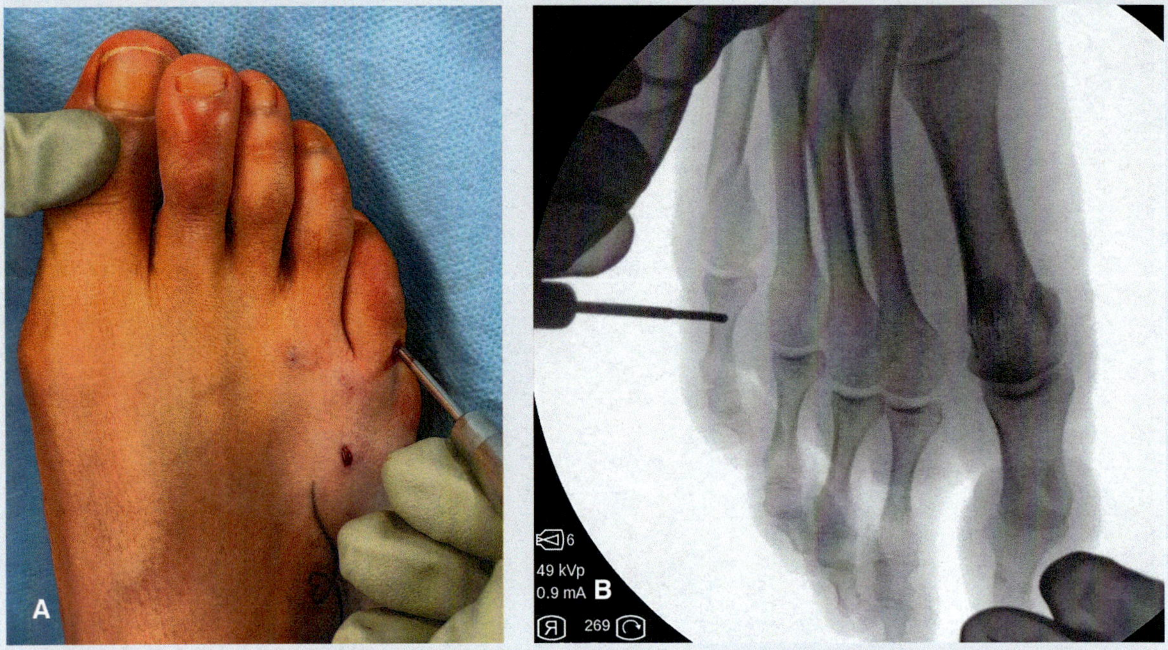

Figure 9.17 Basal P1 osteotomy, **(A)** lateral approach and **(B)** fluoroscopic checking.

◆ POSTOPERATIVE MANAGEMENT

The skin incisions may be sutured or simply left to close under the dressing. The placement of the surgical dressings is extremely important, using gauze, elastic bandages, and taping. A transversal gauze and taping are placed to promote medial translation of the M5 head (Figure 9.18A). Dressing and sutures are removed between the 12th and 14th days. At that time, transverse tape pushing the M5 head medially is placed (Figure 9.18B), and if the fifth toe was surgically treated, additional taping to hold the fourth and fifth toes is required. Patients are instructed to renew the taping at home until the 6th postoperative week. A flat sole full weight-bearing shoe is used unless another procedure has been performed, such as a bunion procedure that may require a heel weight-bearing shoe. The postoperative shoe is worn for 2 to 3 weeks. After that, patients may transition to comfortable shoes or sneakers. Running is permitted at 3 months postoperative. Radiograph images of the foot should be taken at 6 weeks and 3 months to confirm progression of healing. Frequently, radiological images without evidence of complete bone healing may be noted in patients clinically doing very well. In those cases, patients are advised to return at 6 months postoperatively if they have complaints.

◆ OUTCOMES

Complications in the bunionette percutaneous treatment performed with an isolated M5 osteotomy are not frequent. The most common complication is delayed union, which is usually well tolerated by the patients. In these cases, usually there is no pain after 2 or 3 months, and patients are still able to return to sports at 3 months. The very rare symptomatic patients are advised to restrain from high-impact activities, and usually, complaints disappear after 6 months. Other minor and transient complications include wound healing problems secondary to thermal damage to the skin. Saline irrigation during the osteotomy is critical to avoid this type of complication. The M5 osteotomy is a simple technique that is ideal for starting the percutaneous surgery practice.

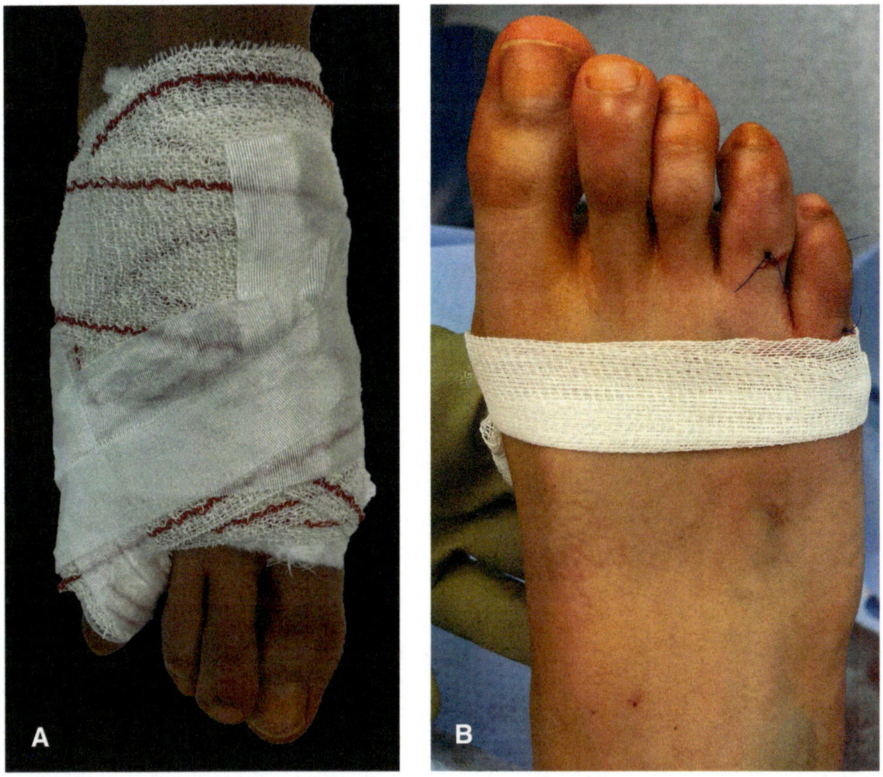

Figure 9.18 A. Intraoperative dressing with gauzes and taping pushing fifth metatarsal (M5) head. **B.** After removing the dressing, a transversal tape maintains M5 head medialization.

REFERENCES

1. Davies H. Metatarsus quintus valgus. *BMJ.* 1949;1(4606):664-665.
2. Fallat LM, Buckholz J. An analysis of the tailor's bunion by radiographic and anatomical display. *J Am Podiatr Med Assoc.* 1980;70(12):597-603.
3. DuVries HL. *Surgery of the Foot.* 3rd ed. CV Mosby; 1973.
4. Coughlin MJ. Etiology and treatment of the bunionette deformity. *Instr Course Lect.* 1990;39:37-48.
5. Coughlin MJ. Treatment of bunionette deformity with longitudinal diaphyseal osteotomy with distal soft tissue repair. *Foot Ankle.* 1991;11(4):195-203.
6. Shimobayashi M, Tanaka Y, Taniguchi A, et al. Radiographic morphologic characteristics of bunionette deformity. *Foot Ankle Int.* 2016;37(3):320-326.
7. Kitaoka HB, Holiday AD, Campbell DC. Distal chevron metatarsal osteotomy for bunionette. *Foot Ankle.* 1991;12(2):80-85.
8. Michels F, van der Bauwhede J, Guillo S, et al. Percutaneous bunionette correction. *Foot Ankle Surg.* 2013;19(1):9-14.
9. Laffenêtre O, Millet-Barbé B, Darcel V, et al. Percutaneous bunionette correction: results of a 49-case retrospective study at a mean 34 months' follow-up. *Orthop Traumatol Surg Res.* 2015;101(2):179-184.
10. Nestor BJ, Kitaoka HB, Ilstrup DM, et al. Radiologic anatomy of the painful bunionette. *Foot Ankle.* 1990;11(1):6-11.
11. Schoenhaus H, Rotman S, Meshon AL. A review of normal inter-metatarsal angles. *J Am Podiatr Med Assoc.* 1973;63(3):88-95.
12. Lau BC, Allahabadi S, Palanca A, Oji DE. Understanding radiographic measurements used in foot and ankle surgery. *J Am Acad Orthop Surg.* 2022;30(2):e139-e154.
13. Steel MW, Johnson KA, DeWitz MA, Ilstrup DM. Radiographic measurements of the normal adult foot. *Foot Ankle.* 1980;1(3):151-158.
14. Bishop J, Kahn A, Turba JE. Surgical correction of the splayfoot: the Giannestras procedure. *Clin Orthop Relat Res.* 1980;146:234-238.
15. Kitaoka HB, Holiday AD. Metatarsal head resection for bunionette: long-term follow-up. *Foot Ankle.* 1991;11(6):345-349.
16. Dorris MF, Mandel LM. Fifth metatarsal head resection for correction of tailor's bunions and sub-fifth metatarsal head keratoma: a retrospective analysis. *J Foot Surg.* 1991;30(3):269-275.
17. Kitaoka HB, Holiday AD. Lateral condylar resection for bunionette. *Clin Orthop Relat Res.* 1992;278:183-192.
18. Shi GG, Humayun A, Whalen JL, Kitaoka HB. Management of bunionette deformity. *J Am Acad Orthop Surg.* 2018;26(19):E393-E404.
19. Martijn HA, Sierevelt IN, Wassink S, Nolte PA. Fifth metatarsal osteotomies for treatment of bunionette deformity: a meta-analysis of angle correction and clinical condition. *J Foot Ankle Surg.* 2018;57(1):140-148.
20. Buchbinder IJ. DRATO procedure for tailor's bunion. *J Foot Surg.* 1982;21(3):177-180.
21. Diebold PF, Bejjani FJ. Basal osteotomy of the fifth metatarsal with intermetatarsal pinning: a new approach to Tailor's bunion. *Foot Ankle.* 1987;8(1):40-45.
22. Okuda R, Kinoshita M, Morikawa J, et al. Proximal dome-shaped osteotomy for symptomatic bunionette. *Clin Orthop Relat Res.* 2002;396:173-178.
23. Shereff MJ, Yang QM, Kummer FJ, et al. Vascular anatomy of the fifth metatarsal. *Foot Ankle.* 1991;11(6):350-353.
24. Sponsel KH. Bunionette correction by metatarsal osteotomy: preliminary report. *Orthop Clin North Am.* 1976;7(4):809-819.
25. Coughlin MJ. Bunionette repair with midshaft oblique osteotomy and distal soft tissue repair. *Tech Foot Ankle Surg.* 2010;9(1):14-19.
26. London BP, Stern SF, Quist MA, et al. Long oblique distal osteotomy of the fifth metatarsal for correction of tailor's bunion: a retrospective review. *J Foot Ankle Surg.* 2003;42(1):36-42.
27. Heckman JD, Harkless LB, Wirth MA, Higgins KR. The Sponsel oblique fifth metatarsal osteotomy: evaluation with long-term follow-up. *The Foot.* 1991;1(1):37-44.
28. Maher AJ, Kilmartin TE. Scarf osteotomy for correction of Tailor's bunion: mid- to long-term followup. *Foot Ankle Int.* 2010;31(8):676-682.
29. Necas L, Hrubina M, Skotak M, et al. Bunionette deformity corrected with "shortening" scarf osteotomy of the fifth metatarsal: mid-term results of a 34-cases. *Foot Ankle Surg.* 2020;26(5):541-546.
30. Weitzel S, Trnka HJ, Petroutsas J. Transverse medial slide osteotomy for bunionette deformity: long-term results. *Foot Ankle Int.* 2007;28(7):794-798.
31. Keating SE, DeVincentis A, Goller WL. Oblique fifth metatarsal osteotomy: a follow-up study. *J Foot Surg.* 1982;21(2):104-107.

32. Pontious J, Brook J, Hillstrom H, Tailor's bunion. Is fixation necessary? *J Am Podiatr Med Assoc.* 1996;86(2):63-73.
33. Martinelli B, Valentini R. Correction of valgus of fifth metatarsal and varus of the fifth toes by percutaneous distal osteotomy. *Foot Ankle Surg.* 2007;13(3):136-139.
34. Giannini S, Faldini C, Vannini F, et al. The minimally invasive osteotomy "S.E.R.I." (Simple, Effective, Rapid, Inexpensive) for correction of bunionette deformity. *Foot Ankle Int.* 2008;29(3): 282-286.
35. Magnan B, Samaila E, Bartolozzi P, et al. Percutaneous distal osteotomy of the fifth metatarsal for correction of bunionette. *J Bone Joint Surg A.* 2011;93(22):2116-2122.
36. De Prado M, Ripoll PL, Golano P. *Minimally Invasive Foot Surgery: Surgical Techniques, Indications, Anatomical Basis.* About Your Health; 2009.
37. Nunes G, Baumfeld T, Nery C, Carvalho P, et al. Percutaneous bunionette correction: retrospective case series. *Foot Ankle Spec.* 2022;15(1):36-42.
38. Lui TH. Percutaneous osteotomy of the fifth metatarsal for symptomatic bunionette. *J Foot Ankle Surg.* 2014;53(6):747-752.
39. Frederick Michels SG, Nikita Stevens GC, Burssens A. Percutaneous bunionette correction: a cadaveric study. *Clin Res Foot Ankle.* 2015;3(2):
40. Ceccarini P, Rinonapoli G, Caraffa A, et al. Bunionette: minimally invasive and percutaneous techniques: a topical review of the literature. *Foot Ankle Spec.* 2017;10(2):157-161.
41. Ferreira GF, dos Santos TF, Oksman D, et al. Percutaneous oblique distal osteotomy of the fifth metatarsal for bunionette correction. *Foot Ankle Int.* 2020;41(7):811-817.
42. Molenaers B, Vanlommel J, Deprez P. Percutaneous hardware free corrective osteotomy for bunionette deformity. *Acta Orthop Belg.* 2017;83(2):284-291.

10 Freiberg Disease

Serrano Mariano De Prado and Manuel Cuervas-Mons

◆ INTRODUCTION

Freiberg disease is an avascular necrosis[1] affecting the second metatarsal head and, much less commonly, the third and fourth metatarsal heads[2] (Figure 10.1). The condition manifests in young adolescents, mainly women, and has a variable clinical course. It was first described by Albert H. Freiberg in 1914[3] and later by Köhler in 1915; hence, it is also known as Köhler second disease.[4]

◆ PATHOGENESIS

The pathogenetic pattern seen in Freiberg disease is identical to that of avascular necrosis of the femoral head. Several theories have been proposed to explain the development of necrosis localized in the metatarsal heads; the two most widely accepted is as follows:

- Vascular theory
- Mechanical theory (microtraumas)

Vascular and mechanical factors are closely related. Given the specific biomechanical characteristics of the foot, mechanical factors seem more likely, as the second metatarsal head is subject to greater mechanical demands during the normal gait cycle, reason why it was first referred to as Freiberg infraction.[3,4] However, trauma itself could not reliably explain all cases.[5]

It is a degenerative process involving the epiphysis that results in osteonecrosis of the subchondral cancellous bone. By improving the biomechanical and vascular environment, the process can be altered in such a way as to restore normal physiology (followed by regeneration or recalcification).[3] If not, the process continues to subchondral collapse and fragmentation of the joint surface.[6]

According to Gauthier,[2,7] the necrosis progresses through five stages:

- Stage 0: subchondral necrosis of the upper portion of the metatarsal head. The cartilage may be intact or slightly fractured.

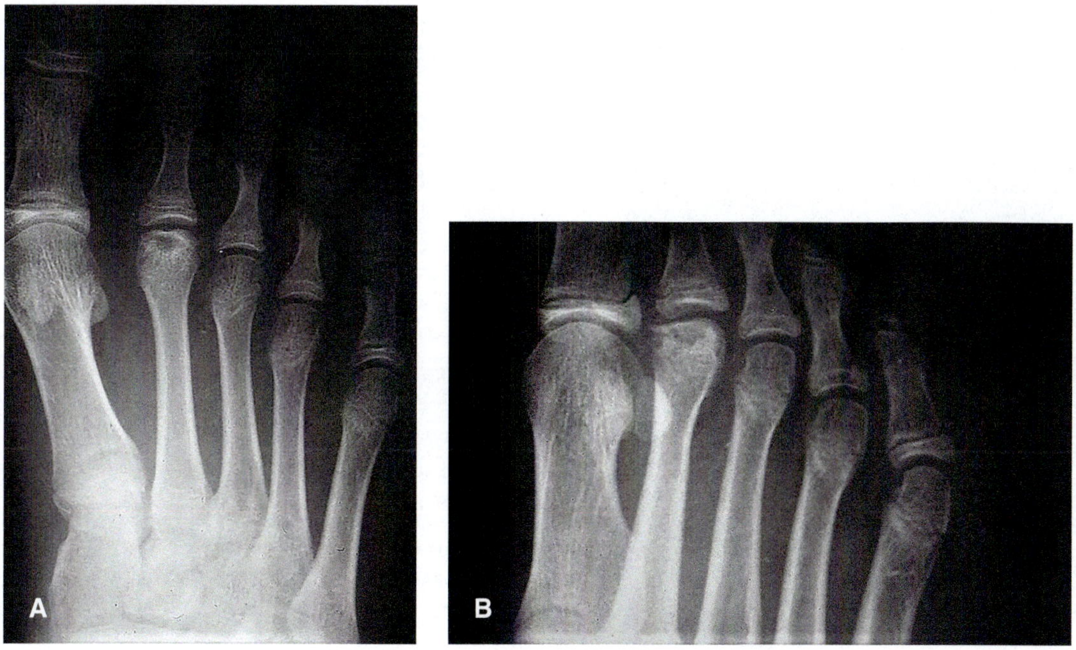

Figure 10.1 A, B. Anteroposterior (AP) and oblique radiographs of Freiberg disease.

- Stage 1: subchondral necrosis progresses to a necrotic osteocartilaginous fragment. The hyaline cartilage remains intact.
- Stage 2: deformation of the necrotic metatarsal head by crushing, accompanied by morphological abnormalities of the metatarsal neck.
- Stage 3: tearing of the cartilage with detachment of the osteocartilaginous sequestrum, leaving the head completely deformed and flat, with a loose intra-articular body.
- Stage 4: sequelae of the deformed head and metatarsophalangeal (MTP) arthrosis.

◆ PATIENT HISTORY AND PHYSICAL EXAMINATION

The individuals most affected range in age from adolescence through the second decade of life.[3]

Patients often present with complaints of activity-related forefoot pain. Walking alone is often enough to trigger pain[3] at the central metatarsal heads, accompanied by claudication that disappears with rest. The patient sometimes may recall a minor trauma, although the onset is more commonly spontaneous with no known cause. Over time, pain becomes more persistent, and dorsal swelling over the injured joint may ultimately develop.

On physical examination, applying dorsoplantar pressure at the painful area easily localizes the affected metatarsal head (Figure 10.2). In early stages of the disease, MTP tenderness may be the only finding.[3]

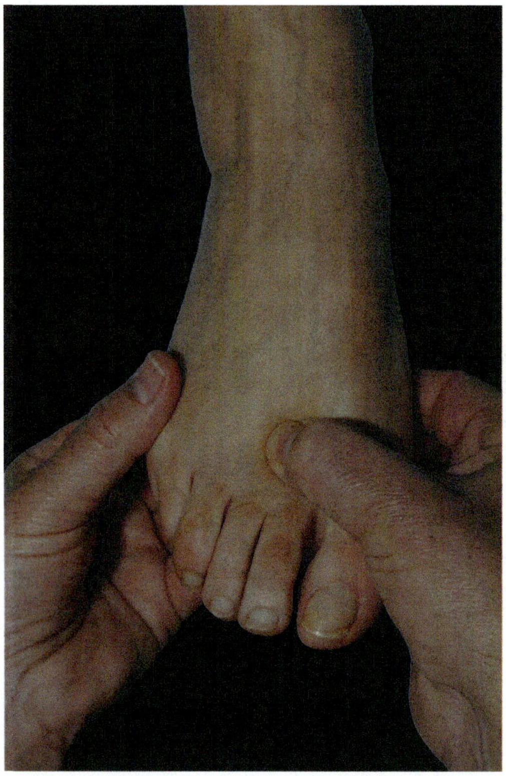

Figure 10.2 Location of the tender spot typical of Freiberg's.

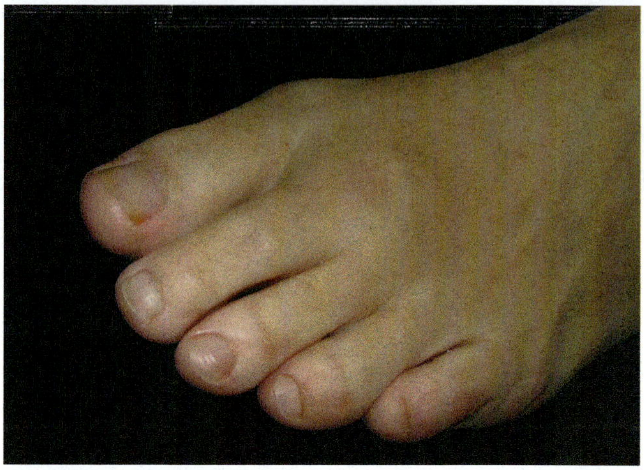

Figure 10.3 Clinical image of a Freiberg case in the final stages with swelling at the dorsal aspect of the second metatarsophalangeal joint.

The subsequent phases are usually seen in middle-aged patients, who have pain at the metatarsal heads, swelling on the dorsal aspect of the forefoot (secondary to exostoses) (Figure 10.3), limited MTP movement, and often hammertoe deformity of the affected toe.

Laboratory Studies

Laboratory studies may be indicated to rule out other etiologies of pain or deformity,[3] such as infectious, rheumatologic, and/or oncologic diseases.

Classification

Several staging schemes have been described. Nevertheless, the classification scheme developed by Smillie in 1967[8] is the most commonly used (Table 10.1).[3]

◆ IMAGING STUDIES

Radiographs

Radiographs provide characteristic images according to the phase of bone necrosis. Weight-bearing anteroposterior (AP), oblique, and lateral radiographs of both feet should be performed. In the first phase, there are no imaging abnormalities, and oblique views may be especially useful for a full appreciation of subtle changes early in the disease[3] (Figures 10.4 and 10.5).

Necrotic areas (osteopenia) gradually appear, alternating with areas of condensation (sclerosis) that progress to osseous sequestrum and joint deformity (like the pattern seen in Perthes disease of the hip) (Figures 10.6 and 10.7).

Nuclear Bone Scans and MRI

When Freiberg disease is suspected clinically despite relatively normal radiographs, nuclear bone scans can help to identify a vascular abnormality at the metatarsal head, although its value as a diagnostic or prognostic tool is still

Table 10.1

Stages of Freiberg Disease

Stage	Findings
I	Fissuring of the epiphysis as earliest sign. Radiographic changes may be so subtle that they are missed with routine radiographs.
II	Later central depression of the articular surface (subchondral cancellous bone is resorbed). The articular cartilage hinges on an intact plantar bridge.
III	Central depression, medial and lateral projections at the margins; the plantar hinge remains intact at its plantar isthmus.
IV	Central portion has sunk below the surface and is free of the plantar hinge (loose body). Fractures of the medial and lateral projections, over the central loose body.
V	Marked flattening and deformity of the metatarsal head with secondary degenerative changes. Central loose body may have been resorbed; metatarsal shaft becomes thickened and dense.

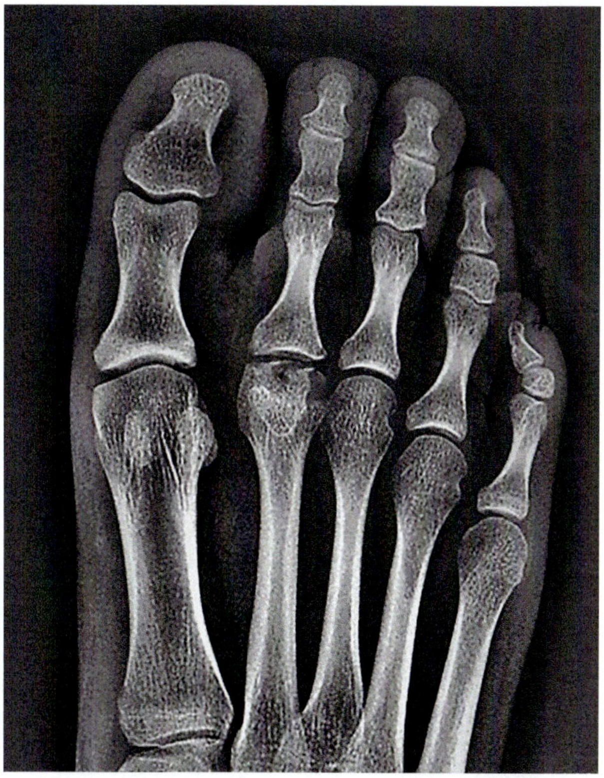

Figure 10.5 Stage 2 radiograph shows rarefaction of the second metatarsal head without subsidence.

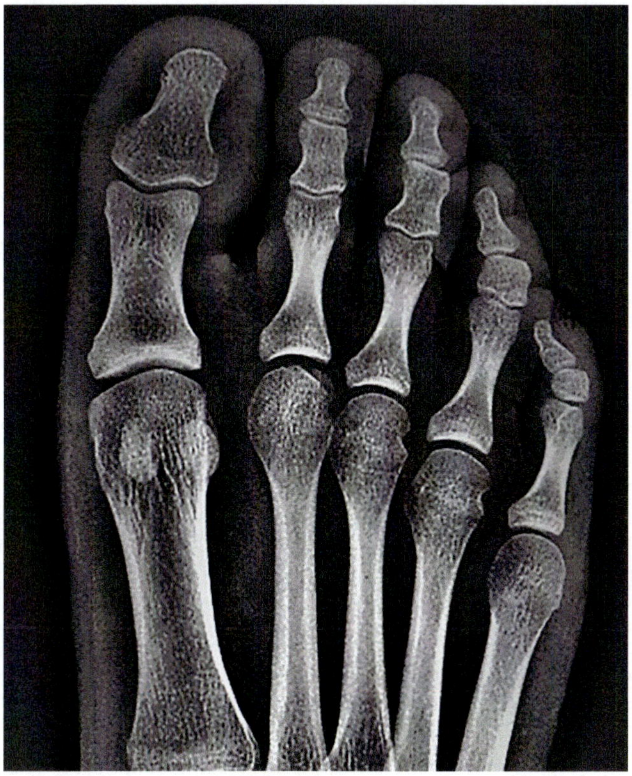

Figure 10.4 Stage 1 radiograph showing very mild flattening of the second metatarsal head as well as a line of increased bone density.

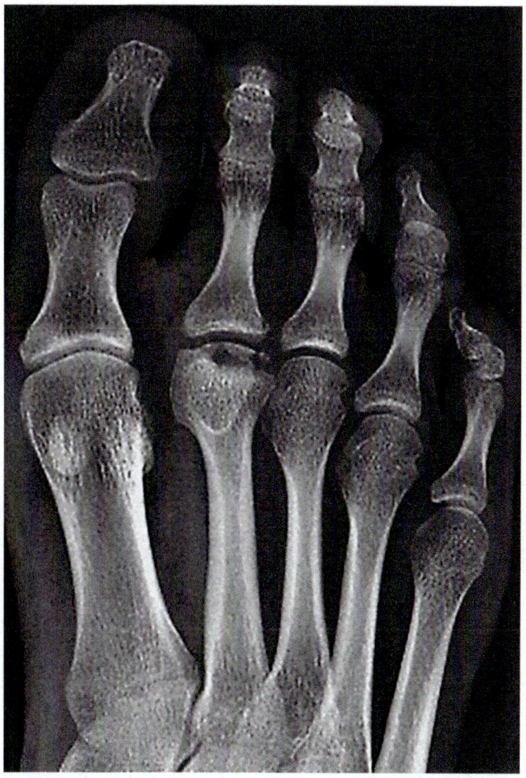

Figure 10.6 Stage 3 radiograph demonstrating subsidence and fragmentation of the second metatarsal head with bone sequestrations.

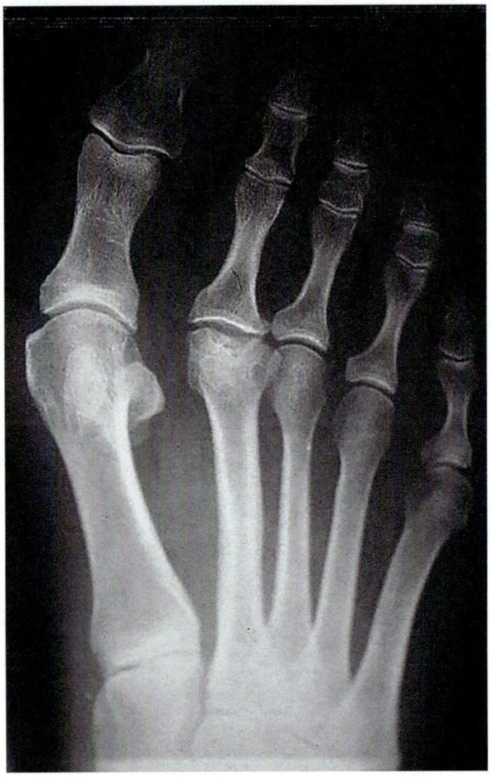

Figure 10.7 Stage 4 radiograph shows sequelae of the disease with deformity and enlargement of the metatarsal head.

debated.[9] MRI may also prove useful in the early diagnostic stages[10] (Figure 10.8).

In the sequel phase, the metatarsal head is flattened and shows multiple osteophytes that may even occupy the base of the corresponding phalanx, which is widened to adapt the size of the head (Figure 10.9).

◆ PREOPERATIVE PLANNING AND PREPARATION

Approach

Although Freiberg disease was originally described more than a century ago, the most appropriate treatment remains controversial.[3] A trial of conservative treatment can be implemented for most patients. Whereas some stage I-III lesions may resolve spontaneously, patients who do not respond to conservative measures may require surgery, as may patients with stage IV-V lesions.

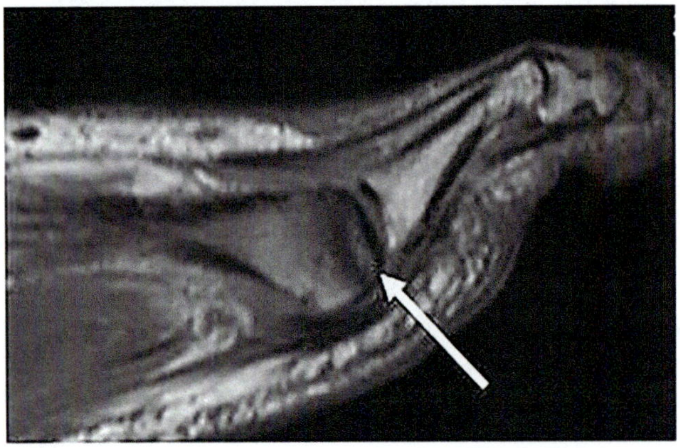

Figure 10.8 MRI showing a case of early stage Freiberg's.

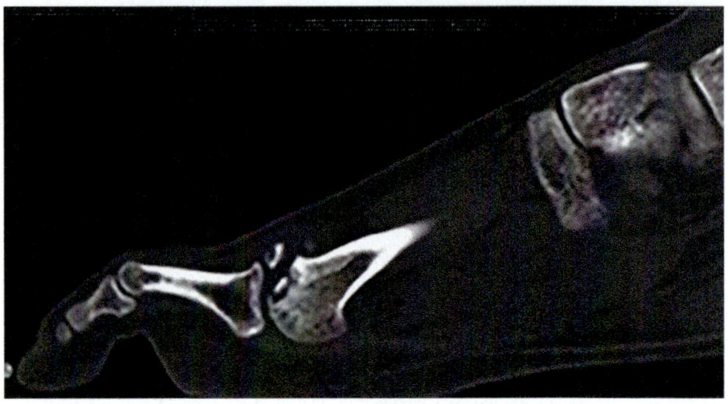

Figure 10.9 CT scan of an advanced case with deformity and dorsal bone sequestration.

Many patients with pain, functional compromise, and abnormal radiographic studies in the initial phases experience gradual, spontaneous recovery of the joint surface. In light of this, prudence is advised when deciding whether or not to operate, although a prompt intervention to optimize the biomechanical environment may prevent further damage to the metatarsal and yield better clinical outcomes.

Medical Treatment

A period of appropriate nonoperative conservative management is indicated for all patients.[3] The goal of the therapy is to rest the joint to allow inflammation and mechanical irritation to resolve.[8]

Medical treatment consists of the following:

- Metatarsal bar-pad to off-load the affected metatarsal head
- Shock-absorbing shoes, with a rigid outer sole
- Oral nonsteroidal anti-inflammatories

Intra-articular corticosteroid injections are contraindicated.

Although good long-term results are reported with medical treatment, many patients complain of limited range of motion.[11]

Surgical Treatment

If medical treatment has proven unsuccessful, surgical treatment may become indicated. Two scenarios are possible:

- Early stage (I-III)
  - Given that the dorsal half of the metatarsal head is typically affected by the condition, treatment entails performing a dorsal closing wedge osteotomy of the metatarsal[12] (Figures 10.10 through 10.12). The procedure aims at reducing the load on the metatarsal head and achieves a functional articular surface by dorsalizing the healthy plantar cartilage.
- Sequelae stage (IV-V)
  - It may be necessary to perform removal of osteophytes and loose bodies, osteotomy of the metatarsal, and treatment of the associated toe deformity (Figures 10.13 through 10.16). Resection of the metatarsal head and base of the proximal phalanx is contraindicated.

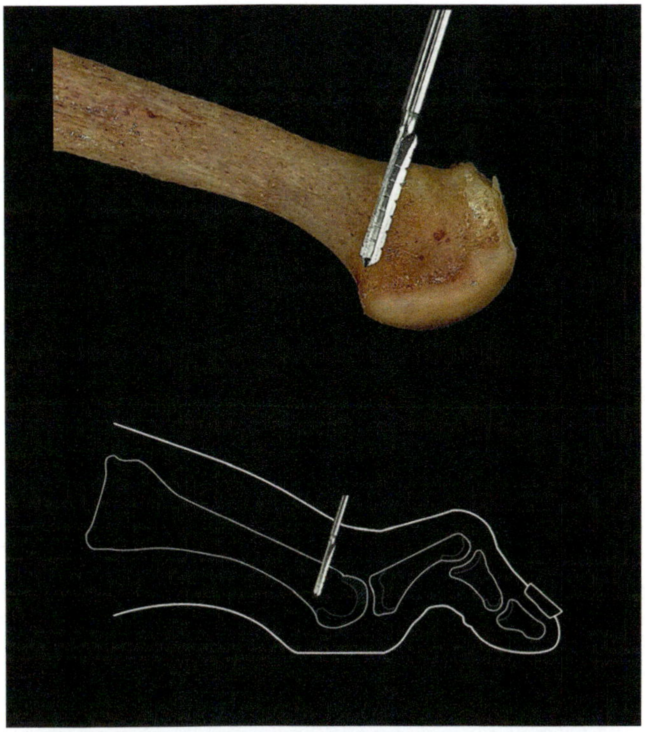

Figure 10.10 Anatomical image and diagram of the location of the distal metatarsal dorsiflexion osteotomy.

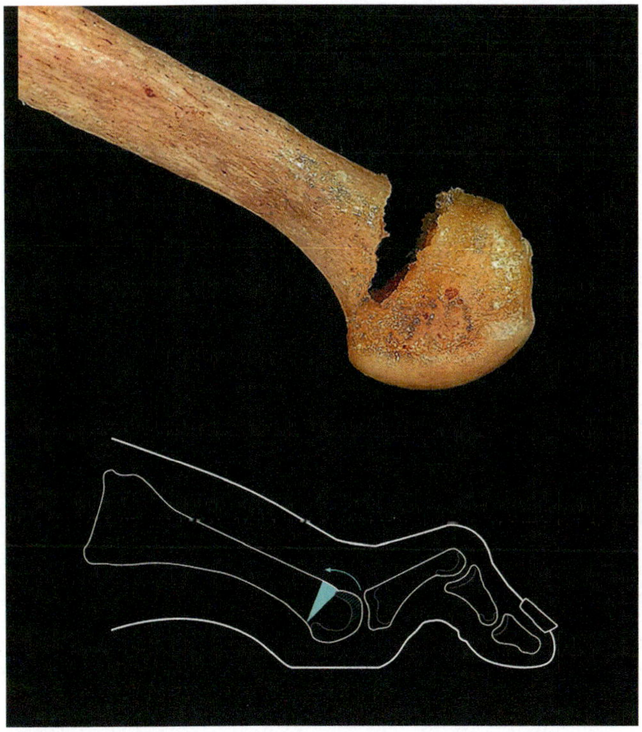

Figure 10.11 Illustration of the dorsiflexion osteotomy and the corrective wedge.

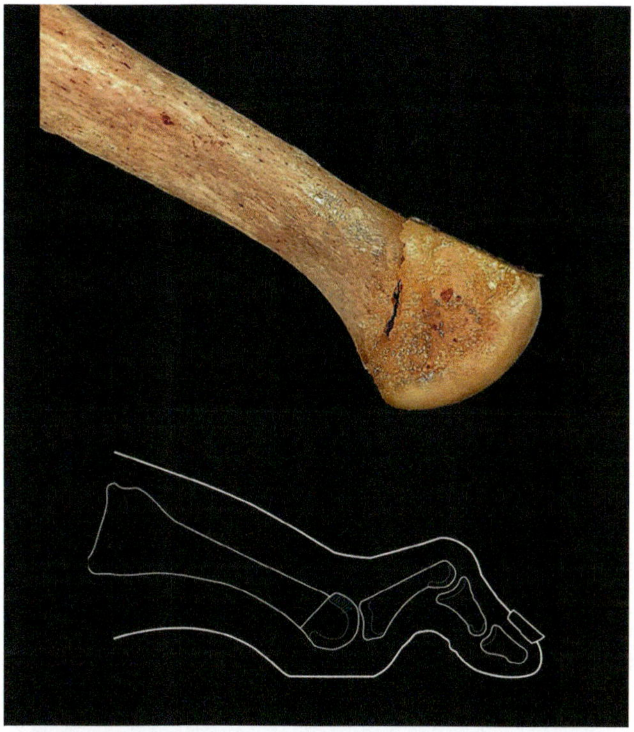

Figure 10.12 Reduction of the dorsiflexion osteotomy with dorsal translation of the articular cartilage.

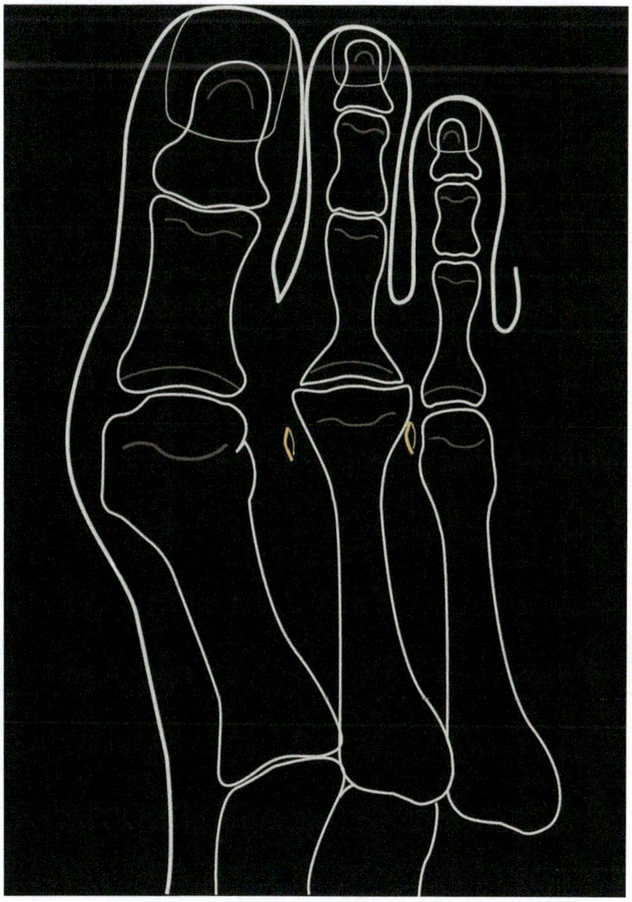

Figure 10.13 Approaches for percutaneous remodeling of the deformed metatarsal head in an advanced Freiberg patient.

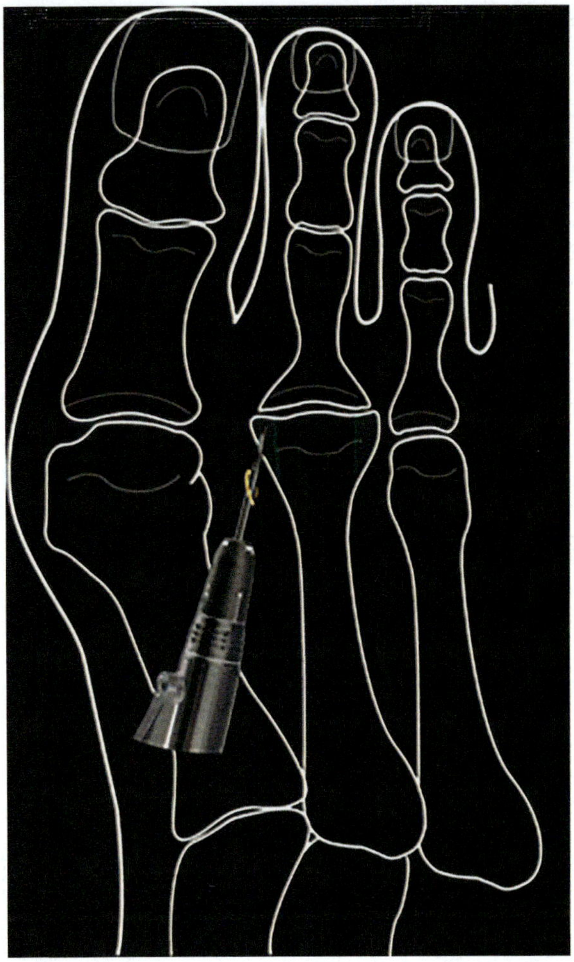

Figure 10.14 Approaches for percutaneous remodeling of the deformed metatarsal head in an advanced Freiberg patient.

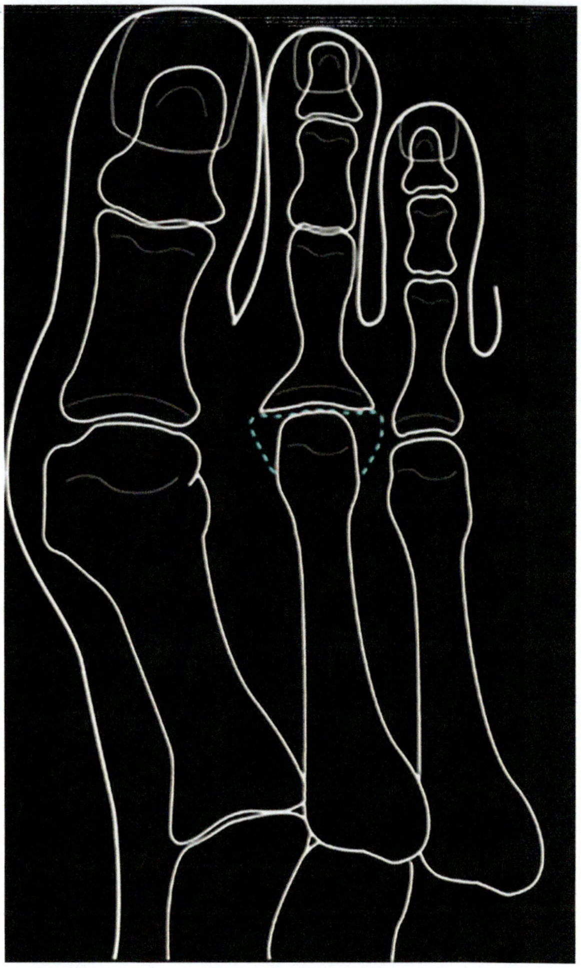

Figure 10.15 Diagram of the remodeling of the metatarsal head in advanced Freiberg's.

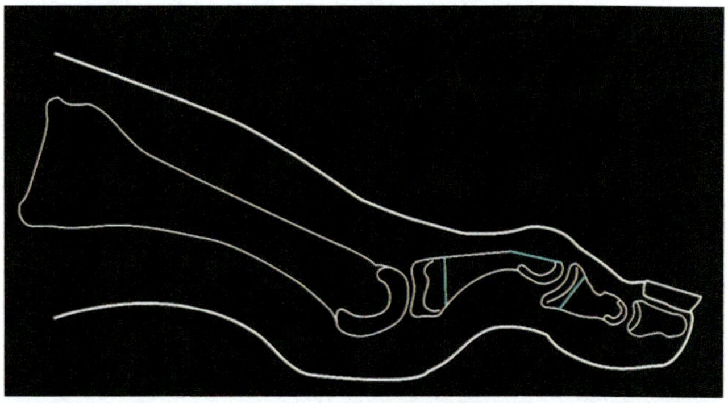

Figure 10.16 Surgical procedures for the correction of concomitant hammertoe correction.

SURGICAL TECHNIQUE

Planning

Instruments

The surgical tools required are those used for percutaneous forefoot procedures:

- Complete general instrument set: elevators, rasp (large and small)
- Beaver blade
- Straight burr 2 × 15 mm, wedge burr 3 × 15 mm, and burr sheath
- Low-speed and high torque drill
- Fluoroscopy

Percutaneous surgery should never be carried out with instruments adapted from conventional surgery as major complications can occur.

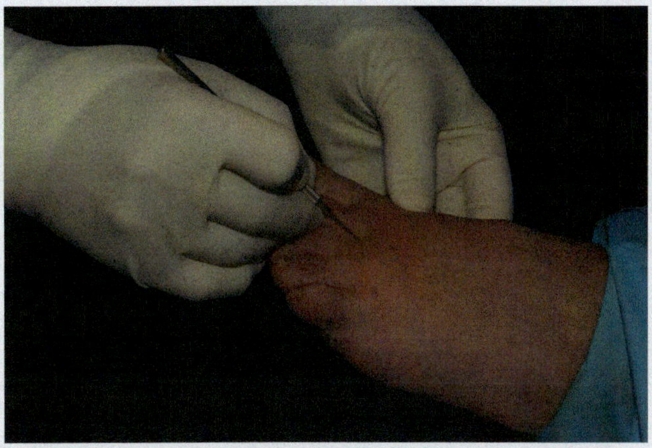

Figure 10.17 Surgical approach for the metatarsal dorsiflexion osteotomy.

Patient Preparation

The patient's foot is scrubbed using disinfectant soap and prepared with antiseptic solution.

Regional anesthesia (ankle block or metatarsal block) is performed, and the patient is placed in the supine position with the foot extending beyond the end of the table.

Lower limb exsanguination and application of a tourniquet to obtain a blood-free working area is never recommended as the cooling effect of bleeding on the burr reduces the risk of thermal injury.

Dorsiflexion Osteotomy[13]

A 5-mm longitudinal incision is made with a Beaver blade in the intermetatarsal space immediately proximal the dorsal interdigital fold (Figure 10.17). Care should be taken to avoid the venous network at this level, which is usually visible owing to vasodilation secondary to the ankle block. The incision is made parallel to the extensor tendon and the neurovascular structures, and the scalpel is advanced until it reaches the dorsal aspect of the second metatarsal neck. A small rasp is then inserted and slid along the lateral or medial cortex of the metatarsal, and the periosteum is elevated over a small area. The absence of soft tissue between the bone and the rasp is verified by scraping the instrument's teeth on the bone. Fluoroscopy is used to confirm the correct osteotomy site on the metatarsal neck (Figures 10.18 and 10.19).

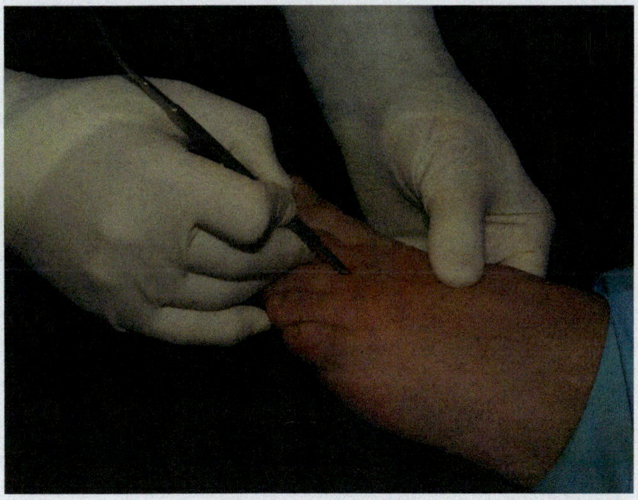

Figure 10.18 Periosteal elevation at the metatarsal neck prior to performing the dorsiflexion osteotomy.

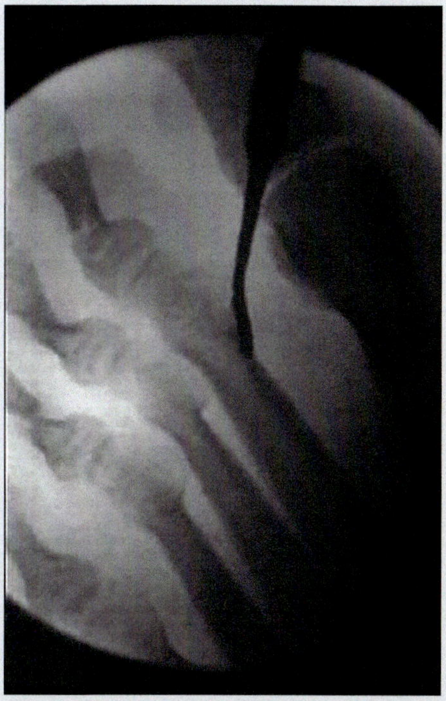

Figure 10.19 Fluoroscopic check of the osteotomy start point.

The straight burr 2 × 15 is then inserted, and the osteotomy is begun perpendicular to the axis of the metatarsal bone. The burr is then withdrawn a few millimeters to spare the plantar surface of the metatarsal (Figure 10.20). The

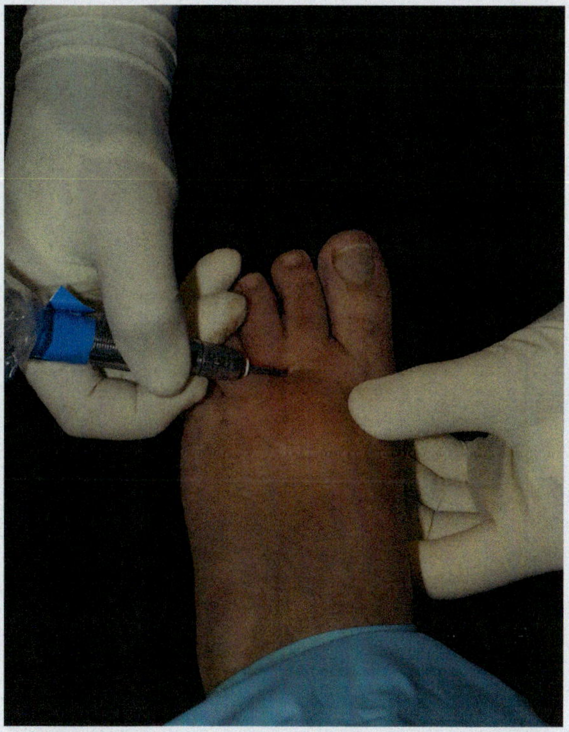

Figure 10.20 Surgical image of the percutaneous osteotomy.

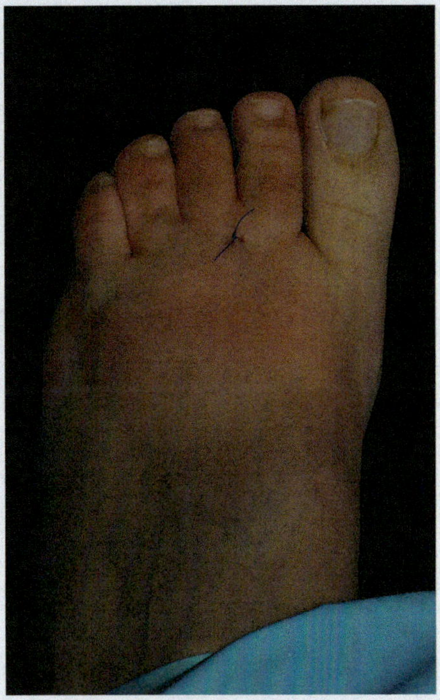

Figure 10.21 Closure and appearance of the foot after percutaneous dorsiflexion osteotomy.

procedure continues toward the medial cortex and finally to the dorsal cortex. Throughout the procedure, care needs to be taken to avoid violating the plantar cortex of the metatarsal. The burr is then positioned at the proximal edge of the osteotomy to remove a wedge. Then, pressure is applied dorsally to the metatarsal head (with counter pressure at the diaphysis), allowing to close the wedge by osteoclasia and allowing to dorsally rotate the head. By doing so, the healthy plantar cartilage will now be articulating with the proximal phalanx.

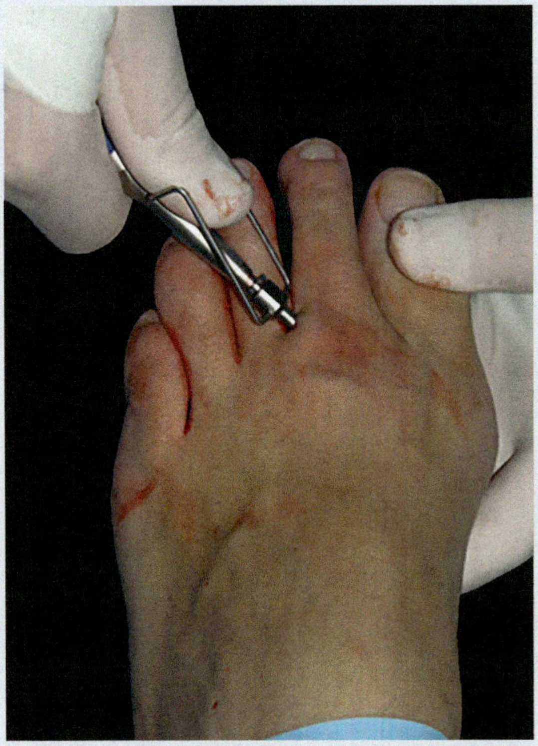

Figure 10.22 Surgical image of the metatarsal head exostectomy.

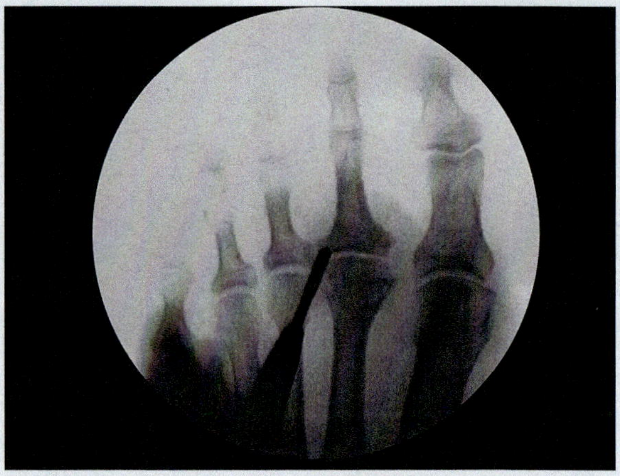

Figure 10.23 Fluoroscopic image during an metatarsal head exostectomy.

Throughout the surgical procedure, the forefoot is held with the other hand (the one not holding the burr), using the thumb to exert a plantarflexion force on the second metatarsal head and placing the other fingers on the plantar surface of metatarsal shaft.

The incisions are closed with a 4-0 monofilament suture, and the forefoot is dressed in a metatarsal strap using a self-adhesive bandage (Figure 10.21).

Exostectomy[13]

The exostosis is usually localized at the dorsal edge of the bone where the cartilage begins. A 0.5-cm incision is made in the second intermetatarsal space at the second metatarsal neck, and the Beaver blade is advanced to the depth of the capsule. As much of the capsule and periosteum as possible is dissected, and a small- or medium-sized rasp is inserted to completely expose the bone spur thus creating a safe working pocket.

The 3-mm wedge burr is advanced into the wound, and the exostectomy is started (Figures 10.22 through 10.24). The motor speed should not exceed 8,000 rpm, and burring

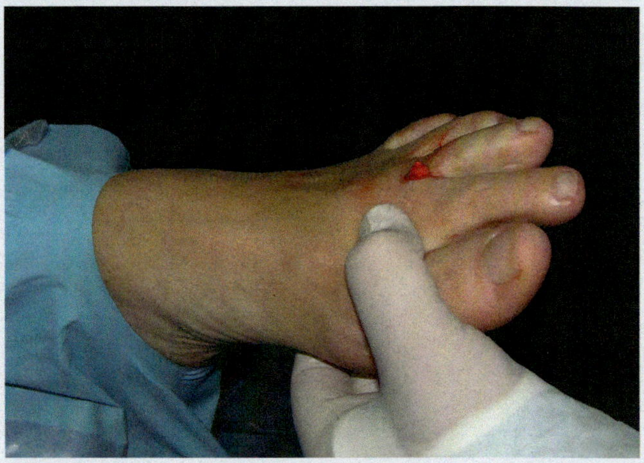

Figure 10.24 Surgical image of the extraction of the debris following exostectomy of the metatarsal head.

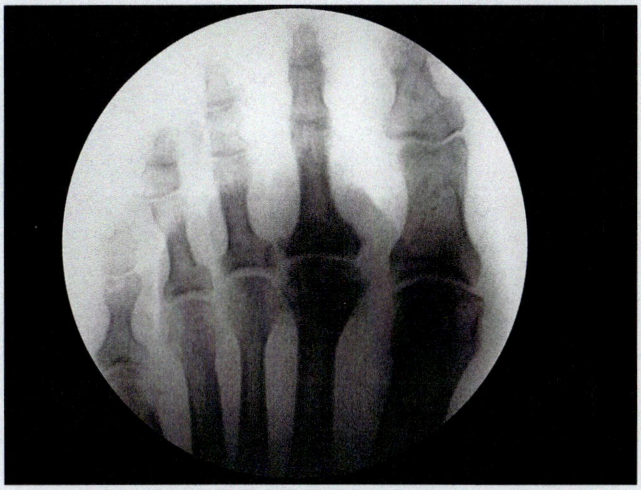

Figure 10.25 Preoperative fluoroscopic image of the metatarsal head deformity.

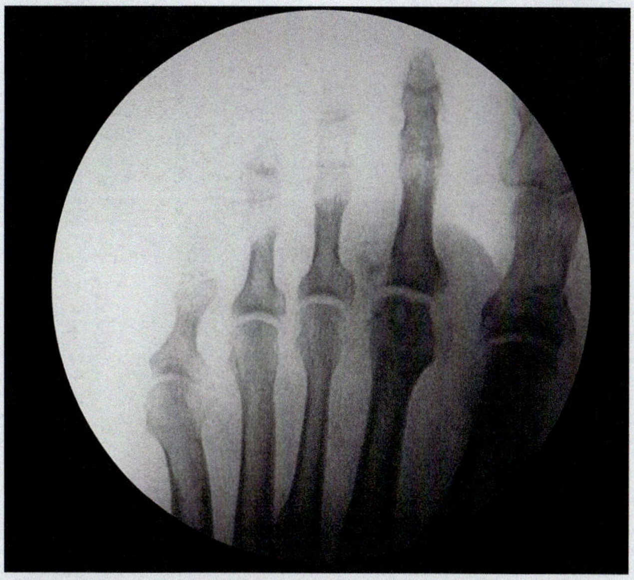

Figure 10.26 Postoperative fluoroscopic image following metatarsal head exostectomy and osteotomy.

should be stopped intermittently for short periods to prevent thermal injury and to flush/débride the wound. This can be performed with the aid of rasps. Once the dorsal exostosis has been completely removed, the surgeon should determine whether a medial/lateral exostectomy of the head is needed. If the decision is to proceed, a new dorsal incision will be necessary via the first or second intermetatarsal space. From this point, the medial/lateral exostectomy can be performed following the same burring and débridement technique described above (Figures 10.25 and 10.26).

After completion of the exostectomy in patients with associated metatarsalgia, the surgeon can proceed with an oblique osteotomy of the metatarsal neck. Likewise, hammertoe correction may also be necessary.

Distal Metatarsal Osteotomy[14]

A 0.5-cm longitudinal incision is made using a Beaver blade at the intermetatarsal space immediately proximal to the dorsal interdigital fold, parallel to the extensor tendon. The blade is advanced at a 45° angle until it reaches the dorsal aspect of the metatarsal neck. A small rasp is then inserted and slid along the lateral or medial cortex of the metatarsal, and the periosteum is elevated accordingly, avoiding excessive stripping beyond the osteotomy area. The absence of soft tissue between the bone and the rasp is verified by scraping the instrument's teeth on the bone. Fluoroscopy is used to confirm the correct location of the osteotomy site on the metatarsal neck. The burr should be oriented at 45° relative to the long axis of the metatarsal, aiming from dorsal distal to proximal plantar. The osteotomy is started at the dorsal cortex where the cartilage of the metatarsal head begins. The straight 2 × 15 burr is introduced into the working pocket, and the burr is activated to start making the osteotomy.

Once the cut has been made, the orientation of the osteotomy cannot be modified without risking breaking the burr. Thus, it is recommended to "twist" the burr rather than shifting it laterally, using the skin incision as a pivot point. The lateral cortex is cut first, followed by the plantar cortex, then medial, and finally the dorsal cortex. During the procedure, the forefoot is held with the nondominant hand, and once the osteotomy is completed, the surgeon will gently push the metatarsal head dorsally. To confirm completion of the osteotomy, the toe associated with the osteotomized metatarsal is pulled in traction under fluoroscopy, demonstrating gapping at the osteotomy site.

◆ POSTOPERATIVE MANAGEMENT

Sterile gauzes are applied over the foot. Crossover taping is then applied in the same direction as the osteotomy in order to reinforce the solidity of the bandage, which, as has already been indicated, is left in slight overcorrection.

The forefoot is then dressed in gauze tube that is held in place with sticking plaster in order to avoid loosening of the bandages. A postoperative shoe is fitted, and weight bearing is allowed immediately.

The first follow-up visit is performed at postoperative day 8. The bandages and the sutures are removed, and a much lighter bandage, which the patient can change daily, is then applied. This consists of a metatarsal strap with a self-adhesive elastic bandage (ie, Coban or similar).

This bandage should be kept in place 24 hours a day for 3 to 4 weeks after the operation. This bandage can be removed during the night.

OUTCOMES

CASE 1

A 22-year-old female patient presented with a 6-month history of forefoot pain at the level of the second metatarsal head. She denied any history of trauma. She noticed worsening of the pain with weight-bearing activities and when using high heels (Figure 10.27).

The initial radiographs appeared to be normal as per her primary care doctor and were ultimately diagnosed with forefoot "overload" (Figure 10.28). She was recommended nonsteroidal anti-inflammatory drugs and rest.

Due to the persistence of the symptoms, she consulted with the authors' foot and ankle unit where an MRI was ordered (Figure 10.29), revealing early-stage Freiberg disease. She was therefore recommended surgery consisting of a dorsiflexion osteotomy of the second metatarsal neck (Figure 10.30). One year postoperatively, the patient reported complete pain relief.

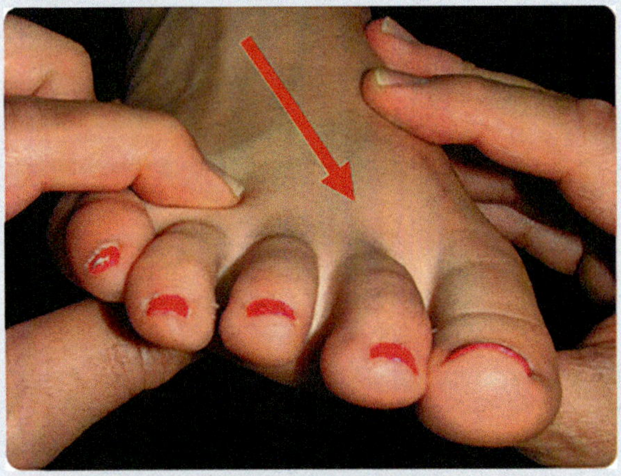

Figure 10.27 Physical examination.

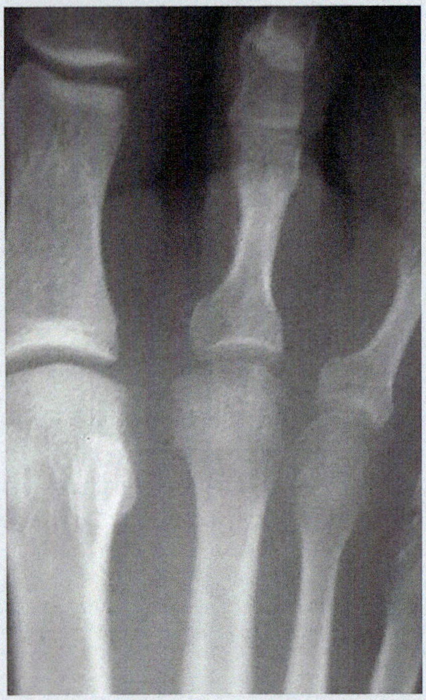

Figure 10.28 Preoperative radiograph of the metatarsal head deformity.

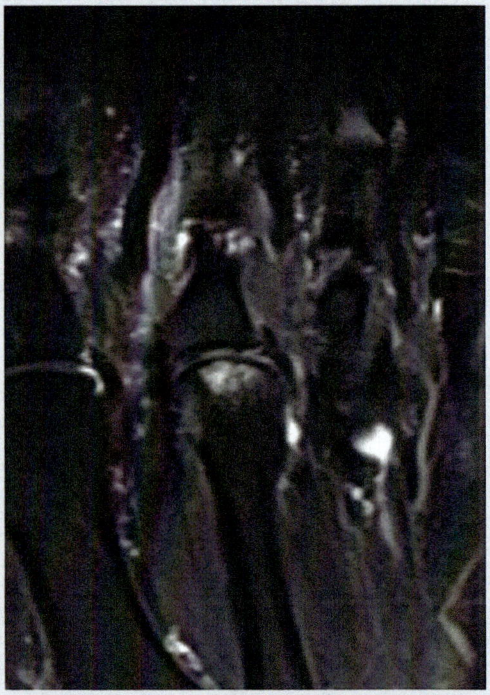

Figure 10.29 Preoperative MRI of the metatarsal head deformity.

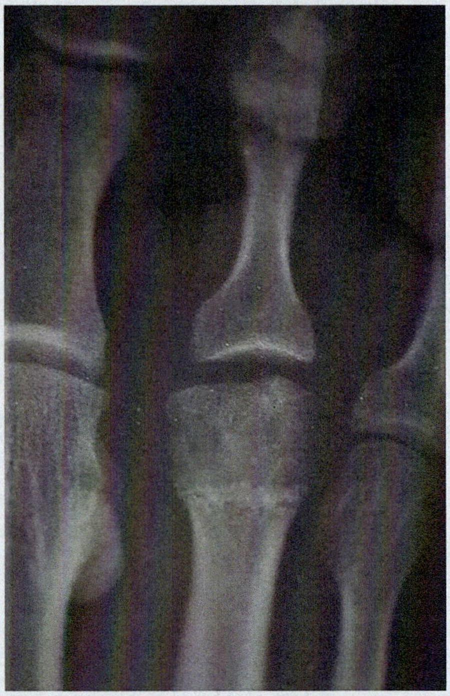

Figure 10.30 Postoperative radiograph of the metatarsal head deformity.

CASE 2

A 53-year-old female presented to the authors' foot and ankle clinic complaining of pain, functional disability, and swelling at the second metatarsophalangeal joint that had developed over several years (Figure 10.31). Radiographs revealed typical features of advanced Freiberg disease, with osteophytes at the metatarsal head and base of the proximal phalanx, flattening of the articular surface, narrowing of the joint space, stiff range of motion, and metatarsalgia with plantar callosity (Figure 10.32). The patient underwent exostectomy to remodel the second metatarsal head as well as a second metatarsal osteotomy. At 1 year postoperatively, the patient reported significant pain relief with no radiographic signs of disease progression (Figure 10.33).

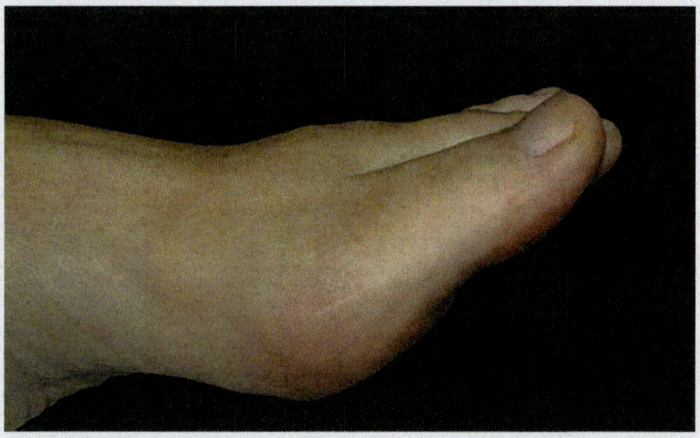

Figure 10.31 Physical examination.

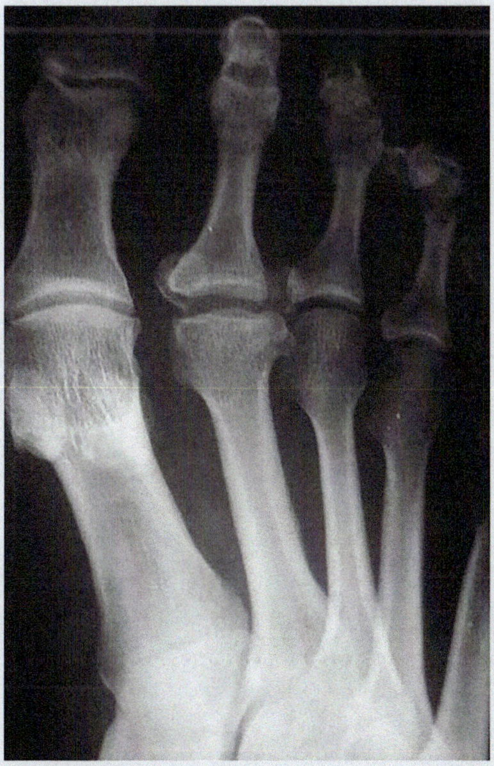

Figure 10.32 Preoperative MRI of the metatarsal head deformity.

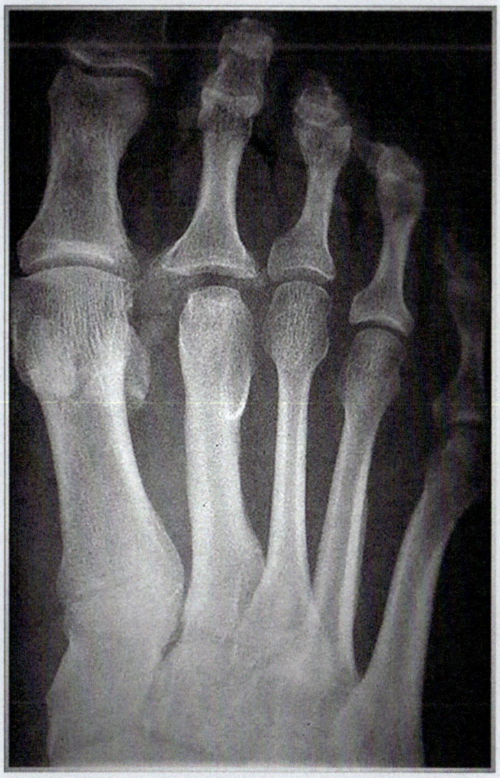

Figure 10.33 Postoperative radiograph of the metatarsal head deformity.

References

1. Wax A, Leland R. Freiberg disease and avascular necrosis of the metatarsal heads. *Foot Ankle Clin.* 2019;24(1):69-82.
2. Gauthier G, Elbaz R. Freiberg's infraction: a subchondral bone fatigue fracture. *Clin Orthop.* 1979;142:93.
3. Fehr DS, Walter KD. *Freiberg Disease (Infraction) [Internet].* Medscape; 2015. Accessed April 13, 2021. http://emedicine.medscape.com/article/1236085-overview
4. Smillie IS. Friedberg's infraction (Köhler's second diseases). *J Bone Joint Surg (Br).* 1957;39:580.
5. Friedberg AH. The so-called infraction of the second metatarsal bone. *J Bone Joint Surg (Am).* 1926;8:257.
6. Murphy GA. Lesser toe abnormalities. In: Azar FM, Beaty JH, eds. *Campbell's Operative Orthopaedics.* Vol. 4. 14th ed. Elsevier; 2021:4227-4283.
7. Gauthier G. Maladie de Freidberg ou 2e maladie de Koler. Proposition d´un traitement de reconstruction au stade évolué de l´affection. 48e Réunion annuelle de la SOFCOT. *Rev Chir Orthop.* 1974;60(II):337-342.
8. DiGiovanni CW, Patel A, Calfee R, Nickisch F. Osteonecrosis in the foot. *J Am Acad Orthop Surg.* 2007;15(4):208-217.
9. Mandell GA, Harcke HT. Scintigraphic manifestations of infraction of the second metatarsal (Freiberg's disease). *J Nucl Med.* 1987;28(2):249-251.
10. Mifune Y, Matsumoto T, Mizuno T, Ikuta S, Kurosaka M, Kuroda R. Idiopathic osteonecrosis of the second metatarsal head. *Clin Imaging.* 2007;31(6):431-433.
11. Hoskinson J. Freiberg's disease: a review of the long-term results. *Proc R Soc Med.* 1974;67(2):106-107.
12. Kinnard P, Lirette R. Dorsiflexion osteotomy in Friedberg's disease. *Foot Ankle.* 1989;9:226-231.
13. De Prado M. Freiberg disease. In: De Prado M, Ripoll PL, Golanó P, eds. *Minimally Invasive Foot Surgery.* 1st ed. AYH; 2009:209-217.
14. De Prado M, Cuervas-Mons M, Golanó P, Vaquero J. Distal metatarsal minimal invasive osteotomy (DMMO) for the treatment of metatarsalgia. *Tech Foot Ankle Surg.* 2016;15(1):12-18.

11 Percutaneous Distal Metatarsal Osteotomy for Morton Neuroma

Alirio J. deMeireles and Ettore Vulcano

◆ INTRODUCTION

Morton neuroma is a compression neuropathy of an interdigital nerve, entrapped by the deep transverse intermetatarsal ligament at roughly the level of the metatarsal heads. The disease frequently affects the third web space and is most commonly found in middle-aged females, where it presents as pain at the plantar surface of the affected web space and is worse with weight bearing or palpation.[1-4]

Initially, Morton neuroma is treated conservatively with a combination of wide toe box shoes, orthoses, and/or nonsteroidal anti-inflammatory drugs, although these methods are rarely curative. Efficacy and longevity of these noninvasive methods are varied—with temporary improvement of symptoms in 28% to 80% of patients.[5-8] Corticosteroid injections are also utilized as a nonoperative treatment option though the authors do not frequently recommend these to the patients due to concern regarding inconvenient side effects such as fat pad atrophy, skin necrosis, long-lasting injection site pain, ligament tear, etc.

◆ SURGICAL TREATMENTS

If symptoms persist after exhaustion of nonoperative modalities, more invasive methods, including chemical neurolysis and the surgical neurectomy, are considered.[9,10] While satisfactory results have been reported, both of these approaches have demonstrated several limitations. Current literature regarding percutaneous chemical neurolysis has demonstrated a wide range of efficacy, with complete resolution of symptoms in 21% to 84% of cases.[7,11,12] In contrast, neurectomy successfully treats the symptoms in 70% to 90% of cases but has a higher complication rate as compared to the relatively low morbidity of neurolysis.[13-15] The most common complications of neurectomy include impaired wound healing, sensory deficits, and traumatic amputation of the neuroma.[10] Thus, given the varied efficacy of chemical neurolysis and the potential morbidity of neurectomy, the development of an effective, minimally invasive procedure to treat Morton neuroma with an equal or lower complication rate would be clinically impactful.

Distal Metatarsal Osteotomy

de Prado et al. described a percutaneous distal metatarsal extra-articular osteotomy of lesser metatarsals (DMMO) for the treatment of Morton neuroma.[16,17] The premise of this technique is to spare the nerve by dorsalizing and shortening the third and fourth metatarsal heads.[16,17] The authors have developed a modification of the de Prado technique, which relies on release of the deep transverse intermetatarsal ligament coupled with a DMMO of the fourth metatarsal, leading to widening of the third web space with decompression of the interdigital nerve.

The objective of this chapter is to describe the basic indications, recommended workup, and in-depth surgical technique for the novel operative intervention for the treatment of Morton neuroma.

◆ INDICATIONS AND CONTRAINDICATIONS

Any patient with a diagnosis of a third web space neuroma who has failed 3 months of nonoperative treatment is a candidate for the procedure. Nonoperative treatments consist of metatarsal pads and wide toe box shoes as described in the Introduction section. Injections of any sort, with the exception of diagnostic lidocaine injections, are not recommended by the authors as they are unlikely to treat the condition and might have inconvenient side effects such as fat pad atrophy, skin necrosis, long-lasting injection site pain, ligament tear, etc.

Contraindications include stump neuromas resulting from a previous neurectomy, active forefoot infections, neuropathy, chronic regional pain syndrome, and recent injections (<3 months) in the affected area.

◆ PATIENT HISTORY AND PHYSICAL EXAMINATION

Patients typically complain of electrical or stabbing pain at the affected web space, often radiating to the third to fourth toes. Pain is usually worse when wearing tighter shoes but is relieved by walking bare foot or in wide toe box shoes. On clinical examination, patients will frequently complain of tenderness to palpation in the third web space but will have little or no pain at the third or fourth metatarsal heads. A Mulder click might be present on physical examination. A diagnostic lidocaine injection in the third web space will eliminate the pain. Partial or no response to the injection likely suggests a different etiology of the metatarsalgia.

◆ IMAGING STUDIES

Ultrasonography or magnetic resonance imaging (MRI) is recommended when there is a high clinical suspicion for a neuroma. The studies will often times identify an enlargement of the interdigital nerve greater than 10 mm. In the senior author's opinion, "neuromas" smaller than 10 mm are unlikely to be responsible for pain.

◆ PREOPERATIVE PLANNING AND PREPARATION

Weight-bearing three-view foot radiographs are obtained for all patients. The osteotomy is planned at the level of the fourth metatarsal neck. The osteotomy should be extracapsular and at the level of the intermetatarsal ligament.

Room Setup

The authors routinely place the patient supine with the surgical foot at or over the edge of the table. The contralateral leg is frog-legged to avoid interference with the mini C-arm and/or the operator. The power box and the scrub technician are always at the left side of the patient, whereas the mini C-arm is always at the right side of the patient, regardless of surgical site laterality. The power box should be set at 6,000 rpm. The use of a tourniquet is highly discouraged as the intraosseous bleeding may help cool down the burr during the procedure, thus reducing the risk of heat necrosis.

Saline irrigation of the burr throughout the procedure is also crucial to reduce the risk of thermal injury to the soft tissues. This may be in the form of automated irrigation systems provided by several manufacturers distributing minimally invasive surgery instrumentation or manually by the surgical assistant with the use of a bulb syringe.

SURGICAL TECHNIQUE

If right handed, the surgeon will stand at the end of the bed when operating on a right foot, or at the left side of the bed if operating on the left foot. The first step is to release the intermetatarsal ligament. In order to minimize devascularization of the osteotomized fourth metatarsal head, the authors prefer to release the ligament from the third metatarsal neck.

A Beaver blade is used to make a stab incision at the dorsolateral aspect of the third metatarsal neck. Once in the deep tissues, the blade should be placed parallel to the bone with the cutting edge facing dorsal (Figure 11.1). The blade is gently rotated toward the dorsum of the foot while staying as close as possible to bone. The intermetatarsal ligament is released (Figure 11.2).

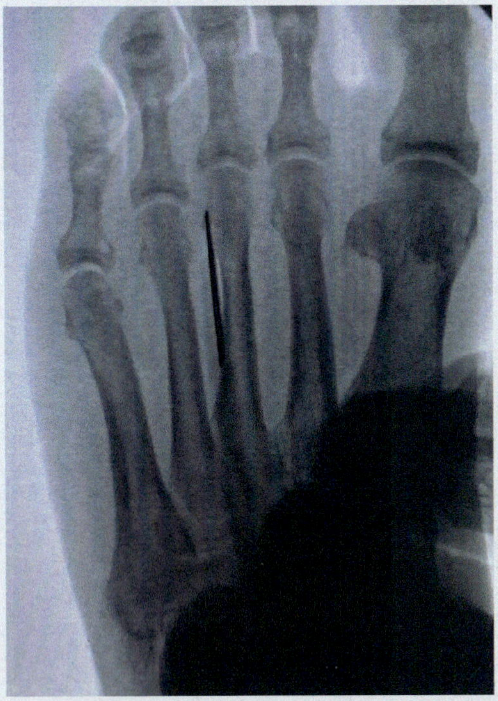

Figure 11.1 Insert the scalpel with the blade facing the toes, in line with the third metatarsal and making sure to stay as close as possible to the lateral cortex.

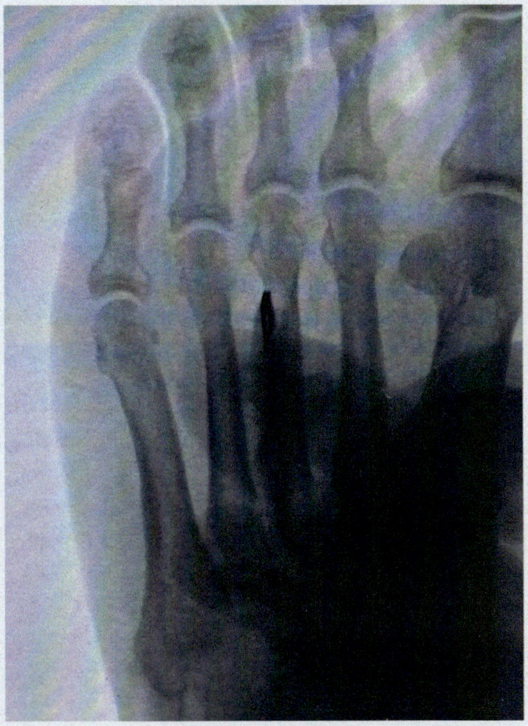

Figure 11.2 Rotate the blade 90° to release the intermetatarsal ligament from the third metatarsal.

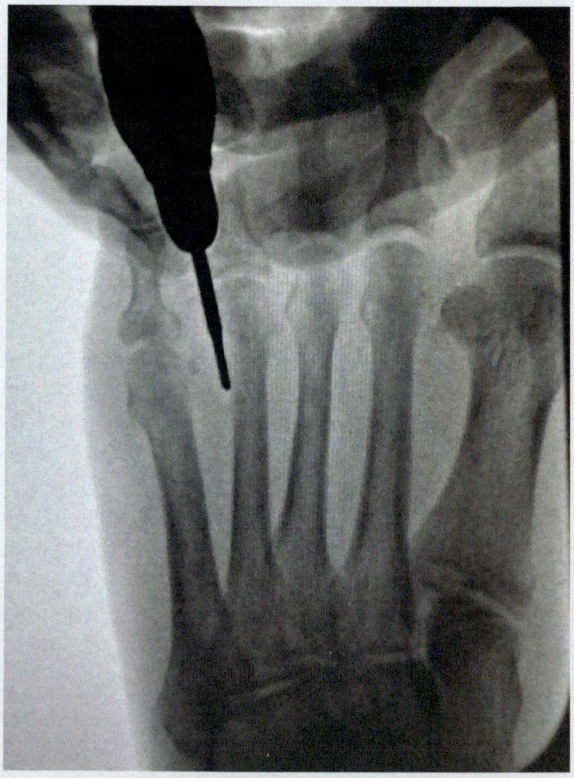

Figure 11.3 Insert the 3 × 12 mm cutting burr at the fourth metatarsal neck (if right handed, the burr will be at the medial cortex [if a right foot] or at the lateral cortex [if a left foot]).

Next, a stab incision is made at the dorsomedial aspect of the fourth metatarsal neck. A periosteal elevator, bone rasp, or a nonactivated cutting burr can be used to elevate the soft tissues from the medial cortex of the metatarsal. A 2 × 12 mm Shannon or cutting burr is advanced in to the wound, angled at 45° to the dorsum of the foot (Figures 11.3 and 11.4). The burr is activated at full speed, and the medial cortex is scored to mark the osteotomy.

Next, the burr is rotated to make the osteotomy. As the burr is advanced more laterally and dorsally, the orientation of the surgeon's hand will change so as for the burr to end at 90° with respect to the longitudinal axis of the metatarsal shaft (Figure 11.5). To confirm the completion of the osteotomy, the surgeon with pull traction on the fourth toe under live fluoroscopy. The metatarsal head should appear to be fully mobile (Figure 11.6).

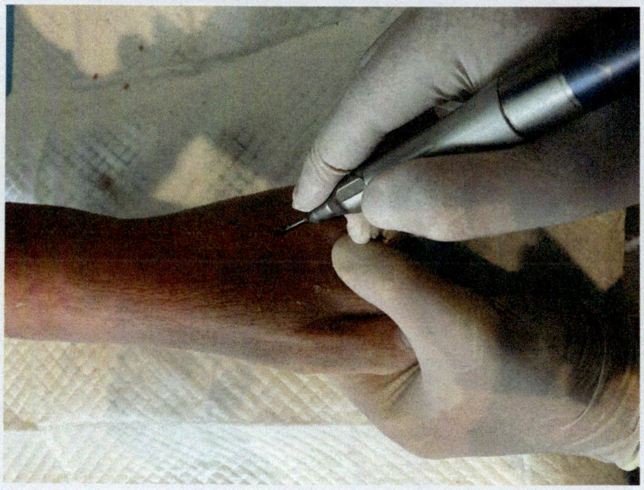

Figure 11.4 The orientation of the burr needs to be at 45° to the foot.

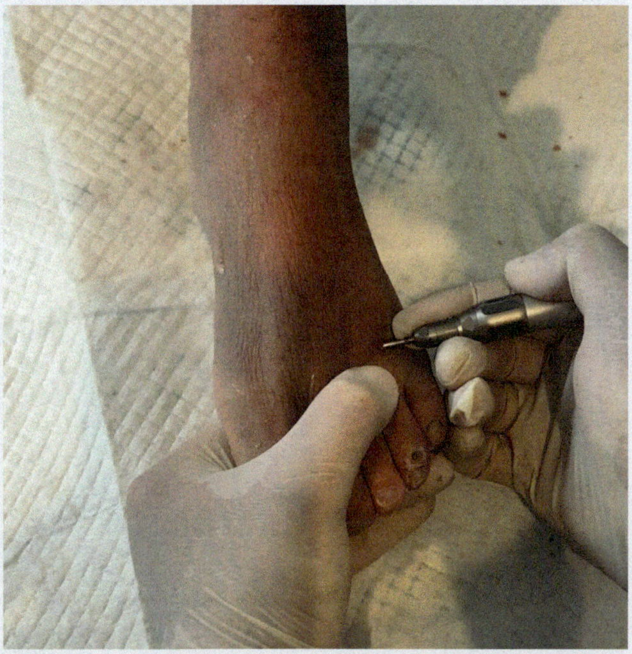

Figure 11.5 As the osteotomy progresses, the orientation of the burr will gradually change to 90° to the long axis of the metatarsal.

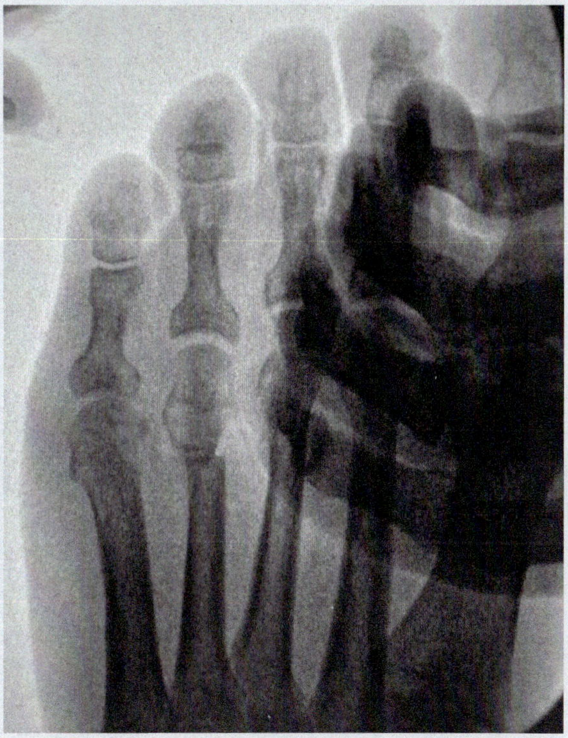

Figure 11.6 Once the osteotomy is completed, the exertion of pressure in the third web space will cause the fourth metatarsal head to shift lateral.

● PEARLS AND PITFALLS

- Do not keep the burr activated for more than 3 to 4 seconds. This might lead to thermal injury to the tissues. Stop the power, allow a few seconds to cool down without removing the burr from its position, and resume the procedure.
- While making the osteotomy, use a gentle sawing motion of the hand to facilitate penetration of the burr into the bone.
- Remember to use a rotational hand movement while making the osteotomy. Imagine the hinge of the burr to be at the skin incision. Ignoring this will cause a widening of the skin incision.

The skin is closed with the surgeon's suture of choice. Soft sterile dressings are applied to the surgical extremity. A hard-soled flat surgical sandal is applied to the surgical extremity.

◆ POSTOPERATIVE MANAGEMENT

Patients are allowed full weight bearing in the surgical sandal. Low-impact activities such as walking, stationary bike, elliptical, upper and several lower body weight-lifting, etc., are allowed in the surgical sandal. Early mobilization is encouraged to cause the lateral shift of the fourth metatarsal head. Deep vein thrombosis chemoprophylaxis is not routinely recommended. Dressings and stitches are removed 2 weeks postoperatively. At that point, patients are allowed to bathe the surgical foot and can wear socks. Two weeks postoperatively, three-view weight-beating radiographs of the foot are obtained to confirm displacement of the osteotomy. Six weeks postoperatively, new radiographs are obtained. Patients are allowed to wear comfortable shoes, avoiding high heels and high-impact activities.

Three months postoperatively, new radiographs are obtained. At this time, most patients will show signs of bone healing. Most patients will already report partial or full resolution of the preoperative symptoms. At 3 months, if comfortable, patients are allowed to return to any shoe and to any activity as tolerated. Remind the patient that postoperative swelling will resolve around 4 months postoperatively.

Most patients will report discomfort at the dorsal aspect of the fourth metatarsal neck during the first 3 to 4 months after surgery, in correspondence to the palpable callus formation. Patients should be reassured that the callus will improve within the first 6 months and may continue to get better during the first year. Patients should be followed every 3 months in their first year, with or without radiographs depending on symptoms and bone healing at the previous visits. Figures 11.7 and 11.8 are representative pre- and postoperative radiographs of two patients who underwent the above procedure.

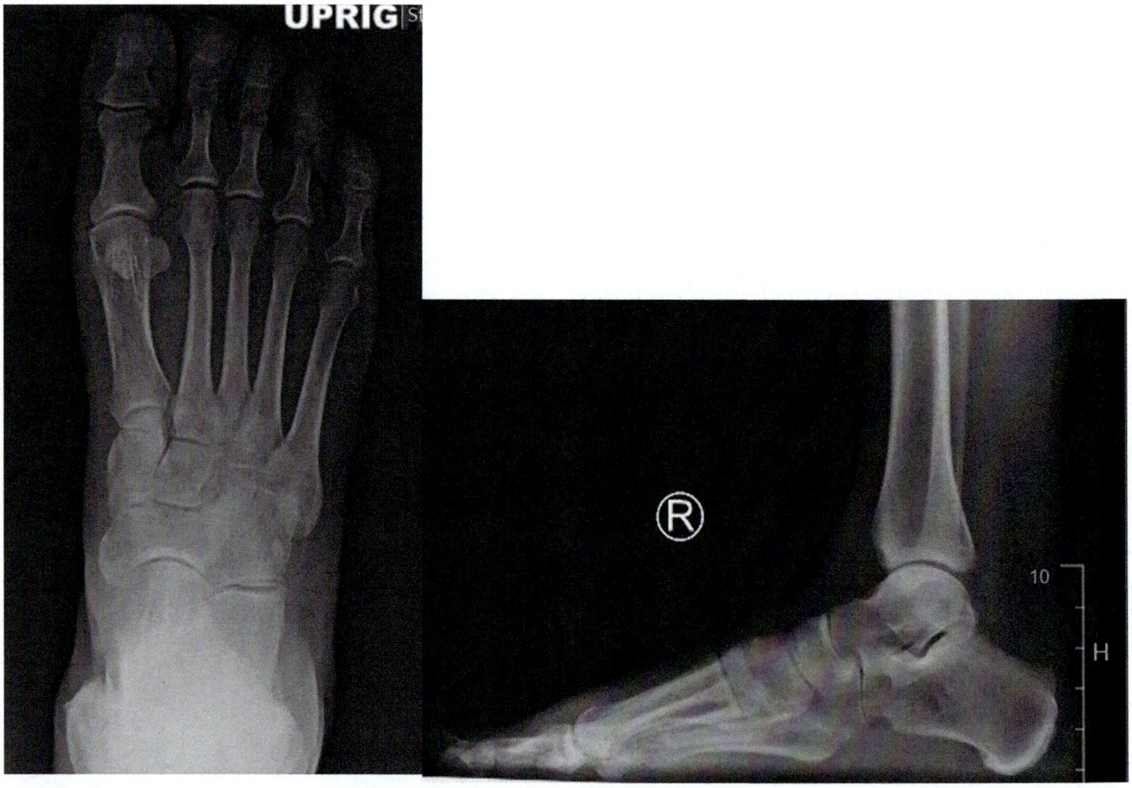

Figure 11.7 Anteroposterior (AP) and lateral weight-bearing radiographs of a 57-year-old female preoperative patient.

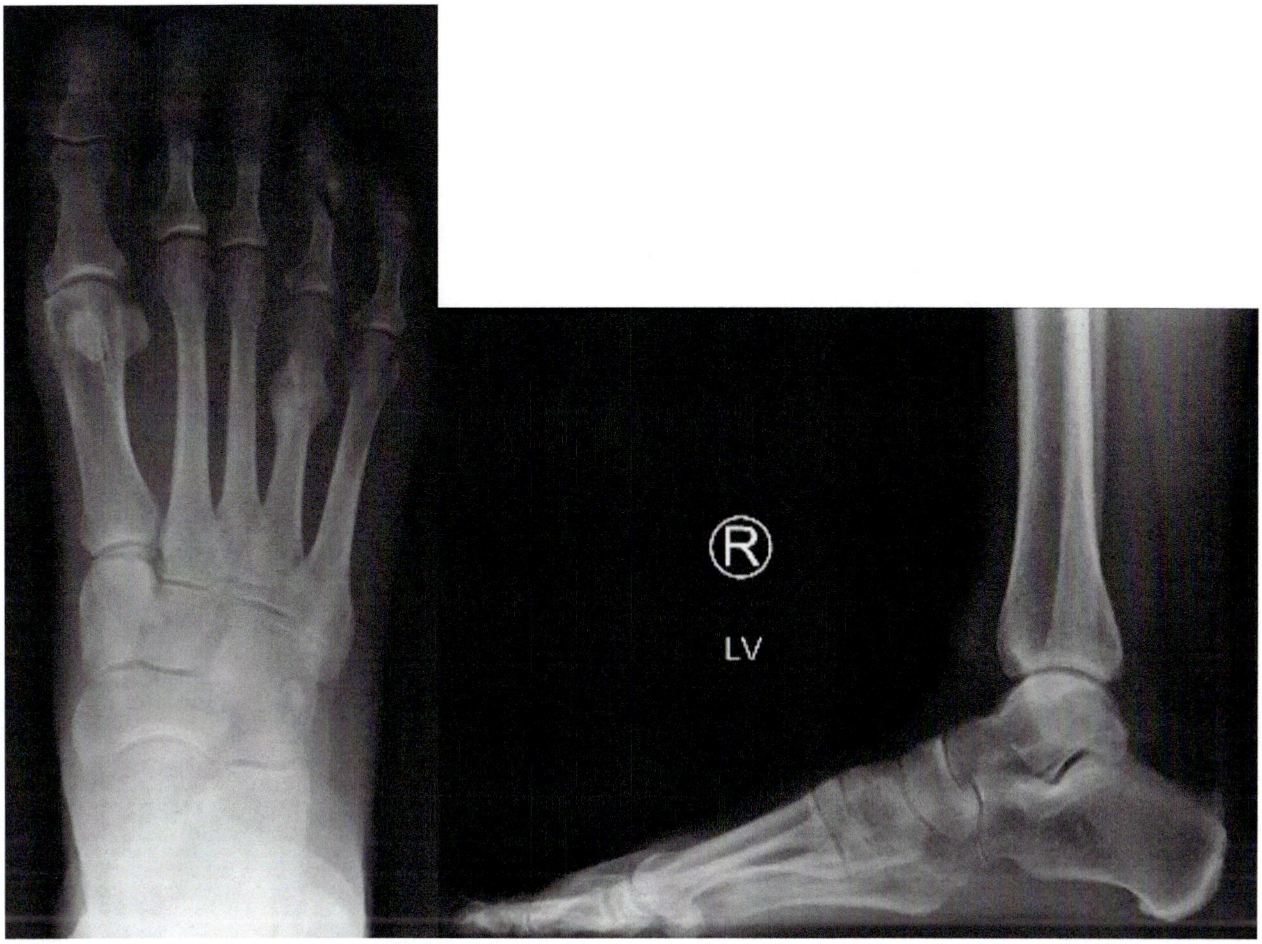

Figure 11.8 Anteroposterior (AP) and lateral weight-bearing radiographs of a 57-year-old female at 13 months after percutaneous distal fourth metatarsal osteotomy and transverse intermetatarsal ligament release.

◆ OUTCOMES

As this is a novel surgical technique, literature regarding outcomes of this specific technique is of course sparse. Early results from the authors' institutional cohort of 22 consecutive patients with a minimum of 1-year follow-up demonstrate significant improvements in patient-reported outcomes measures, irrespective of initial neuroma size, patient sex, or presence of comorbidities and with no surgical complications observed.

The authors' institutional data are consistent with previously published work regarding the operative management of Morton neuroma. Bauer et al. presented a retrospective cohort study of 52 patients comparing open and percutaneous treatment of Morton neuroma. At 2-year follow-up, the authors found substantial improvements in American Orthopedic Foot and Ankle Society Scores after percutaneous treatment. The improvements were noted to be greater than those who underwent open neurectomy. Importantly, they also found a rate of persistent postoperative metatarsalgia at 4% for the percutaneous group as compared to 44% of the open neurectomy group.[18] No patients in the cohort thus far have reported persistent metatarsalgia.

The technique described above differs from that described by Bauer and colleagues in that they elected to perform osteotomies on metatarsals 2 to 4 as opposed to the single metatarsal approach described here. Bauer and colleagues found that in their cohort, the time period for return to normal daily activity and normal shoe wear for the percutaneous cohort was not different than the open cohort, which they attributed to swelling from osteotomy sites.[18] Thus, the authors suggest that minimizing the number of osteotomy sites, when possible, is of particular importance to improve postoperative patient satisfaction.

The authors have had no significant complications to date in the institutional cohort. One patient with diabetes had mild serous drainage from the surgical site with no signs of infection—this resolved by 3 weeks from the procedure. More generally, the main complications noted with percutaneous approach to Morton neuroma have been persistent Morton neuroma symptoms, likely due to incomplete intermetatarsal ligament release.[19,20] Additionally, authors have reported iatrogenic injuries to the interdigital nerve or metatarsophalangeal tendons after percutaneous intervention; however, none of those complications were noted in the cohort.[19]

References

1. Thomas J, Blitch E. Diagnosis and treatment of forefoot disorders. Section 3. Morton's intermetatarsal neuroma. *J Foot Ankle Surg.* 2009;48(2):251-256.
2. Gougoulias N, Lampridis V, Sakellariou A. Morton's interdigital neuroma: instructional review. *EFORT Open Rev.* 2019;4(1):14-24.
3. Mulder JD. The causative mechanism in Morton's metatarsalgia. *J Bone Joint Surg Br.* 1951;33-B(1):94-95.
4. Pastides P, El-Sallakh S, Charalambides C. Morton's neuroma: a clinical versus radiological diagnosis. *Foot Ankle Surg.* 2012;18(1):22-24.
5. Bennett GL, Graham CE, Mauldin DM. Morton's interdigital neuroma: a comprehensive treatment protocol. *Foot Ankle Int.* 1995;16(12):760-763.
6. Matthews BG, Hurn SE, Harding MP, Henry RA, Ware RS. The effectiveness of non-surgical interventions for common plantar digital compressive neuropathy (Morton's neuroma): a systematic review and meta-analysis. *J Foot Ankle Res.* 2019;12:12.
7. Perini L, Perini C, Tagliapietra M. Percutaneous alcohol injection under sonographic guidance in Morton's neuroma: follow-up in 220 treated lesions. *Radiol Med.* 2016;121(7):597-604.
8. Samaila E, Colo G, Rava A. Effectiveness of corticosteroid injections in Civinini-Morton's syndrome: a systematic review. *Foot Ankle Surg.* 2021;27(4):357-365.
9. Peters PG, Adams SB Jr, Schon LC. Interdigital neuralgia. *Foot Ankle Clin.* 2011;16(2):305-315.
10. Weinfeld SB, Myerson MS. Interdigital neuritis: diagnosis and treatment. *J Am Acad Orthop Surg.* 1996;4(6):328-335.
11. Espinosa N, Seybold JD, Jankauskas L, Erschbamer M. Alcohol sclerosing therapy is not an effective treatment for interdigital neuroma. *Foot Ankle Int.* 2011;32(6):576-580.
12. Samaila EM, Ambrosini C, Negri S, Maluta T, Valentini R, Magnan B. Can percutaneous alcoholization of Morton's neuroma with phenol by electrostimulation guidance be an alternative to surgical excision? *Long-term results. Foot Ankle Surg.* 2020;26(3):314-319.
13. Adams SB Jr, Peters PG, Schon LC. Persistent or recurrent interdigital neuromas. *Foot Ankle Clin.* 2011;16(2):317-325.
14. Giannini S, Bacchini P, Ceccarelli F, Vannini F. Interdigital neuroma: clinical examination and histopathologic results in 63 cases treated with excision. *Foot Ankle Int.* 2004;25(2):79-84.
15. Kasparek M, Schneider W. Surgical treatment of Morton's neuroma: clinical results after open excision. *Int Orthop.* 2013;37(9):1857-1861.
16. de Prado M, Ripoll P, Golano P. *Cirugía percutánea del pie: técnicas quirúrgicas, indicaciones, bases anatómicas.* Masson; 2003.
17. de Prado M, Ripoll P, Golano P. *Minimally Invasive Foot Surgery: Surgical Techniques, Indications, Anatomical Basis.* About Your Health; 2009:197-207.
18. Bauer T, Gaumetou E, Klouche S, Hardy P, Maffulli N. Metatarsalgia and Morton's disease: comparison of outcomes between open procedure and neurectomy versus percutaneous metatarsal osteotomies and ligament release with a minimum of 2 years of follow-up. *J Foot Ankle Surg.* 2015;54(3):373-377.
19. Fabié F, Accadbled F, Tricoire J-L, Puget J. Anatomic danger of percutaneous section of the inter-metatarsal ligament for the treatment of Morton's neuroma. *Rev Chir Orthop Reparatrice Appar Mot.* 2007;93(7):720-724.
20. Zelent ME, Kane RM, Neese DJ, Lockner WB. Minimally invasive Morton's intermetatarsal neuroma decompression. *Foot Ankle Int.* 2007;28(2):263-265.

12 Lesser Toes Deformities

Barbara Piclet-Legré and Véronique Darcel

◆ INTRODUCTION

Minimally invasive, percutaneous foot and ankle surgery techniques derive from and borrow the general principles of traditional open surgery. Percutaneous surgical techniques are particularly suitable for correcting lesser toes deformities because they allow targeted tendon, capsular, and bone procedures to be performed "à la carte" according to the different types of deformities and their reducibility. The polymorphism of lesser toes deformities has long been an obstacle to the reliable and reproducible classification schemes.

Physiopathology

Toe deformities usually develop from a disharmony in the musculotendinous balance between the extrinsic and intrinsic muscles of the foot.

As a reminder, the extensors act only on the 1° phalanx (P1) by the suspender effect of the fibro-aponeurotic structure with the extensor sling's transversely oriented fibers (this extensor sling is also called transverse or quadrilateral lamina) and the extensor wing's obliquely oriented fibers; the flexors act on the 2° and 3° phalanges (P2 and P3); the balance between these different tendons is restored only by the interossei and lumbricals (often atrophied in the sedentary) muscles (Tables 12.1 and 12.2).

Passive stabilization of the metatarsophalangeal (MTP), proximal interphalangeal (PIP), and distal interphalangeal (DIP) joints is ensured by the collateral ligaments, the joint capsule, and the plantar plate. Any lesion of these structures may cause or aggravate the deformity.[1,2]

Many hypothesize that a mechanical overload of the joints linked to a retraction of the gastrocnemius, a pathology of the rear, midfoot, or forefoot gradually causes the deformities.

Among the risk factors, female sex, older age, and a high body mass index have been identified[3,4] as well as genetic factors[5] and unsuitable footwear, particularly in the elderly.[6]

Deformities may also be due to central or peripheral neurological disease such as stroke or Charcot-Marie-Tooth disease or rheumatic conditions such as rheumatoid arthritis that may destroy the stabilizing elements of the joint. Iatrogenic and posttraumatic deformities are also caused by malunion, compartment syndrome, or lesion of the tendon apparatus. Harnessing syndrome, due to the presence of an anastomotic slip between the flexor hallucis longus and the flexor digitorum longus (FDL), can cause deformation of the lateral toes in flexion when the first ray is shortened.

Classification of Lesser Toes Deformities

Referenced publications use nonstandardized descriptive international names such as "claw toe," "mallet toe," "hammer toe," "curly toe," or "cross over toe." A Dutch study showed clearly insufficient concordance for the definition of "hammer toe" (24%), "claw toe" (9%), and "mallet toe" (the better with 70%) using as reference the definitions of Coughlin and Mann.[7]

The French Association of Foot Surgery Classification (AFCP)

Almost 10 years ago, the senior author proposed an exhaustive systematic clinical classification deformities of the lesser toes at The French Association of Foot Surgery (*Association Française de Chirurgie du Pied*) spring congress in Lille, France, in 2013. This morphological classification was validated in 2018 and published by Lintz et al.[8] for the second toe. It describes the position of each joint of the toe from proximal to distal in relation to the anatomical

Table 12.1

Global Action of Extrinsic and Intrinsic Pull on the MTP Joints and IP Joints

	Extrinsic	Intrinsic
MTP joints	**Extension**	**Flexion**
IP joints	**Flexion**	**Extension**

IP, Interphalangeal; MTP, metatarsophalangeal.

Table 12.2

Specific Action of the EDL and EDB Tendons on the MTP, PIP, and DIP Joints

	EDL and EDB	FDL	FDB	Interosseous Lumbricals	Plantar Fascia
MTP joints	**Extension**/sling wing			**Flexion**	**Flexion**
PIP joints	**Extension**		**Flexion**	**Extension**	
DIP joints	**Extension**	**Flexion**		**Extension**	

DIP, distal interphalangeal; EDB, extensor digitorum brevis; EDL, extensor digitorum longus; FDB, flexor digitorum brevis; FDL, flexor digitorum longus; MTP, metatarsophalangeal; PIP, proximal interphalangeal.

reference position. Deformities in the sagittal plane take precedence over deformities in the horizontal plane. Each toe is described by its number (from 2 to 5) then by three letters, one for each joint. In the sagittal plane, the position of the segment of the joint is denoted "e" for extension, "n" for neutral, or "f" for flexion (Table 12.3). If there is no deformity in the sagittal plane (ie, the position of the joint is classified as "n"), the deformity in the horizontal plane can be taken into account. It is denoted "m" for medial, "n" for neutral, or "l" for lateral (Table 12.4).

The classification in the only one for which inter- and intra-observer reproducibility and speed have been evaluated (~30 seconds) on second toe deformities.

However, it does not provide information on reducibility, pulp support, joint stability, and radiological characteristics.

This classification may easily be applied to the other toes. Figures 12.1 to 12.6 illustrate examples of the use of the classification.

An additional category of "pulp support score" was added in 2021. It translates the quality of pulp support into passive and active during the foot examination[9] (Table 12.5).

◆ INDICATIONS AND CONTRAINDICATIONS

Indications and contraindications depend on the vascularity of the toe, the goals of the patient, and the overall flexibility of the toe. In an active infection, any surgical intervention other than amputation may be contraindicated. Poor vascularization of the foot may result in delayed bony and soft-tissue healing, and in some cases devascularization of the toe with toe loss. Rigid deformities treated with soft-tissue procedures alone may result in recurrence or worsening deformity. Maintaining patient expectations and careful anatomical understanding will result in better outcomes overall. Other limitations will be exposed in the description below. Meticulous postoperative care is paramount in the first 6 weeks after surgery; if the patient cannot commit to this, surgery may be contraindicated.

Table 12.3

AFCP Classification of Lesser Toes Deformities

Sagittal Deformity			
MTP	e	n	f
PIP	e	n	f
DIP	e	n	f

We proceed in the same way for the PIP and the DIP.

AFCP, French Association of Foot Surgery; DIP, distal interphalangeal; MTP, metatarsophalangeal; PIP, proximal interphalangeal.

◆ PATIENT HISTORY AND PHYSICAL EXAMINATION

What are the decision criteria for a correcting toe deformity?

Analysis of the Functional Impact of the Deformation

The functional impact of pain in the feet on quality of life has been demonstrated as quite significant with an SF-36

Table 12.4

When There Is No Sagittal Deformity (Segment of the Joint in Neutral Position [n]), the Deformity in the Horizontal Plane Can Be Taken Into Account and Denoted "m" When the Segment is Deflected Medially and "l" When Deflected Laterally

Horizontal Deformity		
MTP n	m	l
PIP n	m	l
DIP n	m	l

DIP, distal interphalangeal; MTP, metatarsophalangeal; PIP, proximal interphalangeal.

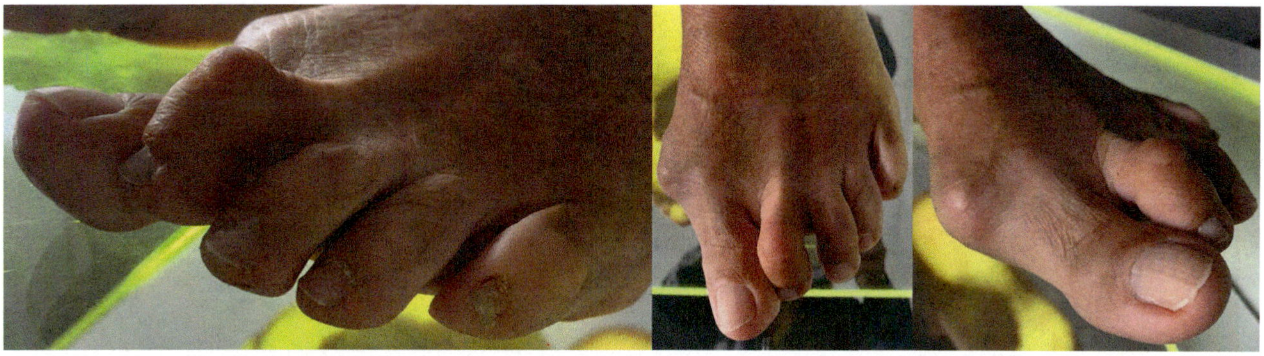

Figure 12.1 2efn deformity according to the French Association of Foot Surgery classification, equivalent of "claw toe."

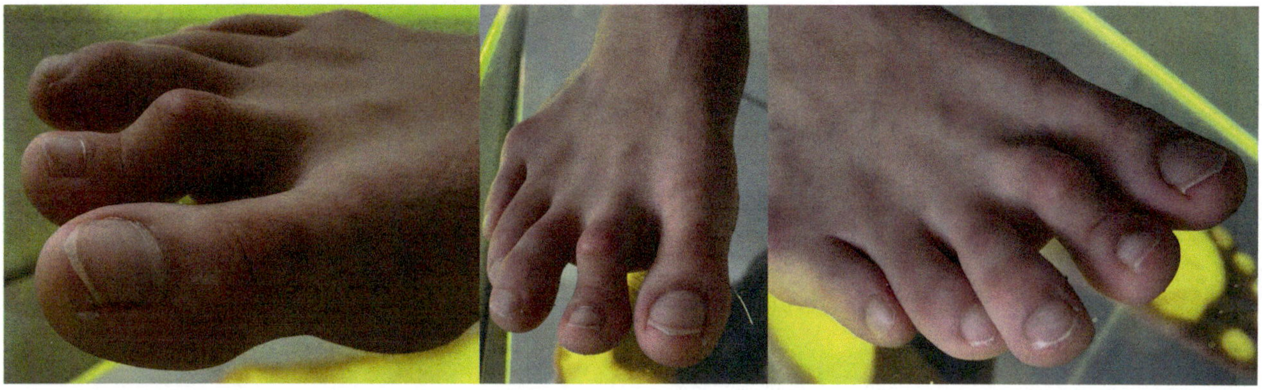

Figure 12.2 2efe deformity according to the French Association of Foot Surgery classification.

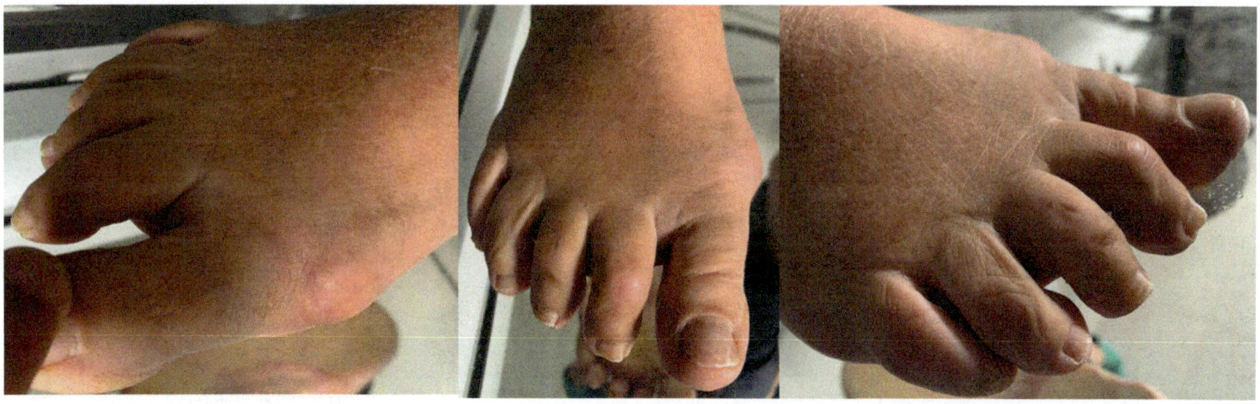

Figure 12.3 2nfn deformity according to the French Association of Foot Surgery equivalent classification of "hammer toe."

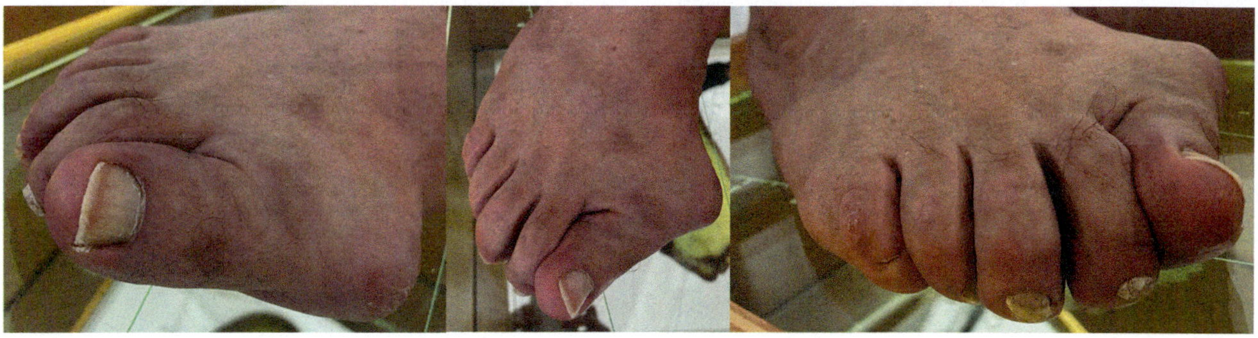

Figure 12.4 2nff deformity according to French Association of Foot Surgery classification equivalent classification to "mallet toe."

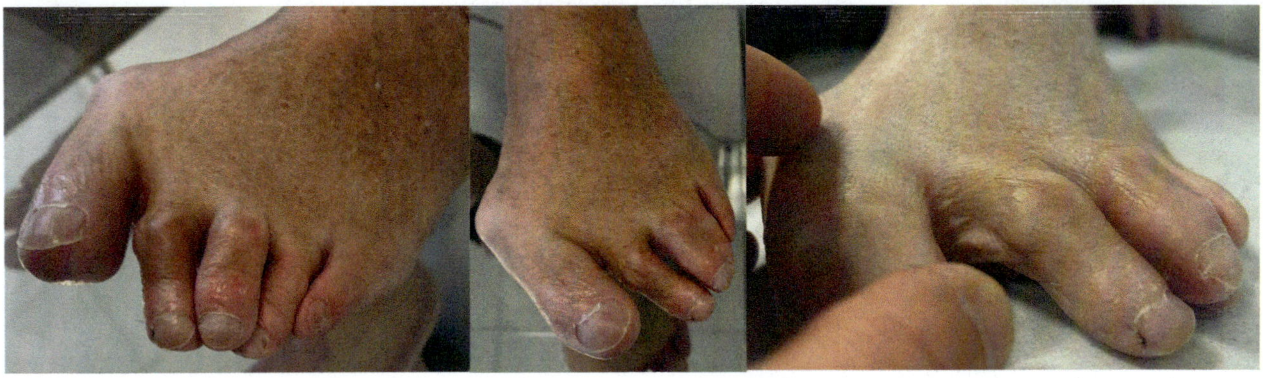

Figure 12.5 2lfn and 3eff according to French Association of Foot Surgery classification.

score being reduced on the physical, social functioning, and mental health components.[3] In the older population, deformities of the lesser toes are associated with an increased risk of falling (67%).[10] The most frequent complaint of toe deformity is the dorsal contact with the shoe, though other complaints such as excess pulp pressure or a metatarsalgia by vertical pressure on the metatarsal head are common.

Pulp Pressure Quality

Pulp pressure can be assessed in weight bearing by the "paper pull-out test" (the patient's ability to hold a sheet of paper on the ground using toe pressure against pull-out) or on the AFCP lesser toe classification of pulp pressure previously described.[9]

Reducibility

The authors test the reducibility of each joint according to the AFCP classification.

One can use the push-off test to qualify the deformation as reducible, semireducible, or nonreducible. In non–weight bearing, the examiner presses under the metatarsal head in question. The deformation is reducible when this support completely corrects the deformation.

The terms used are flexible (f), semirigid (sr), or rigid (r).

In neurological feet, it is not uncommon for the deformity to be reducible in equinus and for an fff (flexible MTP, PIP, DIP) deformity to be observed in dorsal flexion, which testifies to the retraction of the flexors.

The authors usually add reducibility and etiology to the classification description; the reducibility is noted after the description of the deformity of the toe: flexible (f), semirigid (sr), rigid (r) and the cause is noted before: rhumatismal (rh), posttraumatic (pt), neurological (nr), iatrogenic (ic).

If the authors use these descriptors, for instance, they can write (rh)2nfn(r), (pt)3nln(f), or (nr)2345nff(sr) to describe deformities.

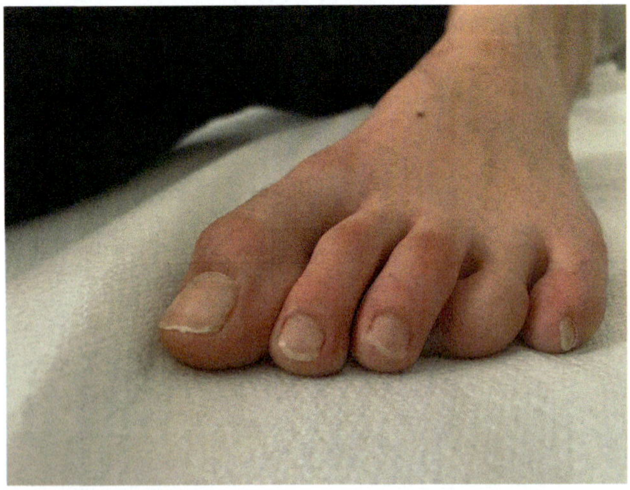

Figure 12.6 4nmn deformity according to French Association of Foot Surgery classification.

Metatarsophalangeal Instability

The evaluate the plantar plate, palpate the MTP and using the drawer test or Lachman test[11]: the foot being off-loaded, the metatarsal head is held between the thumb and index finger, and, with the other hand, move the toe upward; the drawer is positive when the toe subluxates, indicating a lesion of the plantar plate.

Table 12.5

The Score for Each Toe Is 0 When the Pulp Support Is Normal, 1 When Support Is Present Only With Active Flexion, and 2 in the Absence of Support in Passive and Active

Score	State
0	Pulp support at rest, reinforced with active flexion
1	Pulp support only with active flexion (no support passive)
2	Absence of any pulp support on the ground (absence of active and passive support)

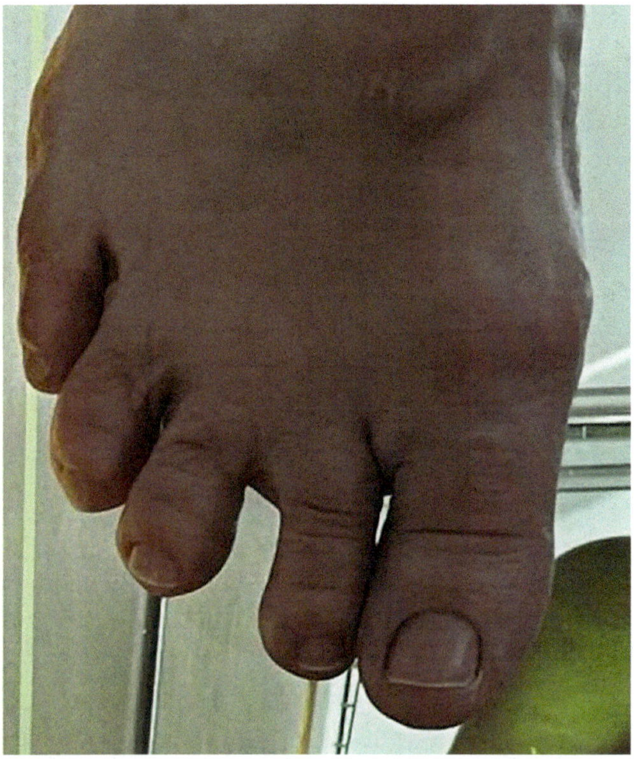

Figure 12.7 "V" sign meaning 2nd MTP (MTP2) synovitis.

At the synovitis stage, the "V" sign is the first seen on clinical examination. Under weight bearing with bare feet, there is an abnormal gap between the affected toe and its neighbor[12] (Figure 12.7).

◆ IMAGING STUDIES

Standard Radiograph

Weight-bearing foot radiographs are useful to analyze phalanx bone morphology and look for osteoarthritic degeneration of the joints. Joint deformities, such as an MTP subluxation or dislocation, may lead to a superposition of the joint spaces of the toes on the standard incidences. Centered or zoomed shots are sometimes necessary. Radiographs also highlight other foot morphology affecting the toes, such as pes cavus or prior traumatic deformity.

Ultrasound

In the hands of a skilled user, ultrasound is extremely helpful in examining the plantar plate[13] as it is dynamic and has the best resolution among all the imaging modalities.

A rupture is noted as a partial- or full-thickness hypoechoic area of the plate, most often distal and lateral with variable propagation proximally and medially. The second ray is most often affected. Toe dorsiflexion improves visualization of lesions. Indirect plantar signs such as phalangeal avulsion and effusion of the flexor tendon sheath in contact with the plate can be visualized. On the dorsal side, ultrasound detects joint synovitis and phalangeal subluxation at the preradiographic stage. The limits of ultrasound are the thickened hyperkeratosis of the anterior pad for the plantar cuts and the fixed and irreducible hyperextension of the MTP for the dorsal cuts.[14]

MRI

MRI has a sensitivity of 96% and a specificity of 95% in the diagnosis of plantar plate lesions.

The lesions usually appear as a discontinuity of the plate in hypersignal T2, which extends toward the base of P1.[15] A trap image is the central and distal pseudodefect of the plantar plate, which causes a physiological T2 hypersignal.

MRI is superior to ultrasound and radiography in the diagnosis of synovitis and subchondral bone changes in arthropathies. It is the reference examination in the differential diagnosis, particularly in the diagnosis of nonmechanical pathologies.[14]

◆ PREOPERATIVE PLANNING AND PREPARATION

Nonsurgical options should be attempted first, although their level of scientific evidence is low.

Physiotherapy for stretching the gastrocnemius muscles or strengthening the intrinsic "foot sheathing" is prescribed depending on the etiology. The osteopathic technique of strain counterstrain, advocated by Masson,[16] acts on the abnormal shortening of the tissues at the level of the deformity responsible for the restriction of movement. Intra-articular steroid injection can be proposed in case of synovitis without lesion of the plantar plate, which is essential to seek.[15] Beware of the risk of plantar plate rupture[17] because it will promote joint instability.

SURGICAL TECHNIQUE

What Surgery Apart From Treating the Cause?

Studies on surgical treatments are mostly level 4 (retrospective case series). In all cases, treating the cause of the deformities allows better results. For instance, in this case, the lengthening of the medial gastrocnemius was necessary in association with the percutaneous gestures of the deformed toes to correct deformity (Figure 12.8). The analysis of the deformity according to the morphological classification of the AFCP[8] aided by the pulp score[9] makes it possible to target the surgical indication. The choice of technique is made from proximal to distal, and the deformity is corrected sequentially at the level of the MTP, then of the PIP, and finally of the DIP if necessary.

Extensor Tenotomy

The remarkable anatomical work of Pao Golano, who sadly passed away in 2014, helped to define the exact points of skin penetration and the trajectories to follow

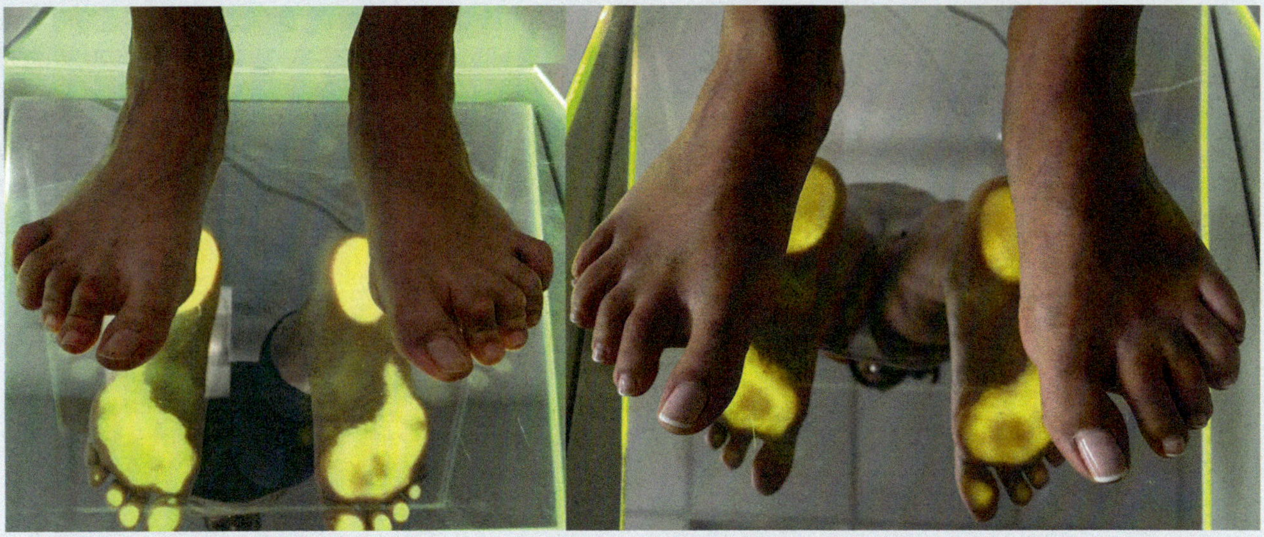

Figure 12.8 Lengthening of the medial gastrocnemius in association with the percutaneous gestures of deformed toes pre- and postoperative aspect after 2.5 years.

in order to avoid noble elements in the absence of direct vision.

Extensors tenotomy should be ideally performed in the area where the two tendons (extensor digitorum longus [EDL] and extensor digitorum brevis [EDB]) are well separated, that is, next to the MTP joint if arthrolysis is necessary or slightly further proximal. When performed within the fibro-aponeurotic sling, a drooping toe may be avoided (Figure 12.9).

Dorsal MTP release may proceed next, if necessary, through the same incision. Toe traction allows the joint to be unloaded in order to facilitate the entry of the "beaver" scalpel in certain cases of dislocated toes.

Flexor Tenotomy

- Selective flexor digitorum brevis (**FDB**) tenotomy by an incision behind the PIP joint (Figure 12.10).

  The incision is lateral or medial depending on the operated foot and the dominant hand of the surgeon. Plantarflex the toe to bring the neurovascular supply plantar to the blade insertion at the joint. The PIP plantar capsule is cut at the base of P2 and then the Beaver blade progresses more

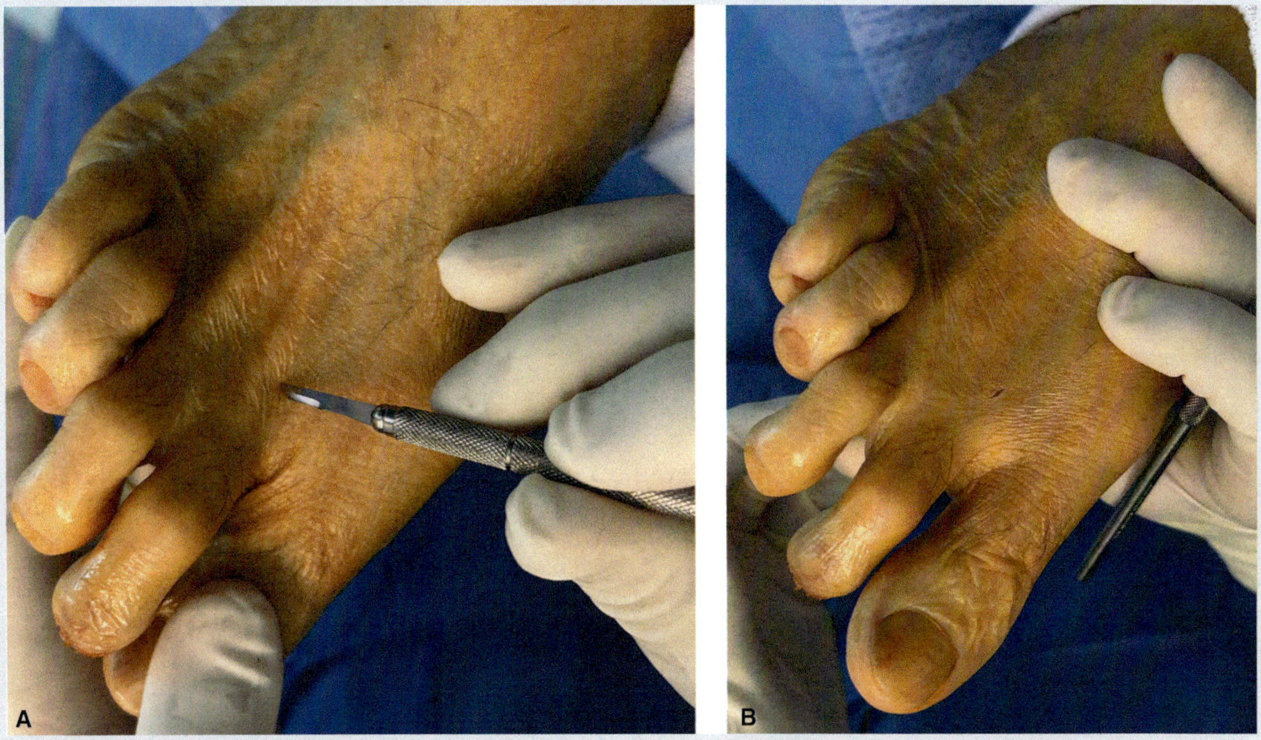

Figure 12.9 Extensor tenotomies before **(A)** and after **(B)**.

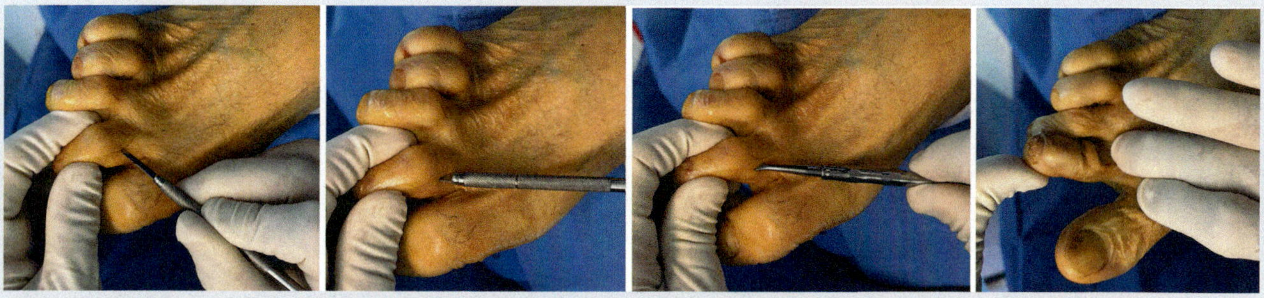

Figure 12.10 Flexor digitorum brevis tenotomy and proximal interphalangeal (PIP) release allowing PIP flexion correction.

distally with a rotational movement allowing the tenotomy of the two tabs of the FDB (Figure 12.11). A rasp or elevator is then introduced to check the complete section. The released toe is brought into dorsal flexion by a passive maneuver. One can also perform the selective FDB tenotomy via the plantar approach at the base of P1 where the FDB is on the surface, but there is a higher risk of not being selective and cutting the FDL as well; moreover, the plantar arthrolysis of the PIP is a significant help for the correction of the deformity.

- Selective tenotomy of the **FDL** is performed by a distal plantar incision next to the DIP joint or lateral as for that of the FDB.
- Complete **FDL + FDB** tenotomy as Mariano de Prado taught us[18,19] by a plantar incision at the base of the toe, next to P1 allows section of both flexor tendons. Neurological deformities (AFCP nff) are often sufficiently relieved by a complete flexor tenotomy.

Proximal Phalanx Osteotomy

- Using the same plantar approach described for the tenotomy of both flexors (Figure 12.12), the osteotomy is best located in the proximal metaphyseal part of P1 to optimize union time. The Shannon burr, typically a short 2 × 8 mm dimension, approaches the bone slightly laterally in relation to the flexor tendons.
- Some surgeons prefer a dorsal lateral approach under the extensors like Michel Bénichou described, the oblique shortening phalangeal osteotomy (OPRO) to shorten P1 (Figure 12.13).
- This OPRO oblique osteotomy can also be performed via the lateral approach used for the FDB tenotomy. The length of shortening can be determined by how oblique the cut is performed (the shorter the cut, the more the toe will move in the opposite direction and shorten) (Figure 12.14).
- A monocortical osteotomy allows flexion or correction of a lateral or medial deviation of the toe (Figure 12.15).
- A bicortical osteotomy allows significant shortening of a toe that is too long or in the event of an old, stiff deformity due to the tendon relaxation effect. The OPRO gives less postoperative edema than the P1 shortening osteotomy via the plantar approach, probably because bone consolidation is faster with this oblique osteotomy allowing more extensive contact between the edges of the osteotomy (Figure 12.16).

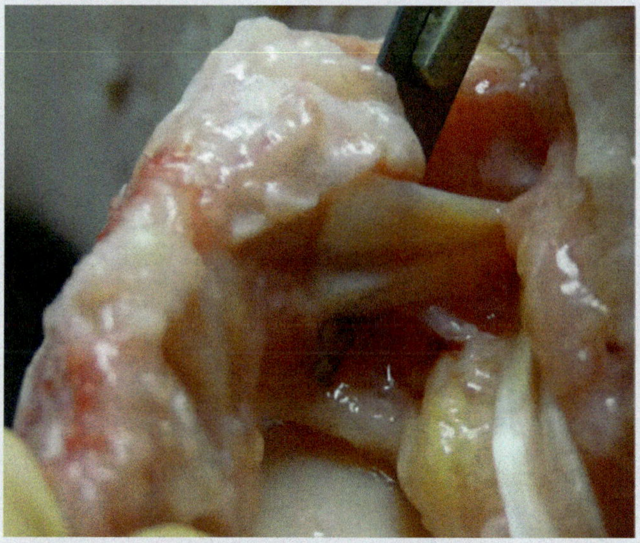

Figure 12.11 Tenotomy of the two tabs of the flexor digitorum brevis, cadaver lab. (Courtesy of Barbara Piclet-Legré.)

P2 Osteotomy

P2 osteotomy is performed via a lateral or medial approach depending on the operated foot and the desired procedure and is mid-diaphyseal to avoid joint invasion.

- Monocortical osteotomy best results in the correction of a lateral deviation of the DIP such as this case with a P2 varus for a 2nnl AFCP classification (Figure 12.17) or for a dorsiflexion deformity.
- Bicortical osteotomy allows the shortening of a long P2 but risks postoperative edema as the toe is unstable. This may be reduced by using temporary percutaneous pinning to avoid any movement in the osteotomy.[20] P2 osteotomy is sometimes a useful complement when the correction of a PIP deformity is insufficient. This is an example of a 73-year-old male with a 2eff, which was also efl with a long P2, and an ultrasound plantar plate rupture causing metatarsalgia; so the authors performed DMMO23, EDL-EDB-FDL tenotomies, and P1-P2 osteotomies with an interphalangeal pinning for 1 month (Figure 12.18).

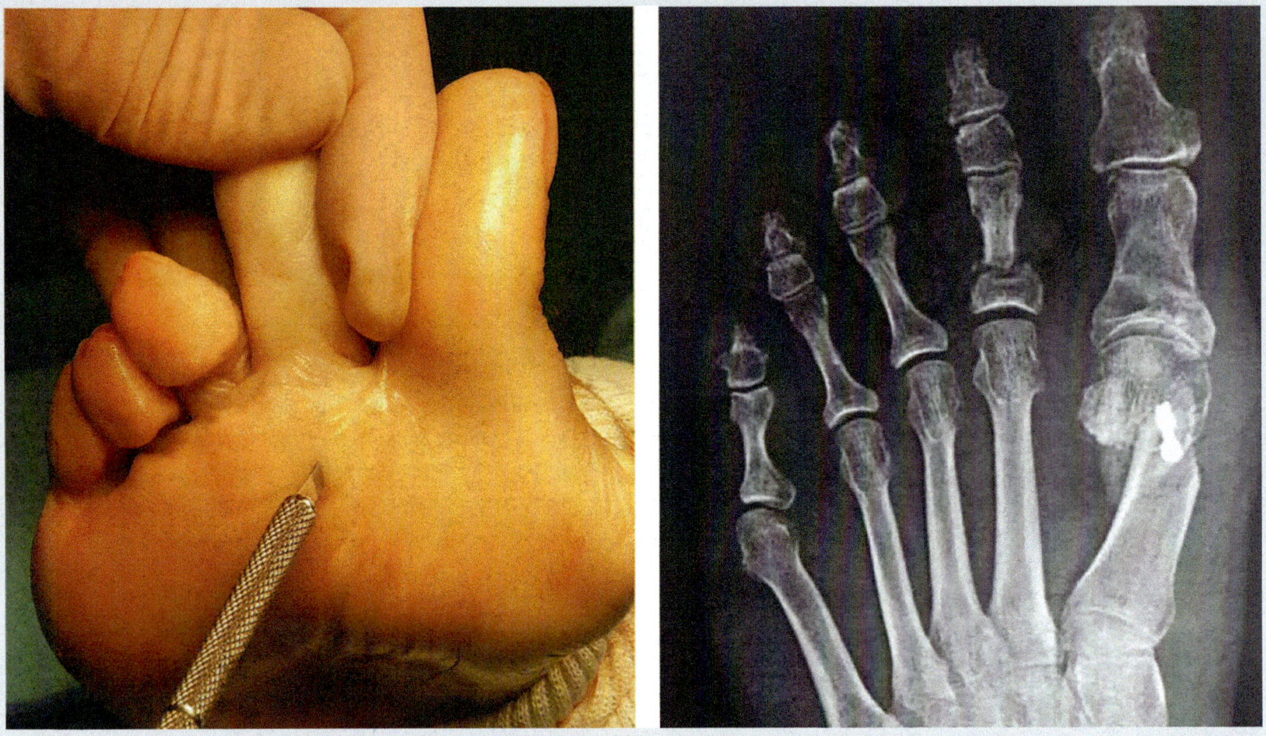

Figure 12.12 Plantar approach for 1° phalanx osteotomy.

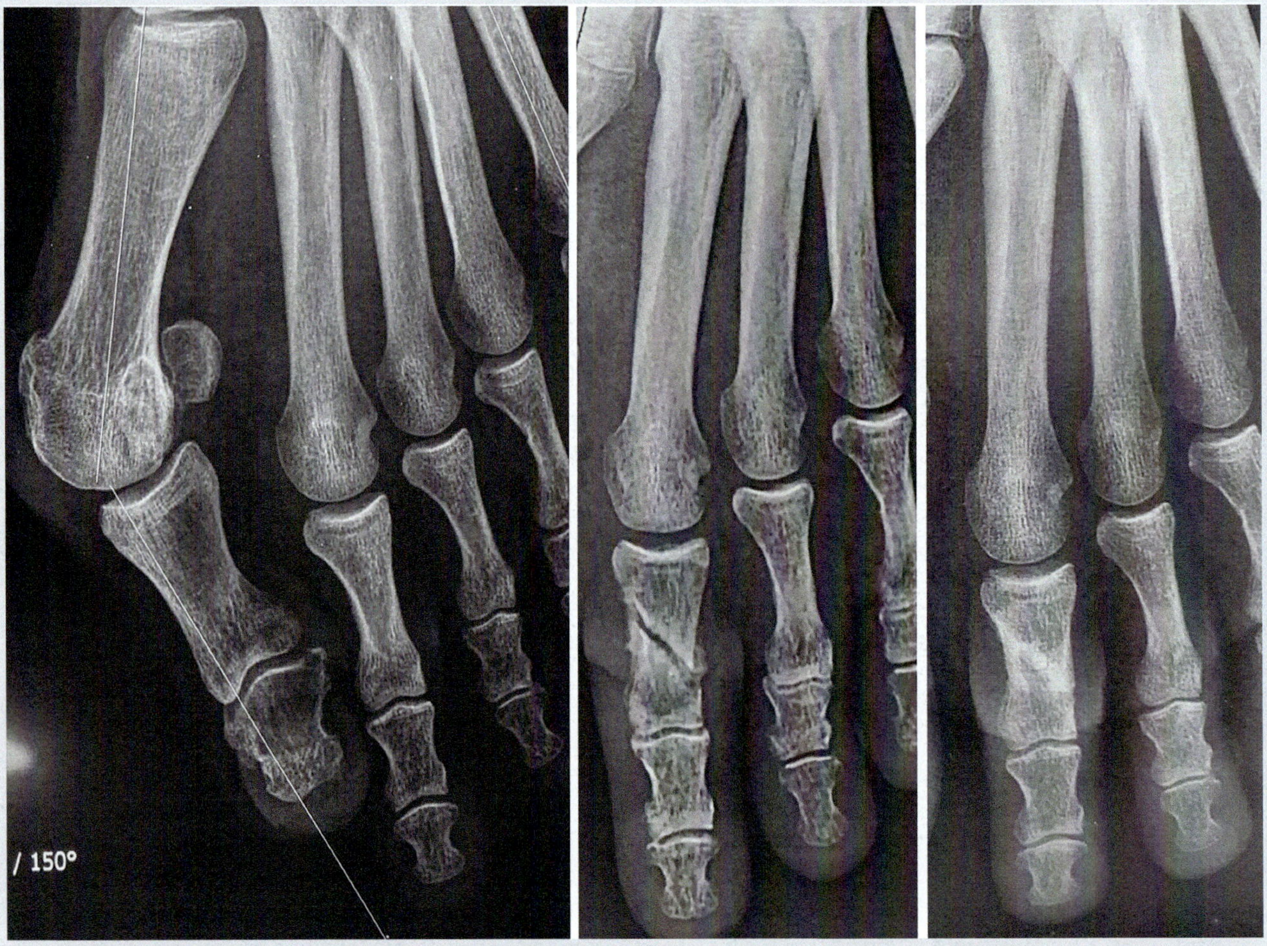

Figure 12.13 Oblique shortening phalangeal osteotomy (OPRO).

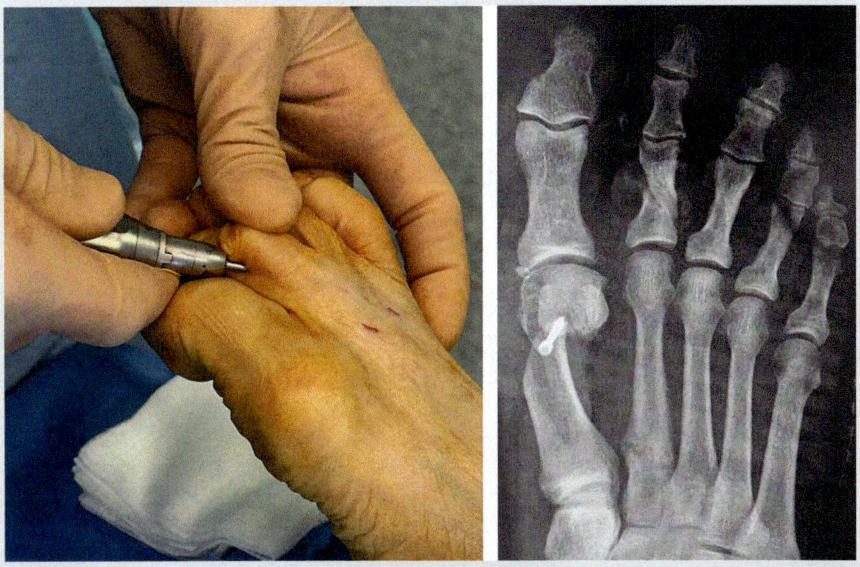

Figure 12.14 The 1° phalanx osteotomy by lateral approach.

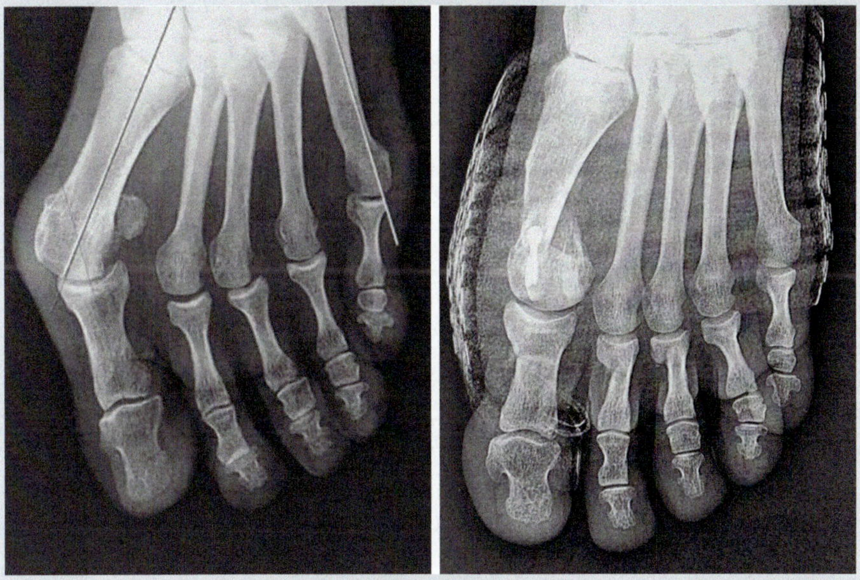

Figure 12.15 The 1° phalanx monocortical osteotomy.

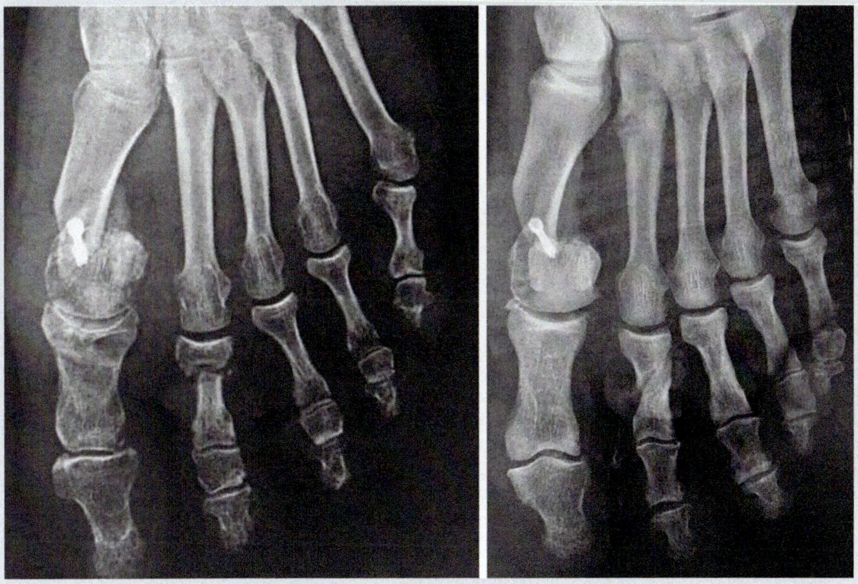

Figure 12.16 The 1° phalanx bicortical osteotomy standard and OPRO.

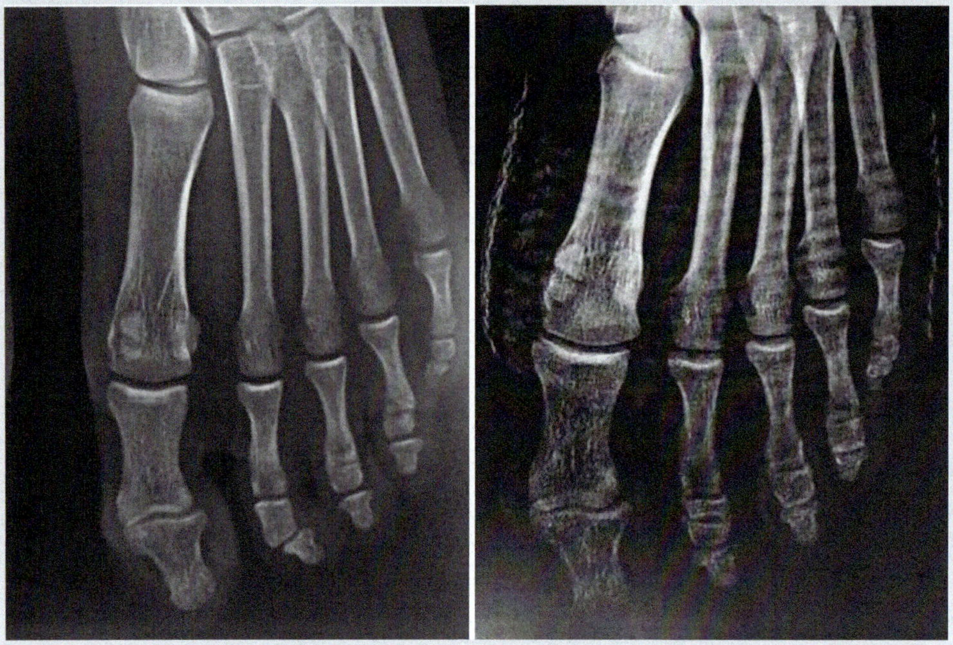

Figure 12.17 Monocortical 2° phalanx variation osteotomy for 2nnl before and after surgery.

Condylectomy

The condylectomy is used to ream the protruding dorsal part of the head of P1, as well as a portion of the base of P2. It is performed by the lateral approach flush with the dorsal face of the neck of P2. Bone debris is removed by pressure around the portal and irrigation to avoid irritation of the soft tissues.

Nonpercutaneous Techniques

In some cases, percutaneous intervention alone is insufficient to correct the toe deformity, and a combination of open and minimally invasive maneuvers is required. Véronique Darcel proposed—in the French Society of Orthopaedic and Traumatological Surgery (SOFCOT) 2022 teaching conference on deformities of the lesser toes—decision-making algorithms based on the latest publications with all their limitations.[21]

Apart from or in addition to percutaneous surgery, tendon transfers[13,22,23] aimed at stabilizing the MTP, repair of plantar plate[21] via the dorsal (with arthrolysis and metatarsal osteotomy) or plantar approach (with the risk of secondary plantar pad atrophy) may be added.[24-26]

For rigid joints, resection of the PIP joint may be performed and stabilized with a temporary pin usually left in place for 3 to 6 weeks or a tenodermodesis. PIP resection may be performed percutaneously, but the risk of leaving some remaining bone residues that causes ongoing swelling and irritation is high.

For PIP arthrodesis,[27-30] there are no prospective randomized studies to compare pin fixation with internal implant fixation. The use of pins would be the only choice if the joint was percutaneously prepared. When the authors need to do a fusion, they prefer open surgery.

DIP arthrodesis can also be stabilized with a pin when combined with other percutaneous gestures, as this case of 2eff treated with EDL-EDB-FDB tenotomies and DIP fusion (Figure 12.19).

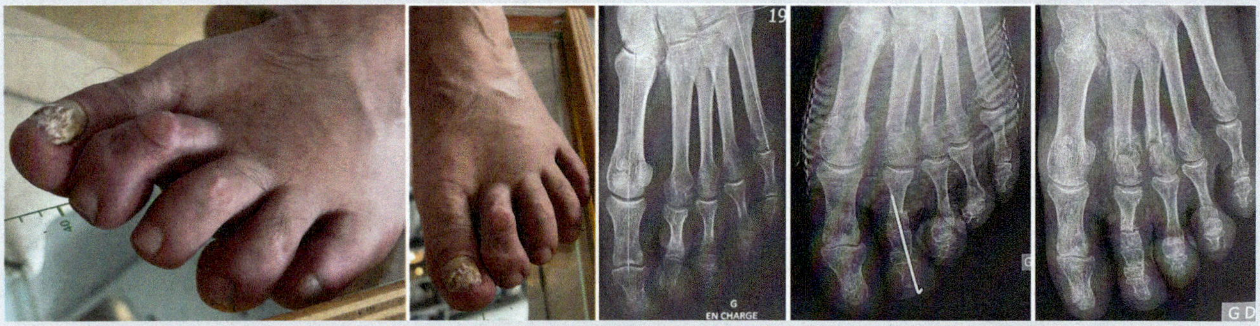

Figure 12.18 2eff according to the French Association of Foot Surgery classification—radiographs before, during, and 45 days after DMMO23, EDB-EDL-FDL, and 1° phalanx osteotomy.

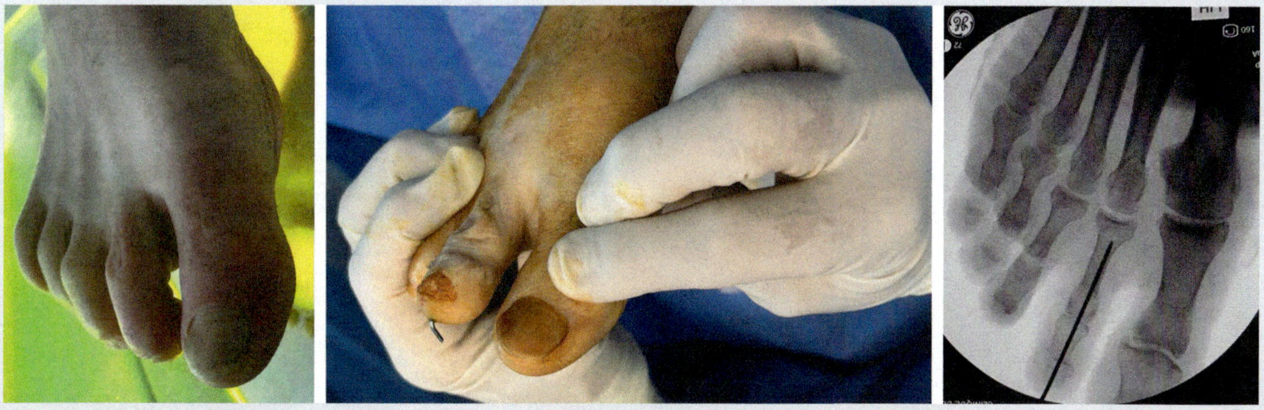

Figure 12.19 Distal interphalangeal fusion and EDL-EDB-FDB tenotomies.

Metatarsal Osteotomy[31]

Apart from the management of an obvious cause of toe deformity such as disharmony in the length of the metatarsals, metatarsal osteotomy is indicated in the event of instability or MTP dislocation. The most frequently used are the percutaneous distal metatarsal metaphyseal osteotomy (DMMO) and the open Weil osteotomy with numerous à la carte variants.

Rarely limited to a single ray, these osteotomies most often address the second and third rays and rarely all of the metatarsals (Figure 12.20).

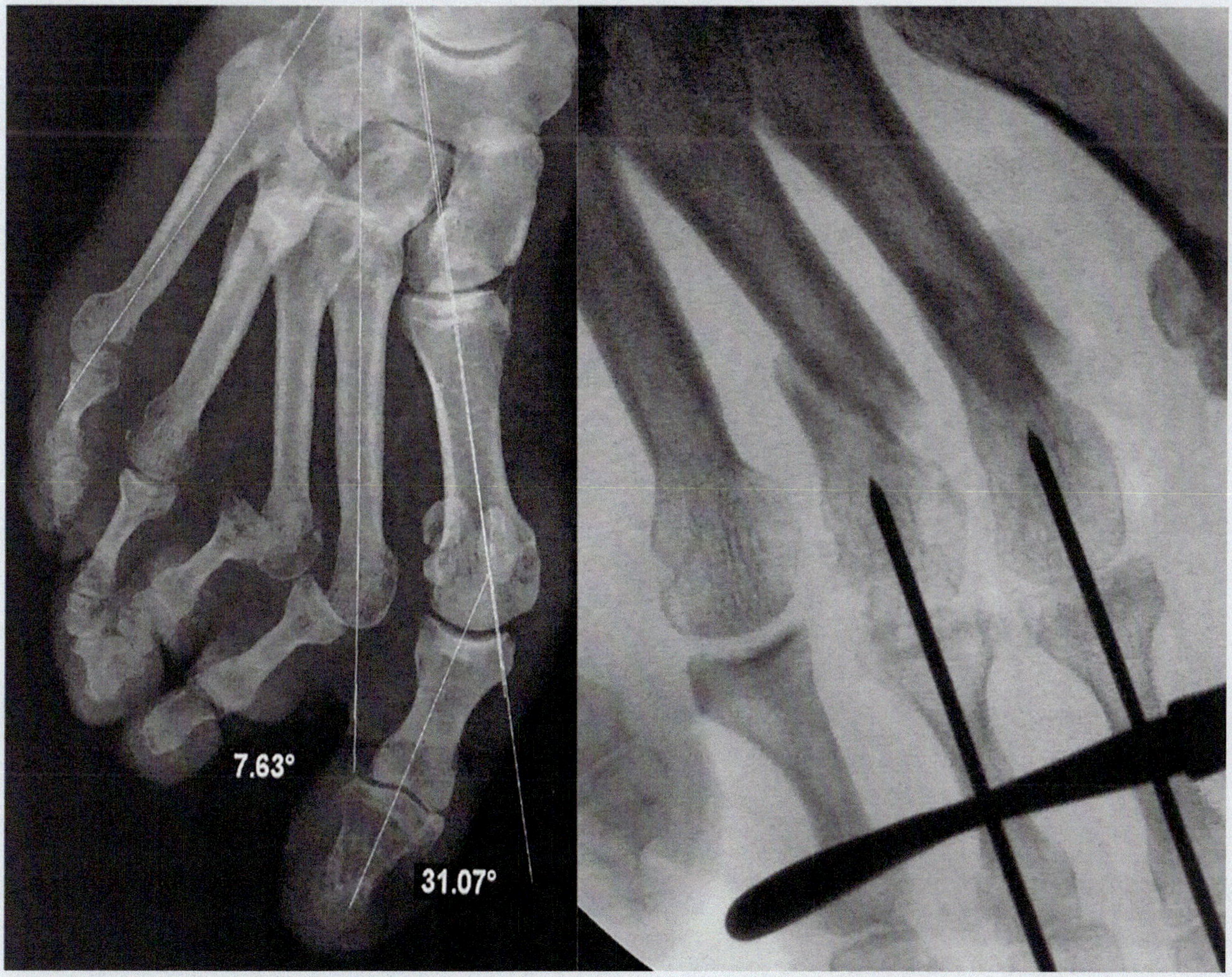

Figure 12.20 Efficiency of distal metatarsal metaphyseal osteotomy associated to 1° phalanx osteotomies for metatarsophalangeal lateral deviation deformities.

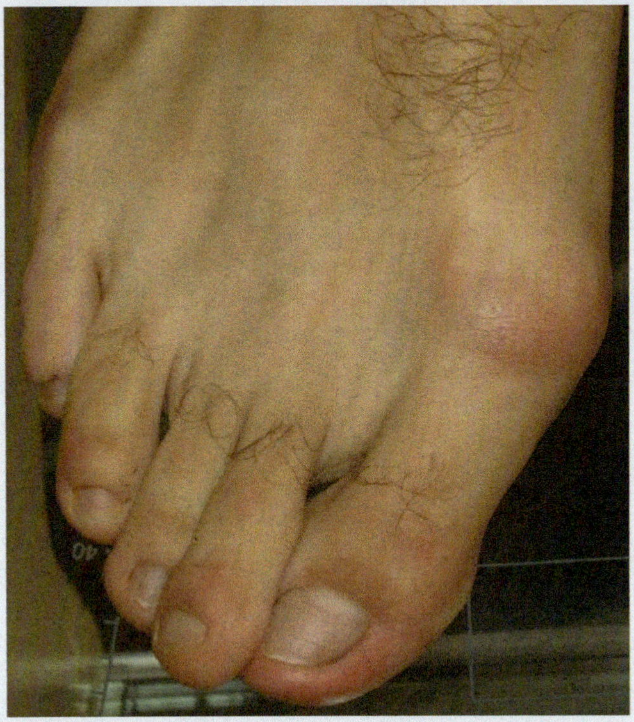

Figure 12.21 Metatarsophalangeal (MTP) pinning in combination with MTT osteotomy (distal oblique minimally invasive metatarsal osteotomy) for MTP dislocation.

When a metatarsal osteotomy is indicated, it is performed first because of the tendon relaxation it allows, sometimes negating procedures initially planned distally. The extent of the dislocation may require associated temporary MTP pinning (Figure 12.21).

Which Techniques for Which Deformities?

The decisional algorithms proposed by Véronique Darcel were presented sequentially according to the analysis of the deformation from proximal to distal with the AFCP classification.

A few examples illustrate the authors' indications.

Deformity in the Sagittal Plane

MTP Dorsiflexion Deformity

Stable MTP deformity in extension (MTPe), without subluxation, requires extensor tenotomies. Monocortical P1 osteotomy for plantarflexion may be indicated as well, even in the case of isolated deformity of the MTP (AFCP: enn) (Figure 12.22; Table 12.6).

When the MTP is unstable, metatarsal (MTT) osteotomies are indicated; percutaneously, the gestures will start with the extensor tenotomy, followed by MTP release depending on the degree of the subluxation, then the MTT osteotomies, and finally the more distal gestures according to the analysis of the deformities.

In the event of MTP dislocation, one can choose combining surgery with open MTT shortening as a Weil osteotomy or stabilize the MTP with pinning after simple resection of a bone cylinder in the metatarsal neck; the diameter of the pin must be at least 1.4 mm to decrease the risk of breaking.

In percutaneous surgery, MTP pinning is possible in combination with a DMMO or a distal oblique minimally invasive metatarsal osteotomy (Figure 12.19).

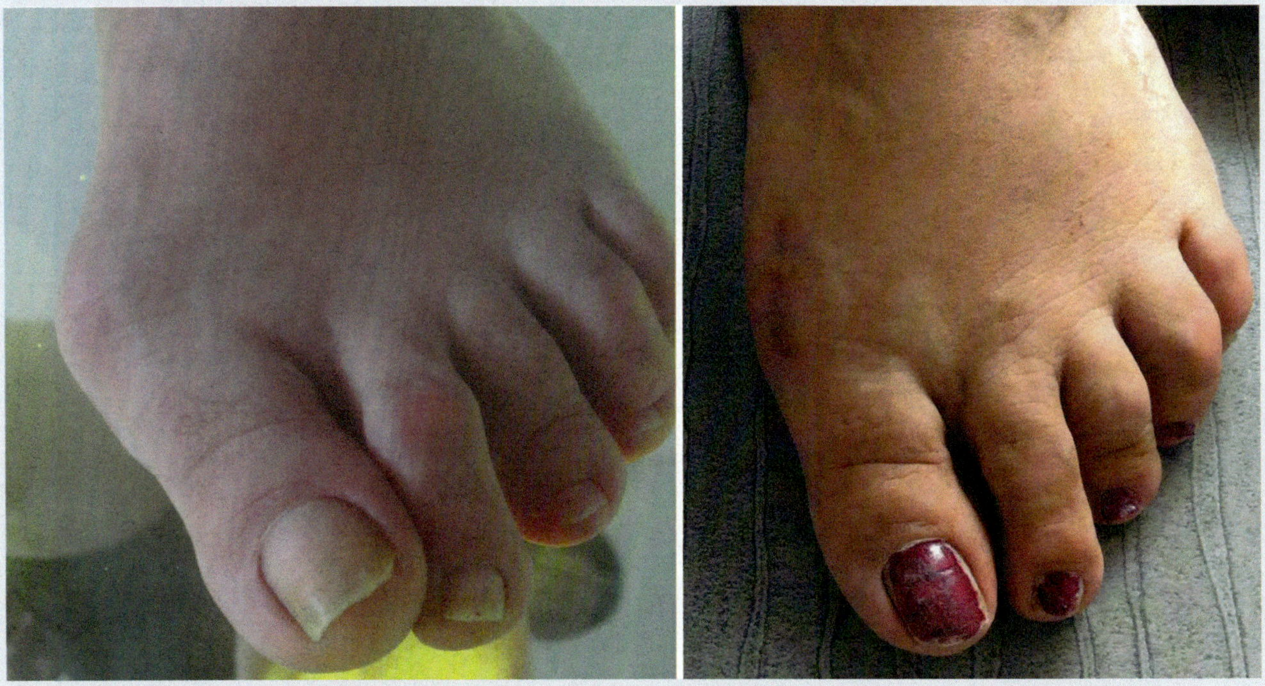

Figure 12.22 2enn deformity according to French Association of Foot Surgery classification.

Table 12.6

MTP Dorsiflexion Deformity

MTPe	Tenotomy	Dorsal MTP Release	MTT Osteotomy	P1 Osteotomy	Others
Stable	EDL-EDB	+/–		+/–	
Unstable	EDL-EDB	+	+	+/–	+/– tendon transfer +/+ PP repair
Dislocated	EDL-EDB	+	+	+/–	+/– tendon transfer +/+ PP repair

EDB, extensor digitorum brevis; EDL, extensor digitorum longus; MTP, metatarsophalangeal; MTPe, MTP deformity in extension; PP, plantar plate; P1, 1° phalanx.

Leaving the MTP dislocated MTP may be decided according to the age and demand of the patient and degree and location of pain.

PIP Plantarflexion Deformity

Faced with a flexible deformity of the PIP in flexion (AFCP nfn), the three associated percutaneous procedures are plantar PIP release, FDB tenotomy, and P1 osteotomy. In case of association with an MTP in extension (AFCP efn), extensors tenotomy is added (Table 12.7).

The authors have studied the effectiveness of these gestures for more than 10 years. The authors' publication in the OTSR in 2015[32] made it possible, with the work of Solenne Frey, to present a prospective series of 57 cases of PIP deformity of the second toe (AFCP nfn or efn). About half of the cases also required extensors tenotomy (efn), but the authors excluded from this study any MTT osteotomy in order to judge the result of these targeted procedures. After 2 years, the authors obtained satisfaction of the patient and the surgeon at almost 90% concerning the correction of the PIP deformity and the active plantarflexion of the toe (Figure 12.23).

FDB tenotomy is not always necessary in a PIP deformity, especially when a possible shortening of P1 allows the shortened tendons to relax.

Table 12.7

PIP Plantar Flexion Deformity

PIPf	Tenotomy	Plantar PIP Release	Phalanx Osteotomy	Others
Flexible	FDB	+	P1	Tendon transfer
Semi rigid	FDB	+	P1	Tendon transfer
Rigid	FDB +/– FDL	+	P1 +/– P2 +/– chondroplasty	Fusion Arthroplasty

FDB, flexor digitorum brevis; FDL, flexor digitorum longus; PIP, proximal interphalangeal; P1, 1° phalanx; P2, 2° phalanx.

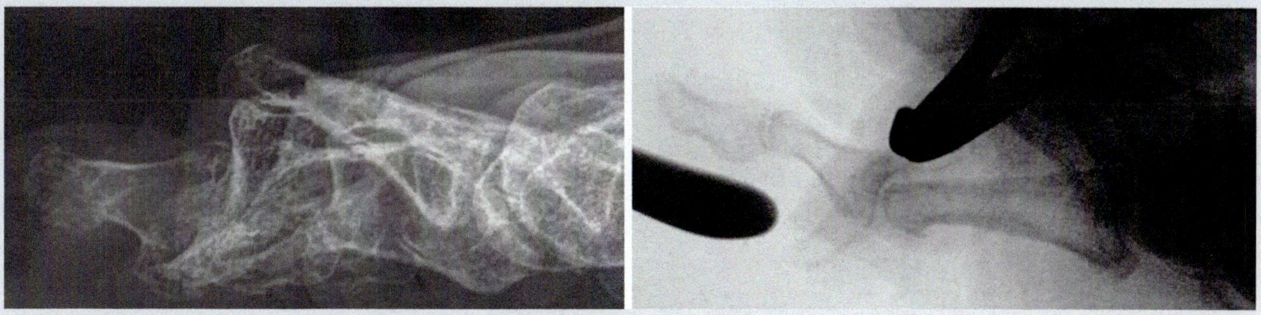

Figure 12.23 Effectiveness of flexor digitorum brevis tenotomy, proximal interphalangeal release, 1° phalanx osteotomy, and EDL-EDB tenotomy for a 2efn according to French Association of Foot Surgery classification.

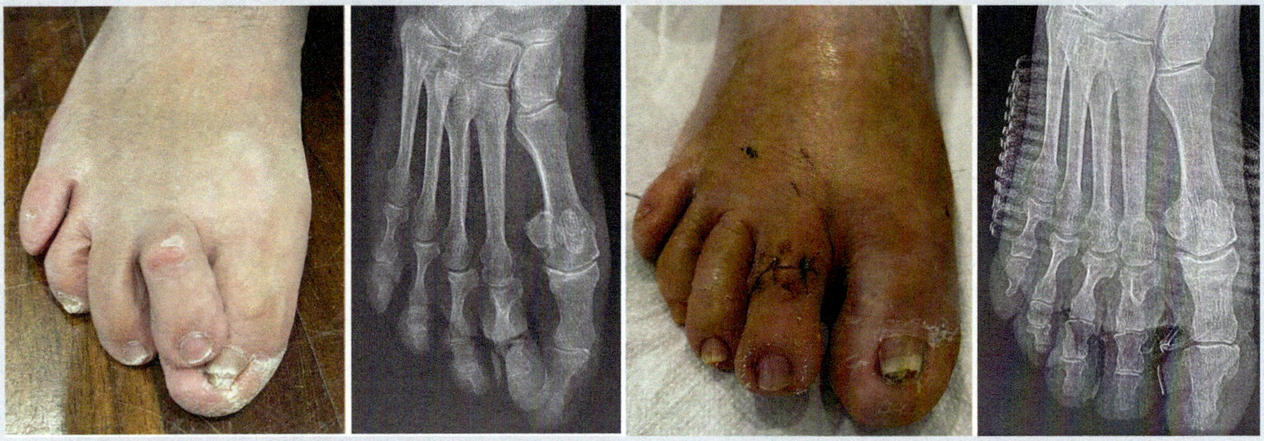

Figure 12.24 Rigid proximal interphalangeal (PIP) deformity. Radiograph before and after flexor digitorum brevis tenotomy and PIP release.

In case of an associated deformity of the DIP in flexion (AFCP nff or eff), FDL tenotomy can be chosen rather than that of the FDB in association with the P1 osteotomy, and EDL-EDB tenotomy is added in case of eff (Figure 12.18).

A recently published study showing connections between the FDL and the FDB on ultrasound described how the tenotomy of the FDL is equivalent to its transfer to the FDB by tensioning these intertendinous structures during the retraction of the FDL at the base of P1.[33]

In case of rigid PIP deformity, fusion is the most practiced technique, often combined with percutaneous tenotomies; many surgeons use resection arthroplasty, which is not the authors' preference due to the risk of lateral deviation.

The authors can push the indications of percutaneous conservative gestures even in case of rigidity of the PIP, whose reducibility can be tested after FDB tenotomy and PIP release under fluoroscopy and in the absence of osteophytes likely to interfere with the shoe (Figure 12.24). For these rigid PIP deformities, a tenodermodesis helps maintain a deformed toe for a long time (Figure 12.25).

Plantarflexion Deformity of the DIP

In case of flexible sagittal deformity of the DIP, FDL tenotomy is performed, while P2 osteotomy is made afterward if necessary (Table 12.8).

In case of stiff, isolated deformity of the DIP, fusion is recommended and fixed by pinning, tenodermodesis, or DIP screw (Figure 12.26).

Deformity in the Horizontal Plane

Medial or Lateral Deviation of the MTP

Lateral deviation of the MTP particularly in the setting of metatarsus adductus is a challenge whatever the chosen technique (open or percutaneous) (Table 12.9).

Horizontal dislocation is treated like a sagittal dislocation.

Instability requires MTT osteotomies; a collateral ligament, extensor, and capsular release is performed first and then the osteotomy of P1 (Figure 12.27).

The authors recommend great caution regarding these releases as excessive release can cause dislocation.

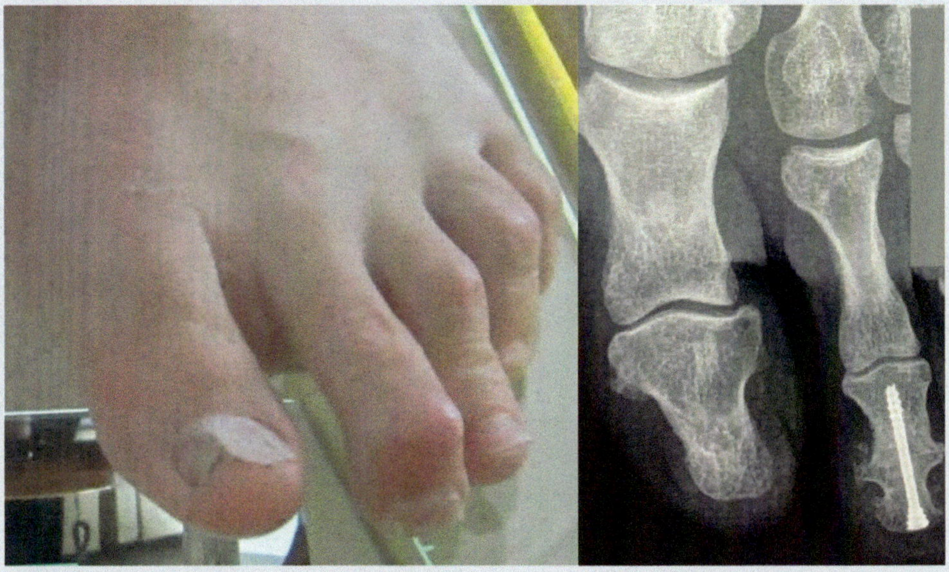

Figure 12.25 Tenodermodesis after reduction of a rigid 2efn.

Table 12.8

Plantarflexion Deformity of the DIP

DIPf	Tenotomy	Osteotomy	Other
Flexible	FDL	+/– P2	
Semirigid	FDL	P2	
Rigid			Arthroplasty Fusion

DIP, distal interphalangeal; FDL, flexor digitorum longus; P2, 2° phalanx.

Without MTP instability, monocortical P1 osteotomy is sometimes sufficient (Figure 12.15).

Medial or Lateral Deviation of PIP

This rare, often posttraumatic deformity is reliably treated by osteotomy if it is a malunion and fusion in the case of rigidity (Table 12.10).

Medial or Lateral Deviation of the DIP

In case of horizontal deformation of the DIP, percutaneous monocortical osteotomy of P2 reorients the oblique surface of an asymmetrical phalanx (Figure 12.17; Table 12.11). Associated tenotomy of the contracted FDL is essential (Figure 12.28).

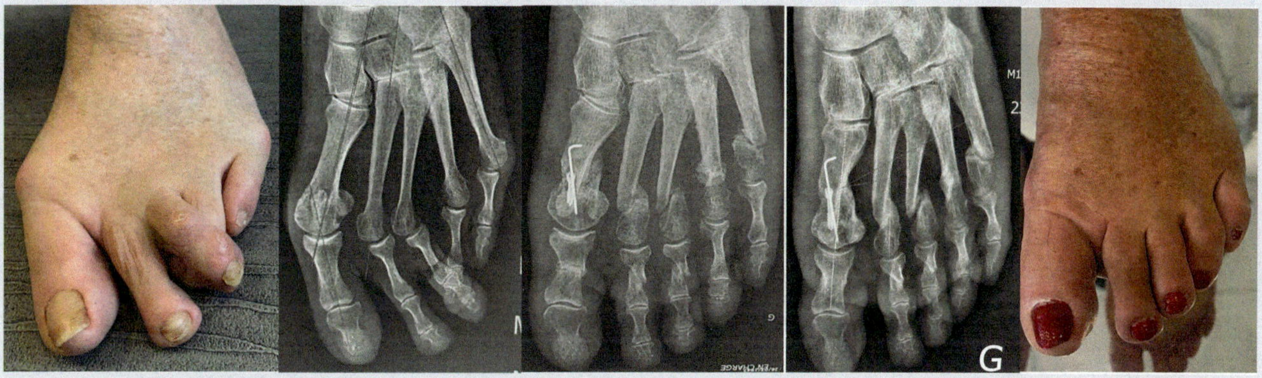

Figure 12.26 Distal interphalangeal fusion with a screw or a 2nnf(r) according to French Association of Foot Surgery classification.

Table 12.9

Medial or Lateral Deviation of the MTP

MTPm MTPl	MTT Osteotomy	P1 Osteotomy	MTP Release	Other
Stable	+/–	+		
Unstable	+	+	+/–	+/– tendon transfer or PP repair
Dislocated	+	+	Dorsal + lateral or medial	+/– tendon transfer or PP repair

MTP, metatarsophalangeal; PP, plantar plate; P1, 1° phalanx.

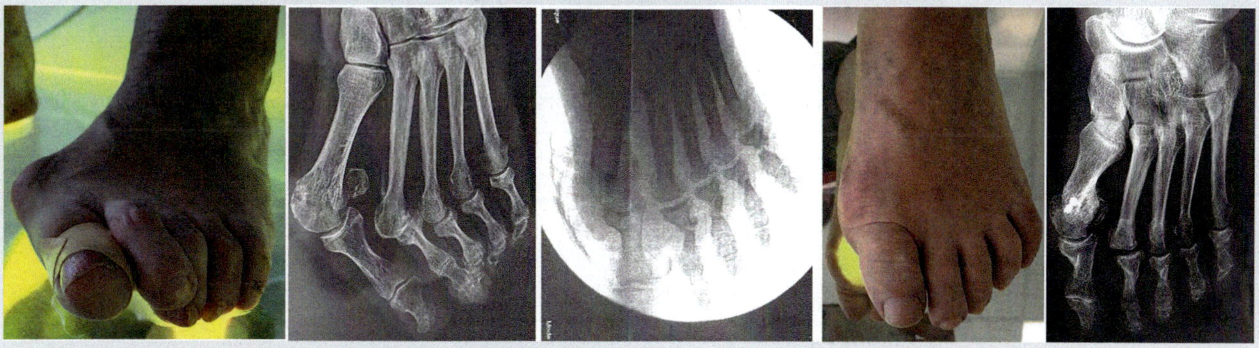

Figure 12.27 Lateral deviation of the metatarsophalangeal (MTP) requiring MTT osteotomies plus lateral MTP release plus phalanx osteotomies.

Table 12.10

Medial or Lateral Deviation of PIP

PIPm PIPl	P1 Osteotomy	PIP Fusion
Flexible	+	
Semirigid	+	+/–
Rigid		+

PIP, proximal interphalangeal; P1, 1° phalanx.

Table 12.11

Medial or Lateral Deviation of the DIP

DIPm DIPl	P2 Osteotomy	DIP Fusion
Flexible	+	
Semirigid	+	+/–
Rigid		+

DIP, distal interphalangeal; P2, 2° phalanx.

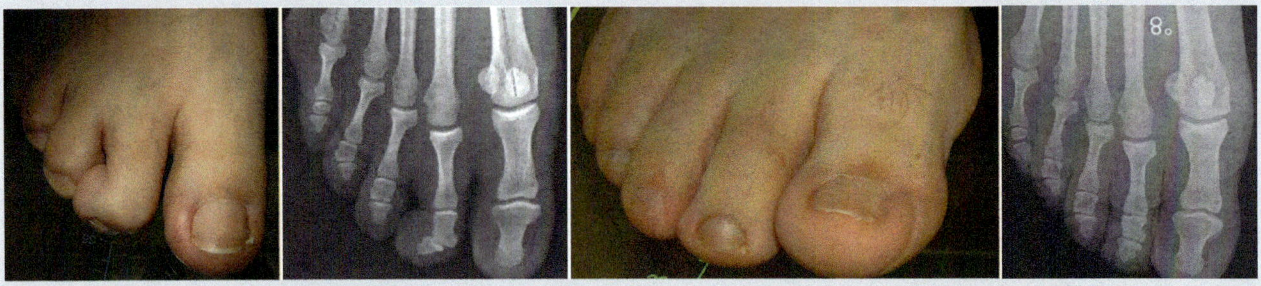

Figure 12.28 Flexor digitorum longus and 2° phalanx osteotomy for 2nnl according to French Association of Foot Surgery classification.

◆ POSTOPERATIVE MANAGEMENT

Percutaneous surgery requires careful follow-up to guide the position of the operated toes and ensure good functional recovery.

The dressing is fundamental. The positioning of a toe operated on percutaneously can easily be modified for 3 weeks (Figure 12.29) but remains possible up to 6 weeks after surgery with taping (Figures 12.30 and 12.31).

Pinning a toe in a noncompliant patient or in the event of a complex deformity is sometimes essential as demonstrated above.

A rigid postoperative shoe or boot is typically maintained for 4 to 6 weeks in the cases of metatarsal osteotomies (Figure 12.32).

Taking the time to educate patients on the ideal positioning and mobilization of the toes help guarantee mutual satisfaction.

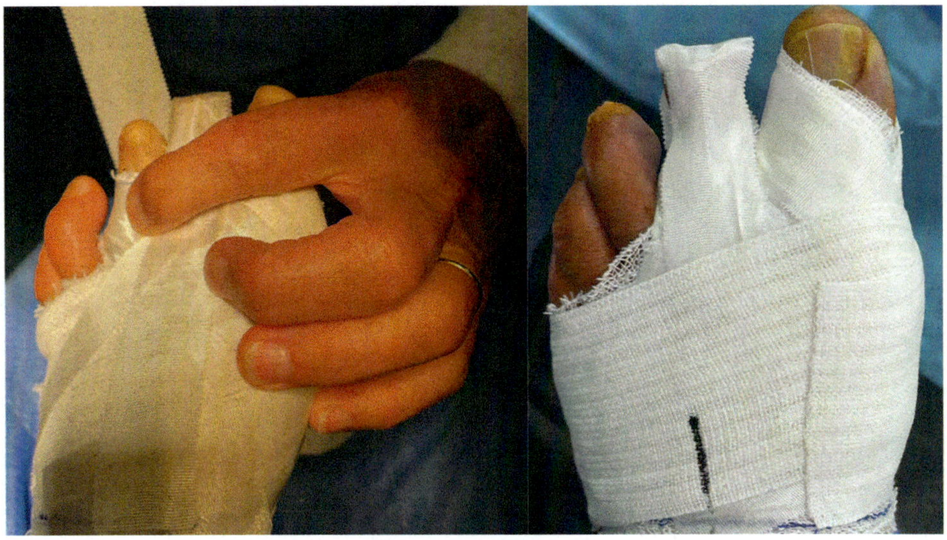

Figure 12.29 Postoperative dressing.

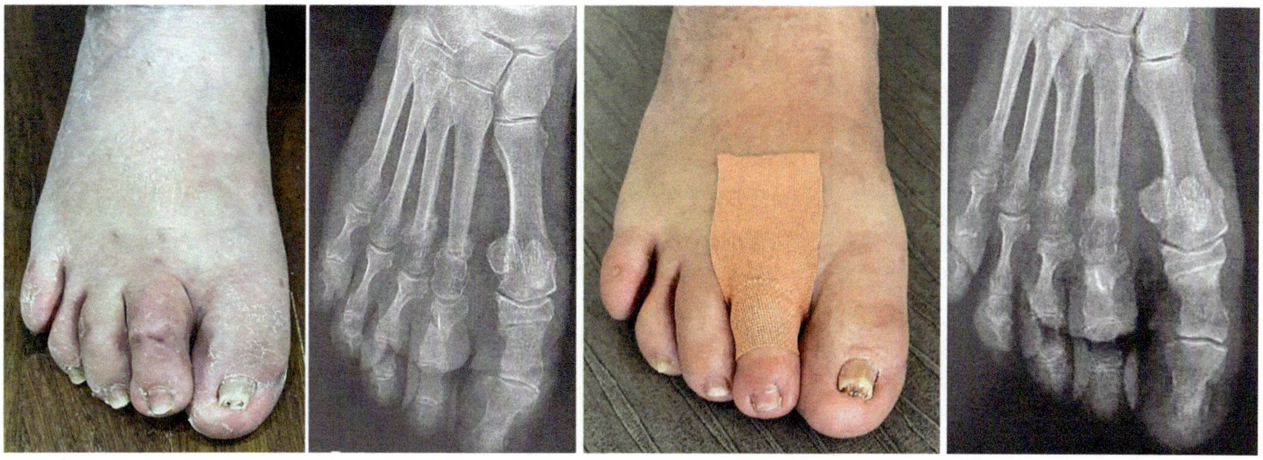

Figure 12.30 Guidance of the second toe seen on image 24 after 45 days with an adhesive tape.

Range of motion exercises for the operated toes are taught after day 45.

◆ TAKE HOME MESSAGES

Treating a toe deformity without treating its cause carries the risks of undercorrection, recurrence, and/or dissatisfaction.

Standardization of the AFCP classification of toe deformity allows collaboration, discussion, and research toward the goal of optimizing techniques for successful treatment of deformity.

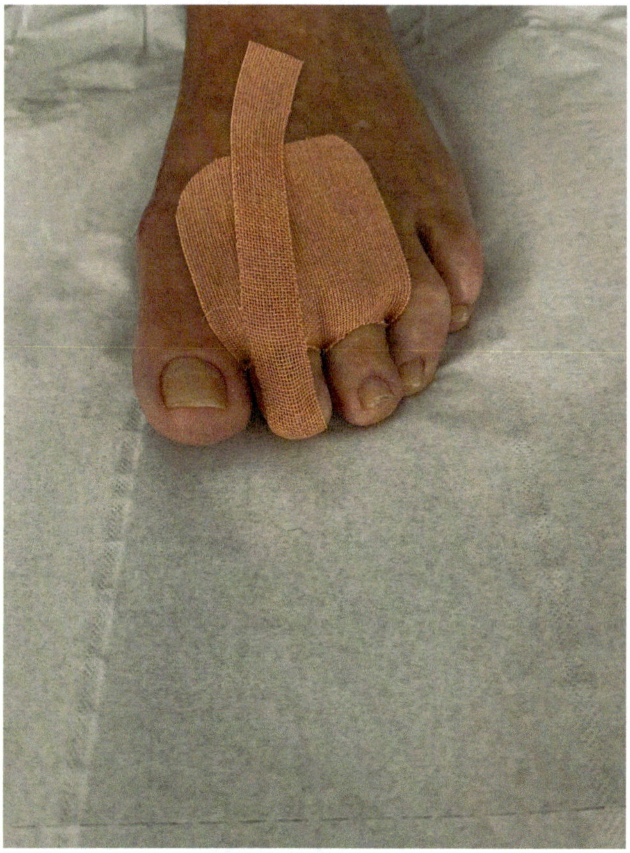

Figure 12.31 Kinesio tape for a rebel second toe.

Begin correction from proximal to distal.

Intraoperative fluoroscopy is necessary in the learning phase or when a specific gesture is indicated.

Extensor tenotomy is not systematic and is only performed if necessary. It is almost mandatory in the event of metatarsophalangeal dislocation.

Dorsal MTP release, also mandatory in case of dislocation, can be dangerous if it is not justified.

Selective tenotomies are the guarantor of maintaining active flexion of the toe.

P2 osteotomy is sometimes a useful complement when the correction of a sagittal PIP deformity is insufficient.

The choice of techniques also depends on the postoperative management; percutaneous surgery requires follow-up to guide the position of the operated toes and ensure their good functional recovery. Pinning a toe in a noncompliant patient or in the event of a complex deformity and taking the time to educate the patients on the ideal positioning and on their mobilization are the guarantees of mutual satisfaction.

Knowing how to master all the open techniques remains essential given the complexity of certain deformities and according to the etiologies, in particular neurological and degenerative.

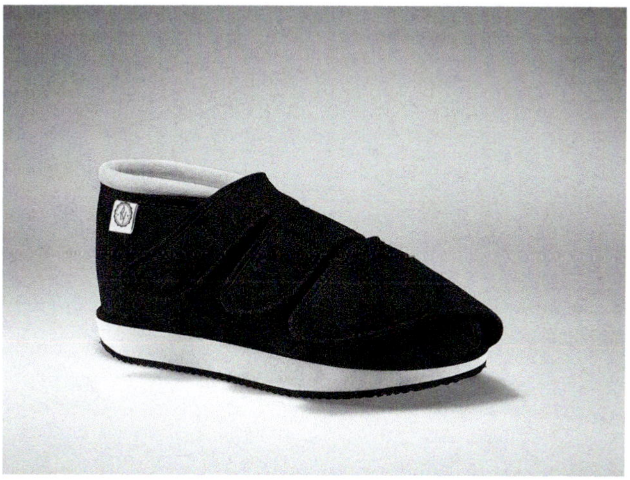

Figure 12.32 Rigid postoperative shoe for 3 to 4 weeks.

References

1. Chalayon O, Chertman C, Guss AD, Saltzman CL, Nickisch F, Bachus KN. Role of plantar plate and surgical reconstruction techniques on static stability of lesser metatarsophalangeal joints: a biomechanical study. *Foot Ankle Int.* 2013;34(10):1436-1442.
2. Barg A, Courville XF, Nickisch F, Bachus KN, Saltzman CL. Role of collateral ligaments in metatarsophalangeal stability: a cadaver study. *Foot Ankle Int.* 2012;33(10):877-882.
3. Hill CL, Gill TK, Menz HB, Taylor AW. Prevalence and correlates of foot pain in a population-based study: the North West Adelaide health study. *J Foot Ankle Res.* 2008;1(1):2.
4. Menz HB, Barr ELM, Brown WJ. Predictors and persistence of foot problems in women aged 70 years and over: a prospective study. *Maturitas.* 2011;68(1):83-87.
5. Hannan MT, Menz HB, Jordan JM, Cupples LA, Cheng C-H, Hsu Y-H. High heritability of hallux valgus and lesser toe deformities in adult men and women. *Arthritis Care Res.* 2013;65(9):1515-1521.
6. Buldt AK, Menz HB. Incorrectly fitted footwear, foot pain and foot disorders: a systematic search and narrative review of the literature. *J Foot Ankle Res.* 2018;11:43.
7. Coughlin MJ. Lesser toe deformities. In: Coughlin M, Saltzman R, Anderson R, eds. *Mann's Surgery of the Foot and Ankle.* 9th ed. Elsevier Saunders; 2014:357-361.
8. Lintz F, Beldame J, Kerhousse G, et al. Intra- and inter-observer reliability of the AFCP classification for sagittal plane deformities of the second toe. *Foot Ankle Surg.* 2020;26(6):650-656.
9. Bernasconi A, Beldame J, Darcel V, et al. Podoscopic classification of second toe deformities. *Foot Ankle Surg.* 2021;27(7):750-754.
10. Menz HB, Auhl M, Spink MJ. Foot problems as a risk factor for falls in community-dwelling older people: a systematic review and meta-analysis. *Maturitas.* 2018;118:7-14.
11. Thompson FM, Hamilton WG. Problems of the second metatarsophalangeal joint. *Orthopedics.* 1987;10(1):83-89.
12. Panchbhavi VK, Trevino S. Clinical tip: a new clinical sign associated with metatarsophalangeal joint synovitis of the lesser toes. *Foot Ankle Int.* 2007;28(5):640-641.
13. Trasposizione del flessore superficiale di II-III-IV-V dito alla falange basale pro interossei. *Chirurgia del Piede.* 2009;33(3): 161-162. Accessed October 31, 2021. https://www.minervamedica.it/it/riviste/chirurgia-piede/articolo.php?cod=R32Y2009N03A0161
14. Thevenin E. Imagerie de la plaque plantaire. EM-Consulte. Accessed February 17, 2022. https://www.em-consulte.com/article/1019280/article/imagerie-de-la-plaque-plantaire
15. Sung W, Weil L, Weil LS, Rolfes RJ. Diagnosis of plantar plate injury by magnetic resonance imaging with reference to intraoperative findings. *J Foot Ankle Surg Off Publ Am Coll Foot Ankle Surg.* 2012;51(5):570-574.
16. Masson E. Place des techniques de « strain-counterstrain » dans l'arsenal du thérapeute manuel en pratique quotidienne. EM-Consulte. Accessed February 17, 2022. https://www.em-consulte.com/article/723129/place-des-techniques-de-strain-counterstrain-dans-
17. Grice J, Marsland D, Smith G, Calder J. Efficacy of foot and ankle corticosteroid injections. *Foot Ankle Int.* 2017;38(1):8-13.
18. Prado MD, Ripoll PL, Golanó P. *Cirugía percutánea del pie: técnicas quirúrgicas, indicaciones, bases anatómicas.* Elsevier-Masson; 2003.
19. *Minimally Invasive Foot Surgery Surgical Techniques Indications.* Accessed February 17, 2022. https://www.citalivres.com/pdf/minimally-invasive-foot-surgery-surgical-techniques-indications-anatomical-basis
20. Frey-Ollivier S, Catena F, Hélix-Giordanino M, Piclet-Legré B. Treatment of flexible lesser toe deformities. *Foot Ankle Clin.* 2018;23(1):69-90.
21. Darcel V. Les deformations des orteils latéraux. *Orthop Traumatol Surg Res.* 2022;108(6):S1-S10.
22. Butterworth M. Tendon transfers for management of digital and lesser metatarsophalangeal joint deformities. *Clin Podiatr Med Surg.* 2016;33(1):71-84.
23. Losa Iglesias ME, Becerro de Bengoa Vallejo R, Jules KT, Trepal MJ. Meta-analysis of flexor tendon transfer for the correction of lesser toe deformities. *J Am Podiatr Med Assoc.* 2012;102(5):359-368.
24. Valtin B, Leemrijse T. Pathologie des orteils: clinique et traitement chirurgical. *Pathologie du pied et de la cheville.* Tsunami. Masson; 2015:227-242.
25. Elmajee M, Shen Z, A'Court J, Pillai A. A systematic review of plantar plate repair in the management of lesser metatarsophalangeal joint instability. *J Foot Ankle Surg.* 2017;56(6):1244-1248.
26. Akoh CC, Phisitkul P. Plantar plate injury and angular toe deformity. *Foot Ankle Clin.* 2018;23(4):703-713.
27. Mirmiran R, Younger M. Lesser digit implants. *Clin Podiatr Med Surg.* 2019;36(4):651-661.
28. Hendrick SE, Kannegieter E. SmartToe, ToeGrip and buried k-wire versus percutaneous k-wire fixation for 2nd PIPJ arthrodesis: a comprehensive review of outcomes. *Foot Edinb Scotl.* 2020;45:101692.
29. Guelfi M, Pantalone A, Daniel JC, Vanni D, Guelfi MGB, Salini V. Arthrodesis of proximal inter-phalangeal joint for hammertoe: intramedullary device options. *J Orthop Traumatol.* 2015;16(4): 269-273.
30. Wei RX, Ling SK, Lui T, Yung PS. Ideal implant choice for proximal interphalangeal joint arthrodesis in hammer toe/claw toe deformity correction: a systematic review. *J Orthop Surg.* 2020;28(1):2309499020911116.
31. Redfern D. Treatment of metatarsalgia with distal osteotomies. *Foot Ankle Clin.* 2018;23(1):21-33.
32. Frey S, Hélix-Giordanino M, Piclet-Legré B. Percutaneous correction of second toe proximal deformity: proximal interphalangeal release, flexor digitorum brevis tenotomy and proximal phalanx osteotomy. *Orthop Traumatol Surg Res.* 2015;101(6):753-758.
33. Beldame J, Lalevée M, Regnard S, et al. Impact of intertendinous connections between the flexor digitorum brevis and longus on percutaneous tenotomy for the treatment of claw toes: an anatomic and ultrasound study. *Surg Radiol Anat.* 2021;43(7): 1067-1073.

PART

2 Midfoot

13 Tarsometatarsal Fusion

Patrick J. Maloney and Adam Lukasiewicz

◆ INTRODUCTION

Arthrodesis is the standard surgical intervention for end-stage arthritis of the tarsometatarsal (TMT) joints. When nonoperative treatment options fail to provide adequate pain relief and restoration of function, then it is time to consider surgical intervention. Minimally invasive approaches to joint preparation are described in the literature for several different areas of the foot and ankle. Common joints that are prepared for arthrodesis through a percutaneous, minimally invasive and/or arthroscopic technique include the ankle, subtalar, hallux, and transverse tarsal joints. With modern techniques and instrumentation, arthrodesis of the TMT joints can also be achieved through minimally invasive techniques.

◆ INDICATIONS AND CONTRAINDICATIONS

Indications for minimally invasive arthrodesis of the TMT joints are similar to indications for traditional open arthrodesis. Arthrodesis is the gold standard surgical intervention for end-stage arthritis of the midfoot. The underlying cause of the arthritis may be primary osteoarthritis, inflammatory, or posttraumatic.

Similar to open arthrodesis, percutaneous arthrodesis should be considered when appropriate nonoperative treatments have failed to provide adequate pain relief and/or return to desired level of function. Nonoperative treatments include shoe modifications, orthotics, immobilization, oral/topical anti-inflammatory medications, and intra-articular injections. Details regarding these interventions are not within the scope of this chapter.

In addition to arthrodesis, surgical cheilectomy of dorsal osteophytes is another operative technique that has some utility in treating midfoot arthritis. This is typically reserved for mild to moderate arthritis and/or in patients who are unable to comply with postoperative weight-bearing restrictions necessary to achieve adequate fusion. Depending upon the location of the osteophyte formation, a percutaneous approach can be utilized. Caution does have to be exercised when considering minimally invasive cheilectomy due to the proximity of neurovascular and tendon structures to the bone being removed (Figures 13.1 and 13.2).

In addition to arthrodesis for osteoarthritis, percutaneous arthrodesis can also be utilized in the setting of acute or subacute fractures and dislocations involving the TMT joints. Primary arthrodesis versus open reduction internal fixation is a topic with numerous comparative studies. The decision to proceed with primary arthrodesis includes a multitude of factors. Anatomic considerations include fracture pattern, joint(s) involved, intra-articular extension, and time since injury. Patient factors include comorbidities, soft-tissue envelope, and desired level of activity postoperatively. Finally, surgeon preference and experience can also play a role in the decision to perform primary arthrodesis.

Contraindications for percutaneous TMT arthrodesis again mirror those of open arthrodesis. These include medical comorbidities that inhibit surgery, active infection, and sepsis. In addition, there are anatomic factors that may force the surgeon to opt for or convert to an open approach for arthrodesis. These factors include large dorsal spurring, which may inhibit access to the joints, chronic dislocated/subluxated joints that are not amenable to closed or limited open reduction, and location of articular surfaces, which may not be accessible to allow for adequate joint preparation. As with preparation of any articular surface for fusion, it is paramount that the surgeon successfully removes all of the articular cartilage surface and prepares a healthy and bleeding bone surface. Then, it is imperative to directly oppose and stabilize the bony surfaces so that arthrodesis may occur.

◆ PATIENT HISTORY AND PHYSICAL EXAMINATION

Patients with TMT arthritis typically present with pain in the middle of the arch, particularly with pushing off. Patients may recall a prior traumatic injury to the foot, but many patients have primary osteoarthritis or inflammatory arthritis without any specific trauma. The pain is usually reduced in stiffer and more built-up shoes. Some patients may notice a dorsal prominence over the midfoot that makes lacing up shoes or wearing tight shoes painful. Occasionally, patients will report burning pain in the first web space due

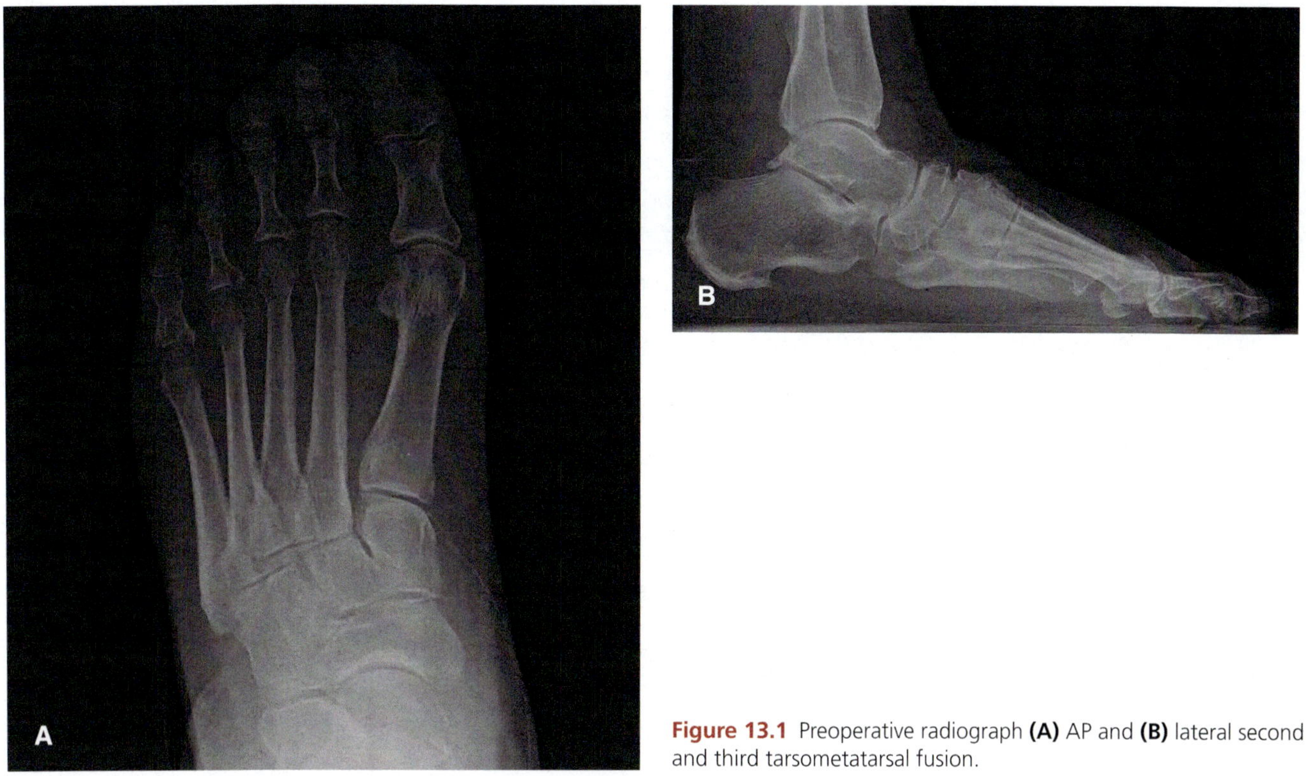

Figure 13.1 Preoperative radiograph **(A)** AP and **(B)** lateral second and third tarsometatarsal fusion.

to irritation and tenting of the deep peroneal nerve over the dorsal midfoot prominence. If there is significant deformity through the TMT joints, such as in Charcot, patients may note collapse of the medial longitudinal arch and abduction of the forefoot.

The most notable examination finding is dorsal tenderness of the involved TMT joints. With careful palpation, the metatarsal shafts, the five TMT joints, and three naviculocuneiform joints can be separately examined. A "piano key" test can be used to help identify the involved joints. To perform this maneuver, the midfoot is stabilized with one hand, and a metatarsal head is moved dorsally and plantarly to stress the corresponding TMT joint. If this provokes pain, arthritis is likely present. Both the dorsalis pedis and posterior tibial arteries should be palpated to ensure adequate pulses. The dorsalis pedis needs to be identified and avoided during surgery, and the posterior tibial artery may be the only major blood supply to the foot in the event of inadvertent iatrogenic injury to the dorsal artery. Moreover, adequate perfusion is required to achieve arthrodesis whether an open or percutaneous technique is used. The patient should be examined while weight bearing to compare the alignment of the foot to the contralateral side to identify deformity. If there is a history of prior surgery or trauma in the midfoot, the extensor tendons, especially the tibialis anterior, should be palpated to ensure that they can be readily identified and avoided during the placement of the bur. A basic neurological examination should be performed. If there is concern for neuropathy, the foot should be examined with a 5.07 Semmes-Weinstein monofilament to check for protective sensation. Occasionally, percussion over the course of the deep peroneal nerve may produce a Tinel sign with tingling in the first web space.

◆ IMAGING STUDIES

Weight-bearing three-view radiographs of the foot can reliably demonstrate deformity and osteoarthritis. On the anterior-posterior view, arthritis is indicated with joint space narrowing, subchondral sclerosis, and periarticular cysts. Instability can be demonstrated by widening of the interspace between the first and second metatarsals. The cuneiforms and metatarsal bases are typically closely aligned, and instability can also be seen with step-off between the cortices of the metatarsal base and cuneiform. Because of the coronal-plane midfoot arch, the third TMT joint is often better visualized on the oblique view. On the lateral view, instability of the TMT joints can be demonstrated by dorsal translation of the metatarsal base or widening of the plantar aspect of the TMT joint compared to the dorsal aspect.

Computed tomography (CT) studies, weight bearing if available, may be helpful in the setting of deformity or comminuted fractures in the midfoot or metatarsal bases. CT may also help to identify exactly which joints are involved and should be incorporated into the fusion, which can be challenging using plain films and examination alone.

Magnetic resonance imaging (MRI) can be used to identify a purely ligamentous Lisfranc injury. MRI may also help clarify which joints are arthritic and should be fused, but CT is usually sufficient for this purpose.

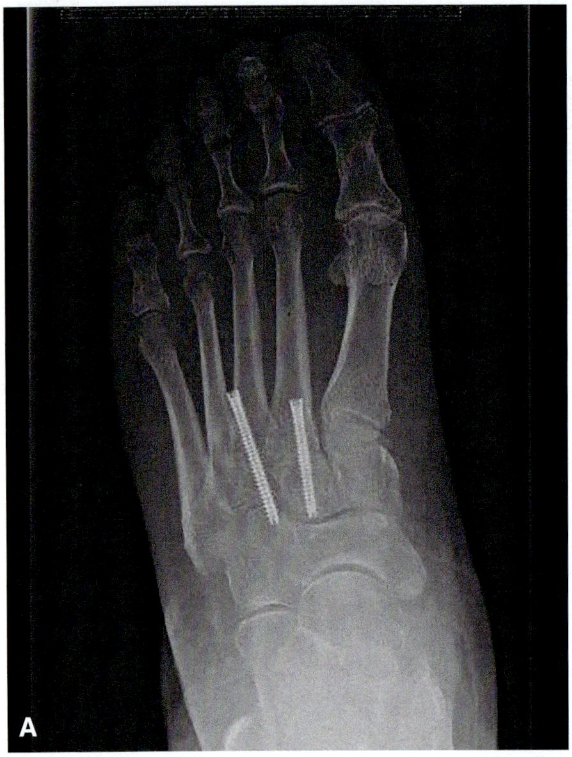

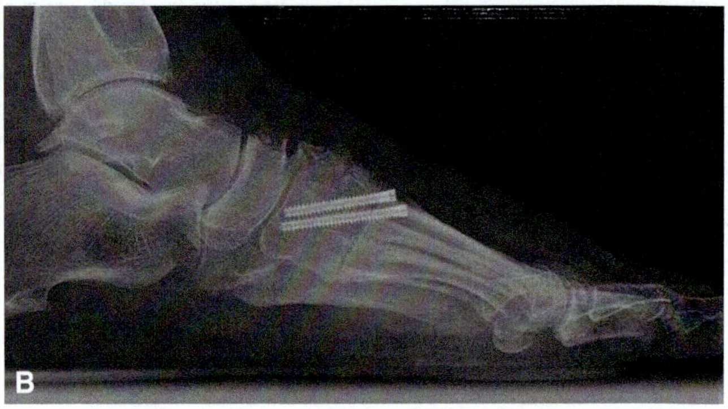

Figure 13.2 Postoperative radiograph **(A)** AP and **(B)** lateral second and third tarsometatarsal fusion.

◆ PREOPERATIVE PLANNING AND PREPARATION

The most critical step in preoperative preparation is to identify the joints to be included in the fusion. The physical examination and imaging studies both contribute to decision-making, and advanced imaging should be obtained to help make a final decision if there is any doubt. At the end of the procedure, the foot should be plantigrade with the first metatarsal in line with the long axis of the talus. In many cases, *in situ* arthrodesis at the TMT joints can maintain an appropriate alignment. In cases with deformity through the TMT joints, preparation of the joint surfaces is often sufficient to allow for reduction of the deformity. In more severe deformities, a wedge resection of the metatarsal base may be necessary to restore alignment and should be planned preoperatively (Figure 13.3).

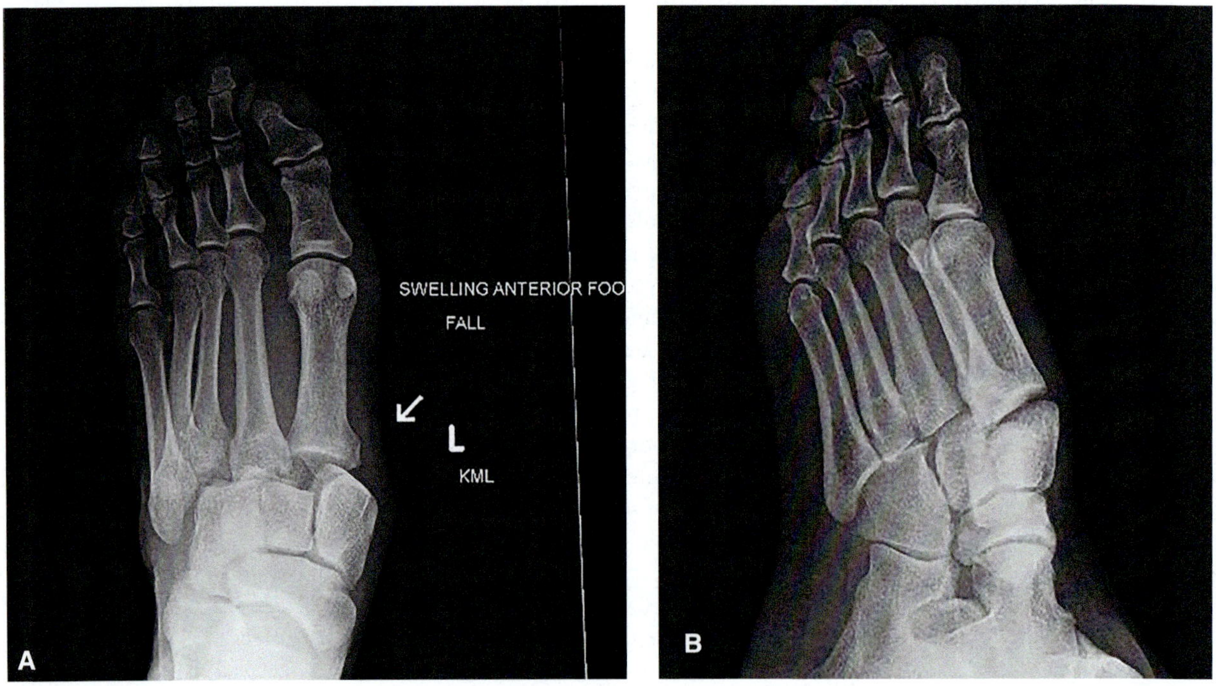

Figure 13.3 Preoperative radiographs **(A)** AP, **(B)** oblique, and **(C)** lateral open reduction and internal fixation (ORIF) midfoot fracture-dislocation with minimally invasive (MIS) tarsometatarsal fusion.

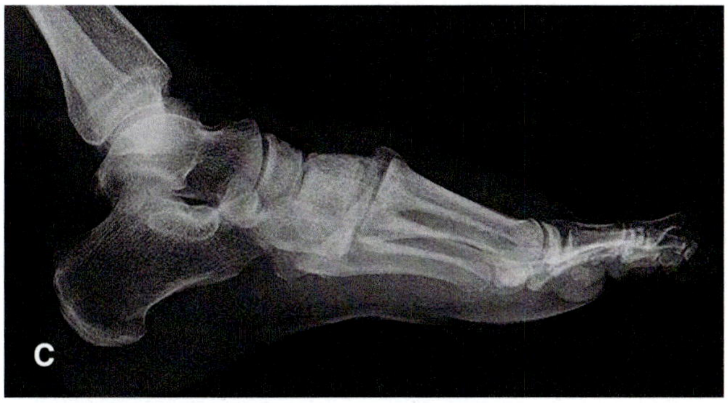

Figure 13.3 *(Continued)*

SURGICAL TECHNIQUE

The first consideration regarding surgical technique is patient and fluoroscopy positioning. Similar to other percutaneous procedures, regular use of fluoroscopy is critical to confirm location of the burr and other tools, as well as to judge the degree of bony resection and joint reduction. The patient is positioned supine on the operative table. The foot needs to be hanging just off the edge of the bed to allow for position of the base of the fluoroscopy unit onto the plantar aspect of the foot. A bump is placed under the ipsilateral hip and proximal thigh so as to position the leg and foot so that the toes are pointed directly up (Figure 13.4). This helps to facilitate access to the dorsal midfoot and appropriate imaging.

The first step of the procedure is gaining access to each joint. For the first TMT, it is typically approached from the dorsomedial aspect. This can minimize potential damage to the extensor hallucis longus tendon straight dorsally, the tibialis anterior insertional fibers medially, and the deep neurovascular bundle dorsolaterally. There is potential for irritation and/or damage to the dorsomedial cutaneous nerve as it extends down toward the hallux. For the second TMT, the joint can be approached from directly dorsal. Care should be taken to avoid the deep neurovascular bundle medially. In addition, superficial peroneal sensory branches are often present in the subcutaneous layer and potentially the second extensor digitorum longus tendon coursing distally from laterally. For the third TMT, a direct dorsal approach is also used. Similar to the approach to the second, superficial peroneal sensory branches as well as the second and third extensor digitorum longus tendons should be avoided. Arthrodesis is not typically performed for the fourth and fifth. However, percutaneous cheilectomy can be considered. The incision and approach are typically made more lateral than dorsal to facilitate the angle of the burr insertion (Figure 13.5).

Once an approach has been selected, the joint is first identified with an 18-gauge spinal needle. Entry into the joint is confirmed with fluoroscopy. Then, a 2-mm incision can be made at the area of the needle insertion with an 11 or 15 blade. This incision should be made through the skin only. Blunt dissection can be continued to and even through the joint capsule with a hemostat. Another option for entry through the joint capsule is the use of either a freer elevator or another straight elevator (Figure 13.6).

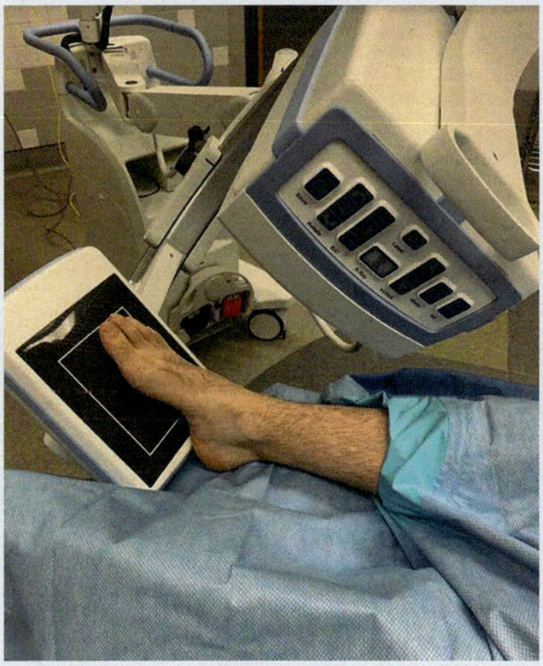

Figure 13.4 Patient positioning.

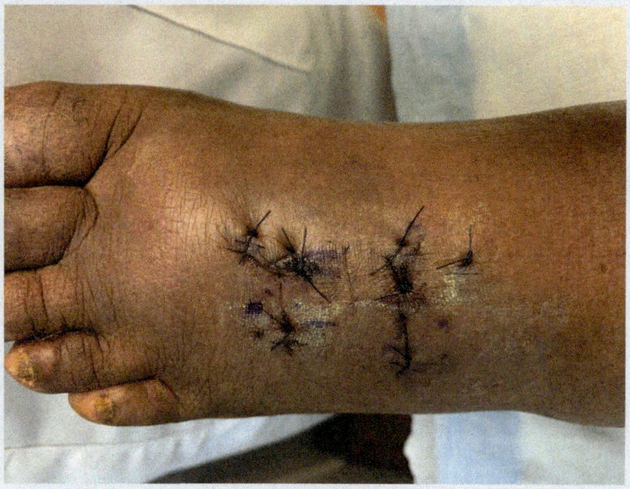

Figure 13.5 Clinical image of incisions 2 weeks postoperative.

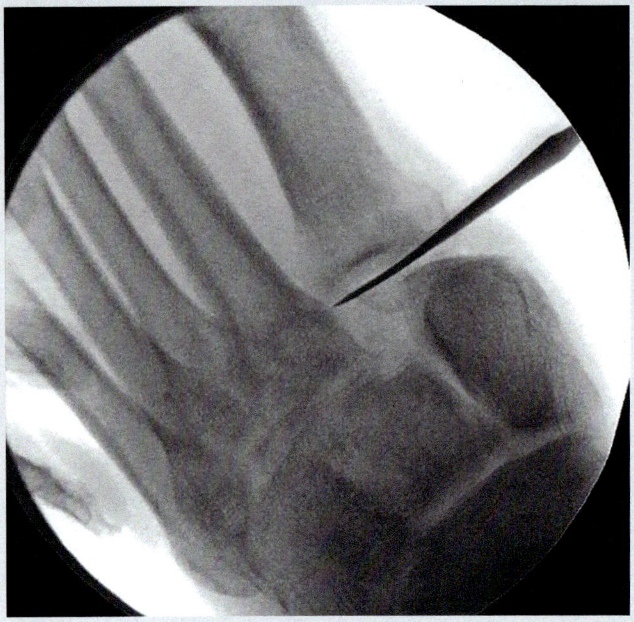

Figure 13.6 Intraoperative fluoroscopy, mobilizing joint with freer elevator.

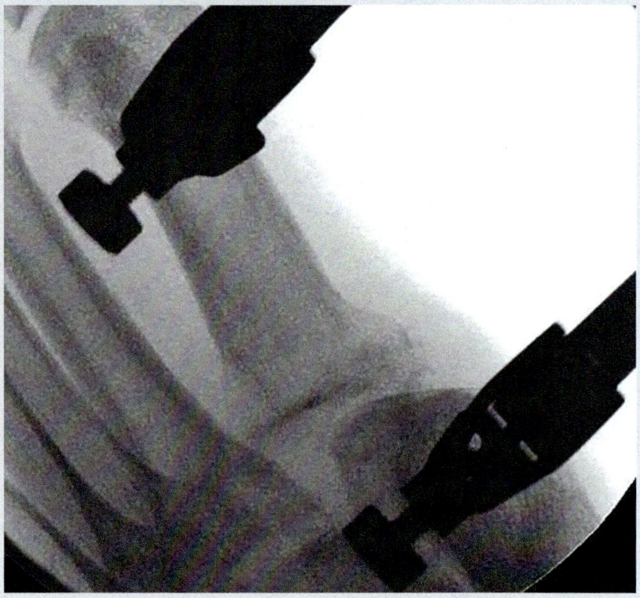

Figure 13.7 Intraoperative fluoroscopy, creating space in the first tarsometatarsal joint with distractor.

To provide adequate space for passage of the burr, it might be necessary to use a pin distractor. K-wires can be placed percutaneously into the cuneiform body and the corresponding metatarsal. Distal pin can be placed either in the proximal metaphysis or into the diaphysis. A pin in the metaphysis may interfere with placement of guidewires for cannulated screw fixation. However, placement of the distractor pin within the diaphysis may potentially put the patient at risk for iatrogenic fracture. Care should be taken to place distractor pins as perpendicular to the long axis of the joints as possible so that if desired, the same distraction device can be used to facilitate compression and reduction of the joint after preparation is completed (Figure 13.7).

Once an entryway into the joint has been established, the burr is inserted to begin joint preparation. The surgeon can utilize different burr tips based upon individual preference (Figure 13.8). A straight Shannon burr is thinner and may be easier to access the joint, especially the more plantar aspects. However, a conical-shaped burr is more adept at resection of the chondral surfaces without removing as much subchondral bone. Both the metatarsal base and cuneiform articular surfaces need to be débrided appropriately down to a subchondral bone level. It is important to understand the shape and contour of the surfaces, as the metatarsal bases tend to be more concave and the cuneiforms more convex. This is especially true of the first TMT. The surgeon must be meticulous with the resection to minimize the risk of overshortening while also adequately débriding to an appropriate depth.

To perform the joint preparation, the burr is rotated and to a lesser extent translated back and forth. This allows for the tip of the burr to débride away the chondral layers down to the subchondral bone. The surgeon can utilize low speeds during joint preparation by only partially depressing the foot pedal, which powers the burr. This can help to minimize overresection. During débridement, serial fluoroscopic images are obtained to repeatedly confirm position of the burr and the degree of any bony resection.

In addition to visual evidence of fluoroscopy, the surgeon can use auditory feedback from the burr to understand when it is débriding away chondral layers versus when it has encountered bone. The pitch of the sounds is different and requires attention as well as experience to accurately distinguish the difference.

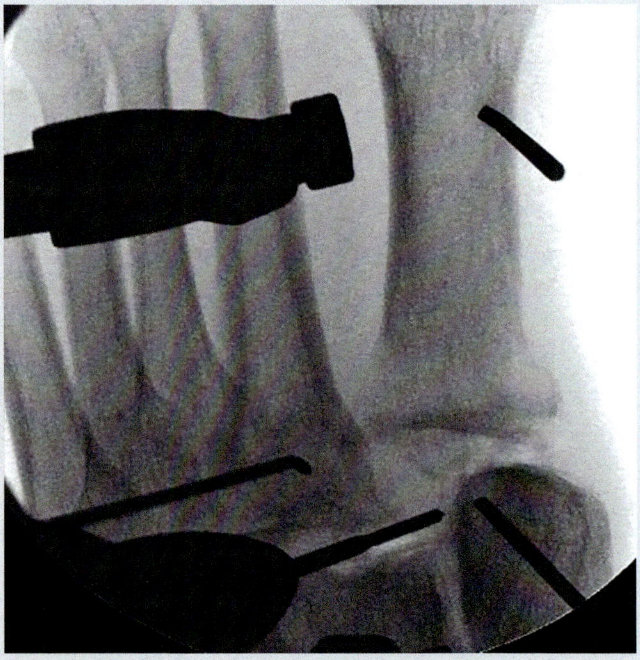

Figure 13.8 Intraoperative fluoroscopy, preparing second tarsometatarsal joint with burr.

Most current burr systems utilize an irrigation mechanism. This serves the dual purpose of keeping the temperature of the burr tip down to minimize the risk of thermal necrosis and to assist with irrigation of the joint. Additional irrigation is also required to adequately remove all chondral debris.

Although not routinely needed, some surgeons might prefer adding a quick arthroscopy concurrently with joint preparation. This can both provide an inflow of irrigation to adequately cleanse the joint as well as providing direct visualization of the bony surfaces. The space within the TMT joints may not be conducive for a 2.7-mm scope. However, a 1.9-mm scope or a single-use disposable scope system can be small enough to fit within the same space occupied and created by the burr.

Once the surgeon is satisfied with débridement of the articular surfaces, perforation of the subchondral bone can be performed. This can be completed with a microfracture pic, a drill, or a K-wire. Depending upon the surgeon's preference, bone graft can then be placed. A mosquito clamp is often useful to insert graft without extending the incision.

At this time, the surgeon can proceed to reduction and fixation. Joint reduction and compression can be performed manually, with percutaneously placed clamps and/or with the compression/distraction device utilized earlier in the procedure. Again, it is critical to use fluoroscopy in multiple angles and views to confirm appropriate reduction and direct bony apposition (Figure 13.9).

Fixation is typically completed with percutaneously placed cannulated screws. Size, design, number, and orientation of screws are dependent upon individual surgeon preferences. Care should be taken during insertion of hardware with delicate technique to minimize damage to soft-tissue structures. For cannulated screw placement, it is important to first ensure adequate placement of the guidewire. The position of the wire should be confirmed on anteroposterior, oblique, and lateral fluoroscopic views. Then, an accurate depth measurement must be obtained to ensure that there is no screw prominence either dorsally or plantarly. Fluoroscopy can be used to assess appropriate seating of the measuring device so that the screw length measurement is accurate. For drilling and screw insertion, soft-tissue retraction is performed with drill sleeves, soft-tissue protectors, and/or manual retraction devices (Figure 13.10).

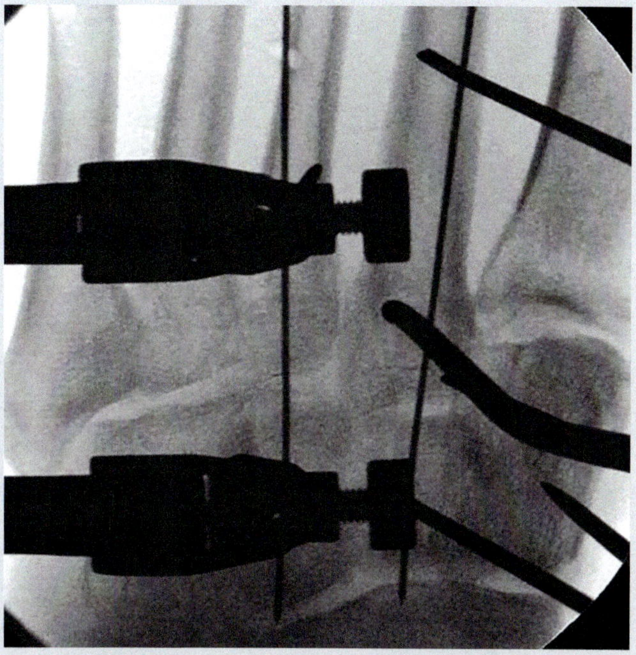

Figure 13.9 Intraoperative fluoroscopy, compression of the third tarsometatarsal joint with device, and placement of cannulated screw guidewire.

Once fixation is completed, guidewires and distractor pins can be removed. At this time, it is critical to assess the construct from multiple fluoroscopic angles. The first TMT is typically best visualized with a more direct AP foot view. This view also allows for visualization of the medial aspect of the second. An oblique view allows for better visualization of the lateral aspect of the second, both aspects of the third, and the medial aspect of the fourth. Then, lateral views are obtained. It may be necessary to slightly rotate the foot in order to view the dorsal and plantar aspects of the joints, as well as the position and length of screws.

Incisions are then closed. Typically, 3-0 nylon can be used to perform closure of all incisions. Following closure, dressings are applied (Figure 13.11). Dressing application is left up to the preference of the individual surgeon. Then, the leg is placed into a well-padded splint in a neutral position at the ankle.

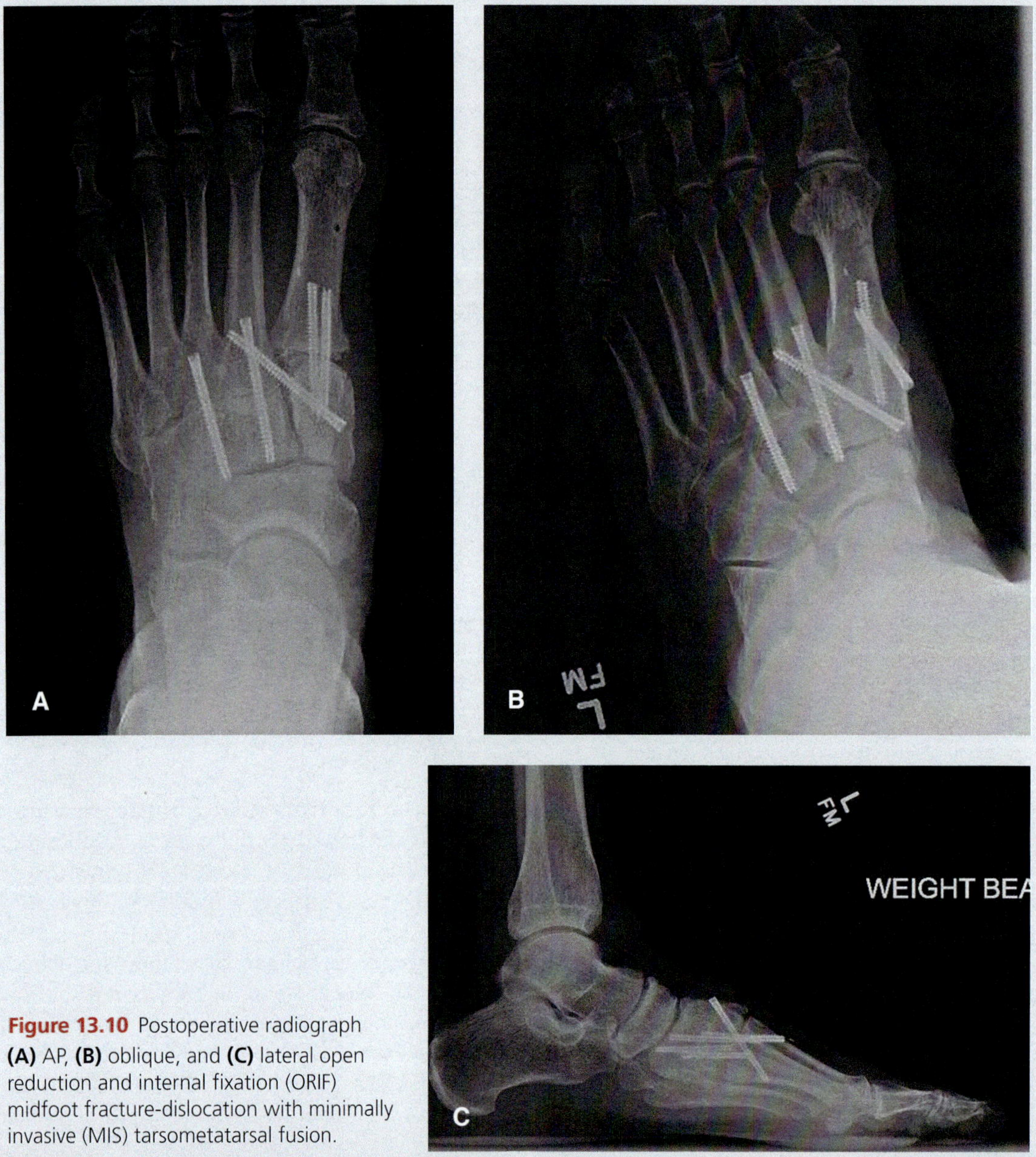

Figure 13.10 Postoperative radiograph **(A)** AP, **(B)** oblique, and **(C)** lateral open reduction and internal fixation (ORIF) midfoot fracture-dislocation with minimally invasive (MIS) tarsometatarsal fusion.

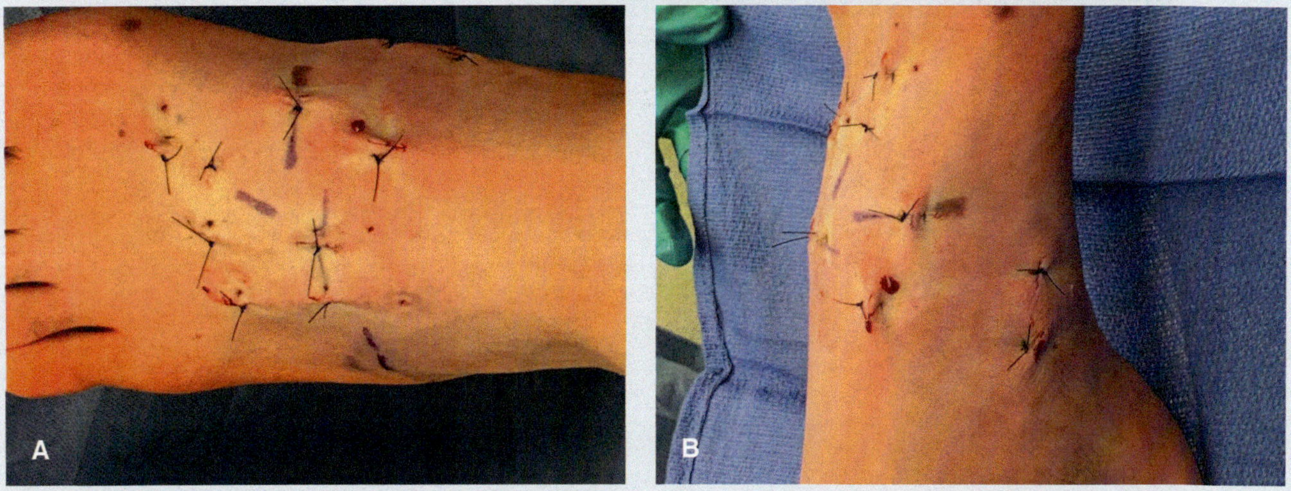

Figure 13.11 Intraoperative clinical photos **(A, B)** after closure.

◆ POSTOPERATIVE MANAGEMENT

Postoperatively, the patient is kept non–weight bearing. Typically, at 10 to 14 days, the patient returns for suture removal. Use of the percutaneous techniques often results in less soft-tissue edema postoperatively. This may allow for transition to a removable boot rather than require a period of cast immobilization. Patients wear the boot for 23 hours each day, removing it for hygiene and gentle active ankle range of motion. Initiation of weight bearing may begin 6 to 8 weeks postoperatively. If indicated, they begin physical therapy. The patient can transition to a regular shoe with the addition of a rigid orthosis at 8 to 10 weeks. By 12 weeks, the patient is able to wean out of the rigid orthosis and resume desired level of activity. Specific postoperative protocols are up to the individual surgeon and may need to be altered depending on various patient factors, which can affect the rate of healing.

Radiographs are obtained at each visit to ensure alignment is alignment is maintained and to assess for consolidation at the fusion sites. A CT scan can be utilized to assess for bony union around 12 weeks postoperatively if plain radiographs are not conclusive.

In patients with diabetes, neuropathy, smoking, tenuous perfusion, or other comorbidities placing them at high risk of nonunion, weight bearing is often delayed until 12 weeks. In this higher-risk population, a CT is often obtained to assess the degree of fusion prior to initiation of weight bearing.

While there is no clear evidence for prophylactic anticoagulation after percutaneous TMT fusion or other foot and ankle procedures, aspirin 81 mg daily for patients without risk factors for thromboembolic disease is typically prescribed.[1,2] In patients at high risk for the development of venous thrombus, low molecular weight heparin or direct oral anticoagulants may be prescribed. Anticoagulation prophylaxis continues until patients begin weight bearing.

Pain is well controlled initially with regional anesthesia, which typically provides 12 to 24 hours of no pain. As sensation does start to return, the pain is managed with oxycodone for the first few days, as well as acetaminophen and nonsteroidal anti-inflammatory medications. Patients are encouraged to elevate in order to minimize swelling and use gabapentin if needed for neuropathic pain.

◆ OUTCOMES

There has been sparse literature to date on the outcomes of TMT fusions using minimally invasive (MIS) techniques. Vernois and Redfern described using a Shannon burr to perform joint preparation for a Lapidus fusion in 70 patients.[3] They had good to excellent satisfaction in 95% of patients and four nonunions. Chaparro and colleagues performed Lapidus fusion in 10 ft in eight patients using a Shannon burr for joint preparation and an intramedullary nail for fixation.[4] In this study, radiographic correction was satisfactory, and the only complication noted at 18 months was a return to the operating room for screw removal. Miller described percutaneous osteotomy for correction of Charcot foot deformities, including 14 midfoot procedures.[5] The procedures were performed using a Shannon burr to make the osteotomy cuts and wedge burr to mill the bone between the cuts. Of the 14 patients with midfoot procedures, 4 had deep infection requiring partial removal of hardware and 3 had hardware failure. There are no reported outcomes in the literature for primary TMT fusion using a percutaneous technique for osteoarthritis.

In the authors' experience, the outcomes of MIS TMT fusion are comparable to the results of open TMT fusion procedures. Historically, the fusion rate for TMT fusion has been reported to be 90% to 95%. Patient satisfaction is generally reported at 90% with marked improvement in outcome measures and visual analog pain scores.[6] Removal of hardware may be required in up to 20% of patients due to persistent irritation.[7]

The authors have used a percutaneous approach to TMT fusion mostly in patients with Charcot arthropathy, lymphedema, or other conditions at high risk for poor wound healing. Wound healing, postoperative swelling, and fusion have all been comparable to published fusion rates using traditional open techniques in these high-risk patients. In this select patient population, the complications have been less than with a more traditional open approach.

References

1. American Orthopedic Foot and Ankle Society. *The Use of Venous Thromboembolic Disease Prophylaxis in Foot and Ankle Surgery Position Statement.* 2020 Feb.
2. The ICM-VTE Foot & Ankle Delegates. International Consensus Meeting on Venous Thromboembolism. *J Bone Joint Surg Am.* 2022;104:163-175.
3. Vernois J, Redfern D. Lapidus, a percutaneous approach. *Foot Ankle Clin.* 2020;25:407-412.
4. Chaparro F, Cárdenas PA, Butteri A, Pellegrini MJ, Carcuro G, Ortiz C. Minimally invasive technique with intramedullary nail for treatment of severe hallux valgus. *J Foot Ankle.* 2020;14(1):3-8.
5. Miller RJ. Neuropathic minimally invasive surgeries (NEMESIS): percutaneous diabetic foot surgery and reconstruction. *Foot Ankle Clin.* 2016;21:595-627.
6. Nemec SA, Habbu RA, Anderson JG, Bohay DR. Outcomes following midfoot arthrodesis for primary arthritis. *Foot Ankle Int.* 2011;32(4):355-361.
7. Dock CC, Freeman KL, Coetzee JC, McGaver RS, Giveans MR. Outcomes of nitinol compression staples in tarsometatarsal fusion. *Foot Ankle Orthop.* 2020;5(3).

14 Charcot Foot

Roslyn J. Miller

◆ INTRODUCTION

Collaborative efforts by multidisciplinary diabetic foot teams have significantly reduced morbidity and mortality from the risks associated with diabetic foot disease.[1-13] High-pressure areas secondary to foot deformity results in recurrent ulceration in patients with Charcot neuroarthropathy (CN). Repeated skin breakdown has a negative impact on their quality of life due to multiple hospital visits to treat or prevent sepsis and amputation.[14-16] Reconstructive surgery has been shown to improve patient-reported outcomes by reducing amputation rates.[3,4,12,17,18]

Orthopedic foot and ankle surgeons are better equipped to address these complex cases.[19] "Superconstruct" internal fixation and extended arthrodesis, with Charcot-specific reconstruction systems, facilitates earlier surgical intervention preventing significant, difficult-to-manage deformities.[20] With percutaneous skin incisions, minimally invasive surgery (MIS) corrects abnormal biomechanics with minimal disruption of the surrounding tissue leading to lower risk of infection.[2] External circular frames can also be used either in isolation or in conjunction with internal fixation.

◆ BACKGROUND

CN leads to loss of foot and ankle sensation in patients most commonly with diabetes. Microfracture and disorganized bone healing results in a rocker bottom deformity of the midfoot.[8] The gradual and progressive destruction of the architecture of the midfoot arch increases the risk of ulceration and osteomyelitis. Initially, the medial column is affected, where deformity may remain static or progress to the lateral column.[21]

Secondary changes in collagen fibers due to glycosylation caused by sensorimotor and autonomic neuropathy result in progressive tightness of the gastrocnemius and soleus muscle complex. The resulting equinus deformity of the ankle and talus, +/− cuneiforms is countered by opposing forces from the tibialis anterior and posterior muscles.[8,12,22] Ultimately, a midfoot break occurs due to failure of the plantar osseous-ligamentous structures. Ulceration occurs due to the increased peak plantar pressures in the forefoot and midfoot caused by the rocker bottom deformity.

Classification systems are important tools for understanding the progression and severity of CN and determining the appropriate treatment approach. Two commonly used classifications for CN are the Eichenholz and Brodsky classifications, based on the disease's clinical, anatomical, and radiological location.[23,24] The Eichenholz classification is a three-stage system based on the degree of osteolysis. In contrast, the Brodsky classification is a four-stage system based on the degree of bone and joint destruction. These classifications are widely used and have been validated in several studies.

The Tiruveedhula classification combines clinical features and radiographic parameters with the anatomic location of the disease to determine which patients would benefit from percutaneous tendo-Achilles lengthening and total contact casting (TCC).[25] This classification system is useful for determining the appropriate surgical intervention for patients with CN.

Sammarco midfoot classification helps to determine which midfoot pattern may benefit from the "superconstruct" fixation method.[26] This classification system helps to identify the specific midfoot pattern and select the appropriate surgical technique to correct the deformity.

Despite the usefulness of these classification systems, there are also limitations, such as the patient's functional status or the presence of ulceration, so each should be used in conjunction with other clinical and functional assessments to ensure accurate diagnosis and management of CN.

◆ INDICATIONS AND CONTRAINDICATIONS

Historically, the management of the acute phase of CN has been TCC. MIS techniques and the development of implants specifically designed for Charcot reconstruction make early surgical intervention in the acute phase to prevent deformity possible.[2]

Neuropathic minimally invasive surgery (NEMISIS) performed via percutaneous incisions under fluoroscopic guidance have certain advantages over traditional TCC. One of the main benefits of NEMISIS is correcting the deformity early on before it becomes severe and difficult to manage. This can improve healing and reduce the risk of reulceration and amputation.

NEMISIS also allows for preserving the patient's mobility and quality of life, as it is less invasive and has a shorter recovery time than traditional open surgery.

MIS exostectomy can be used in the later stages of CN or in patients who are poor candidates for major reconstructive surgery. Bony prominences are removed to redistribute forces across the whole foot, reducing the risk of further ulceration. Exostectomy should only be performed when the foot is stable with fused midfoot joints as there is a risk of exacerbating the deformity otherwise.[27]

With regard to patient selection, there must be adequate skin coverage and sufficient bone stock to support using intramedullary beams, nails, and bolts for reconstruction.[28-30] For single-stage reconstruction, it is important that there is no active infection.

◆ PATIENT HISTORY AND PHYSICAL EXAMINATION

Patient History

Key questions in the patient history include the following:

- Cause of neuropathy?
- How much protective sensation is present?
- Are peripheral pulsed palpable?
- If the patient is diabetic, are they diet, tablet, or insulin controlled?
- Are there any sign of ischemia present?
- Are there any cardiovascular, renal, or other sequelae of diabetes present?
- What is the patient's current mobility?
- Who is at home?
- Do they smoke?
- How do they get around?

Physical Examination

- Check for neuropathy with monofilament test.
- Check peripheral pulses—consider vascular assessment or referral.
- Assess for any Achilles contracture.
- Examine non-weight bearing and weight bearing to determine high-pressure areas from:
  - Bony prominences and rocker bottom on the foot
  - Check for any signs of active infection.
  - Check for temperature difference.
  - Check if any peripheral edema present.

◆ IMAGING STUDIES

- Standard weight-bearing radiographs include an AP ankle and AP, lateral, and oblique foot views to determine deformity.
- MRI to assess for active Charcot, infection, and bone marrow edema.
- CT with 3D reconstructions to aid with surgical planning.

◆ PERIOPERATIVE PLANNING AND PREPARATION

Preoperative Prophylaxis[2,29,30]

Naseptin nasal cream and Hibiscrub use for 5 days before the procedure effectively reduces the risk of infection from *Staphylococcus*. The use of these antibiotics for 5 days before the procedure is found to be sufficient to reduce the bacterial load and prevent postoperative infection.

Anesthesia

Surgery is performed under general or spinal anesthesia, with popliteal block to allow for a reduced dose of an anesthetic agent, decreasing the risk of complications such as respiratory depression or sedation. Regional block also provides additional pain relief. Intravenous antibiotics are administered before, during, and after the surgery.

SURGICAL TECHNIQUE

Setup

The patient is supine with their feet off the end of the operating table.[30] This facilitates access for the mini C-arm, which is used for intraoperative fluoroscopy. The leg is prepared to the knee to allow for the possibility of external fixator application. A calf tourniquet may be applied if pulses are present.

Procedure

Achilles tendon lengthening is an important step in midfoot reconstruction for patients with CN. Patients with Achilles tendon contractures have increased midfoot pressures with increased risk of ulceration.[2,22,25,30] Percutaneous Achilles tendon lengthening allows the calcaneus to become plantigrade with the ground.

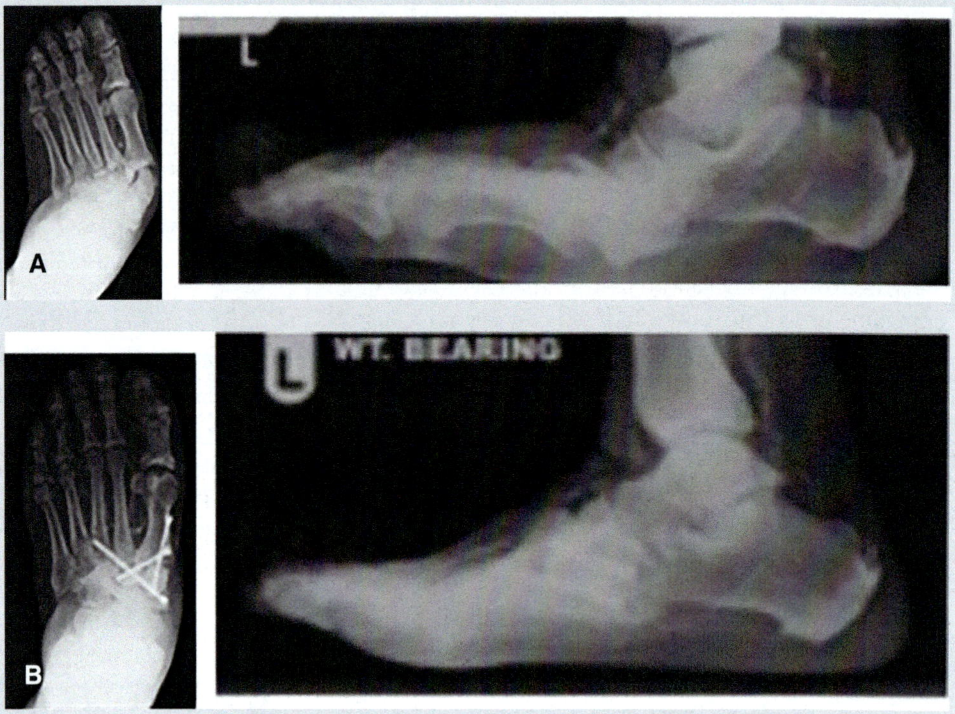

Figure 14.1 Preoperative **(A)** radiographs showing rocker bottom deformity, and postoperative **(B)** radiographs showing midfoot correction.

The midfoot incision is made along the medial column, the central portion of the foot typically affected by CN. The incision is made in a dorsal, medial, and longitudinal direction. This approach allows the surgeon to access the affected area with minimal disruption to the surrounding tissues.[30]

The triplanar closing wedge osteotomy corrects severe Charcot deformities in multiple planes (Figure 14.1). A medially based midfoot osteotomy corrects deformity in the sagittal and transverse planes (Figure 14.2).[29-31] A combination of 3-mm-long Shannon burrs and 3- and 4-mm wedge burrs are used to excise the medial-based wedge. A tourniquet is not used for the procedure. Copious refrigerated saline (37 °F) via a bulb syringe is used to cool the burr in order to reduce the risk of skin and bone thermal necrosis. The burr flutes should be frequently cleaned during the procedure to facilitate cutting, and multiple burrs may be necessary depending on the bone quality.

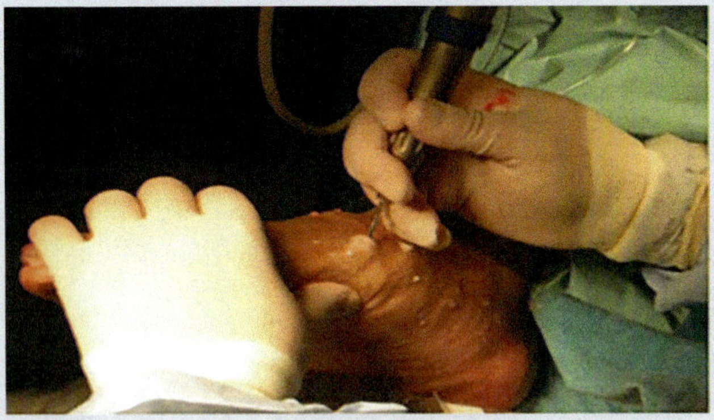

Figure 14.2 Medial percutaneous incision for bone wedge excision.

Two-millimeter K-wires or Steinman pins are inserted medial to lateral, encompassing the apex of the deformity to act as a cutting tract (Figures 14.3 and 14.4).[30]

A second lateral incision may be necessary to allow for proper repositioning of the forefoot relative to the proximal midfoot in any plane.[30]

The concept of the "superconstruct," with beams and bolts, which spans adjacent joints, was first introduced by Grant in 1991 and further developed by Sammarco in 1994.[32,33]

The bone resection shortens the foot allowing adequate reduction of the deformity and reducing tension on the soft-tissue envelope. Internal fixation can be combined with external fixation, if necessary, as described by Lamm et al.[34]

In cases with severe fragmentation of the navicular bone with the involvement of the perinavicular joints, traditional techniques of sparing the talonavicular joint may not be possible. In these situations, arthrodesis (fusion) of the talonavicular joint, and potentially the subtalar joint, is necessary to correct the deformity, properly adhering to the principles of the superconstruct spanning beyond the zone of injury to include unaffected joints for improved fixation.[32]

If dorsal dislocation of the midfoot joint is present at the tarsometatarsal, naviculocuneiform, or talonavicular joints, it is necessary to span the medial column for proper correction. This can be accomplished through an antegrade approach through the first metatarsal head or a retrograde approach from the talus.[27,33-35]

A single beam or bolt to the medial column alone may be insufficient for stability. Additional fixation with a 5-mm bolt into the second and/or third metatarsal and cuneiform

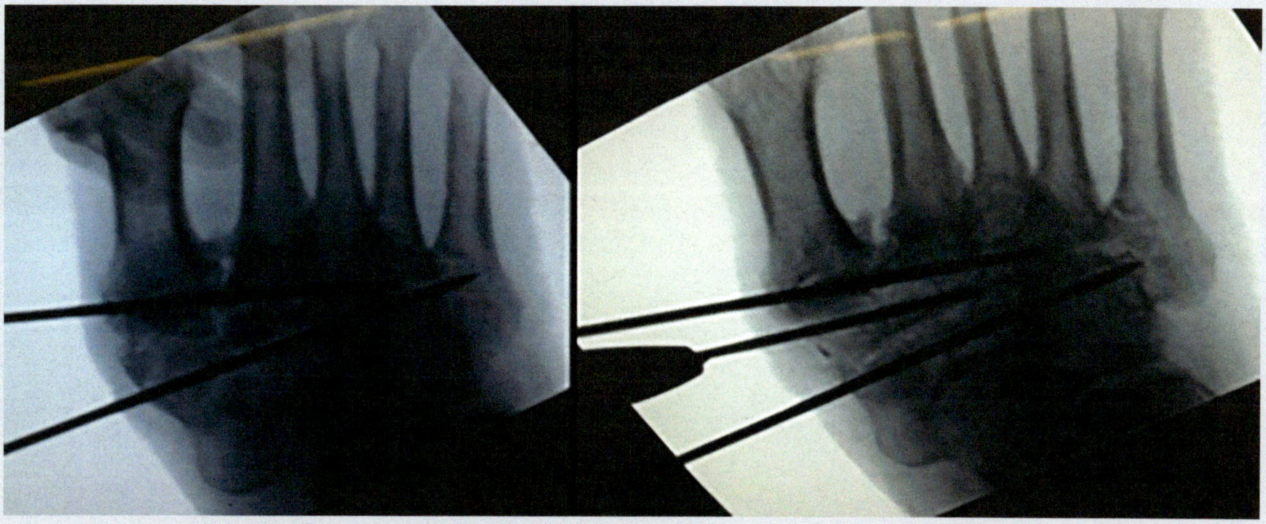

Figure 14.3 Wires placed to guide bone wedge excision.

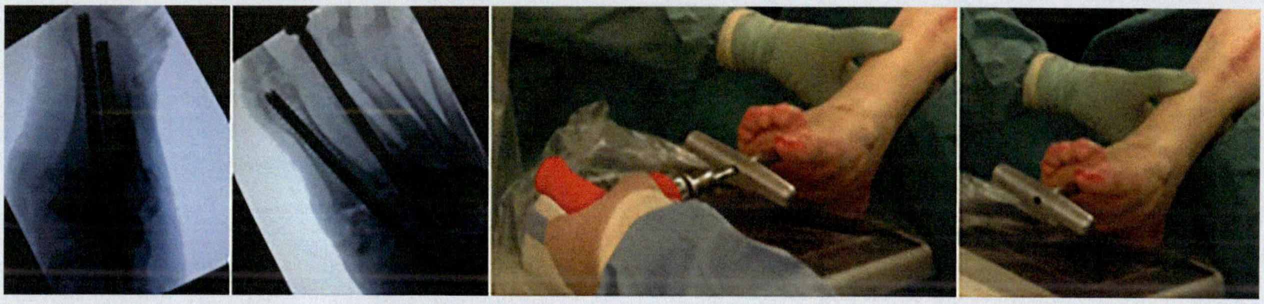

Figure 14.4 Intraoperative and clinical pictures showing Charcot arthropathy "superconstruct."

or talus is recommended. The second metatarsal should be stabilized first and, if significant calcification of the Lisfranc ligament is present, it should be débrided with a 3-mm wedge burr to achieve proper reduction and correction of the deformity (Figure 14.5).[30]

Untreated deformity of the lateral column can lead to recurrence of the rocker bottom deformity. Five-millimeter bolts are typically used to fixate the fourth and/or fifth metatarsals to the cuboid or calcaneus to align and stabilize the foot (Figure 14.6).

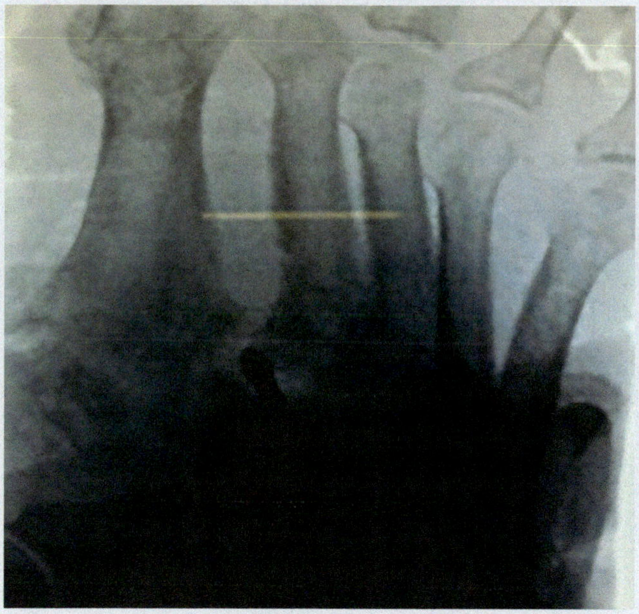

Figure 14.5 Intraoperative AP fluoroscopy view showing débridement of a calcified Lisfranc ligament with a 3-mm wedge burr.

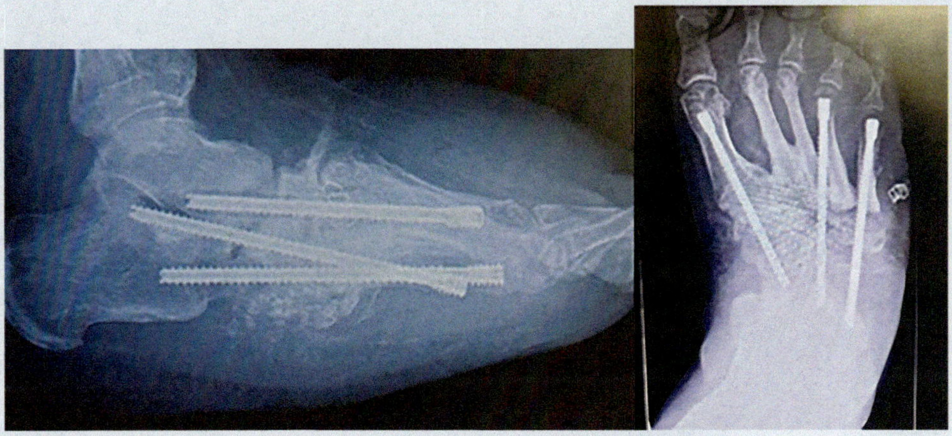

Figure 14.6 Postoperative AP and lateral radiographs showing inclusion of lateral column fixation.

◆ POSTOPERATIVE MANAGMENT

The patient's foot is placed into a below-knee short leg cast that extends beyond the toes. The ankle is dorsiflexed at the hindfoot rather than the forefoot, to prevent stress across the midfoot and reduce the risk of hardware failure. The patient should remain non–weight bearing for typically 3 months postoperatively.

Oral antibiotics are prescribed for 1 week. The first postoperative wound check is at 7 days, at which point the patient is placed in a full cast/plaster with an axial off-loader.

During the early stages of recovery, the foot may become swollen and exhibit erythematous changes similar to the reactivation of CN, which is often caused by extruded bone graft leaking out of the incision. In such cases, the patient will be instructed to remain on oral antibiotics and have weekly check-ups until the foot shows clinical signs of stability.[30]

Once the foot demonstrates signs of stability, such as reduced swelling, temperature, and pain, the patient will be placed into a moonboot with total contact insole until custom footwear is available.

◆ COMPLICATIONS

Arthrodesis is the desired outcome in correcting CN. A fibrous nonunion can still allow for a successful transition to footwear without loss of correction and reulceration. If there is some loss of correction due to nonunion, typically, it is not significant enough to cause the high peak pressure and ulcer formation associated with the initial rocker bottom deformity.[2,29,33,36,37]

Migration and hardware failure are potential complications that can occur when using percutaneous fixation to correct CN (Figure 14.7). Migration occurs when the implants are not securely attached to the bone or when there is insufficient

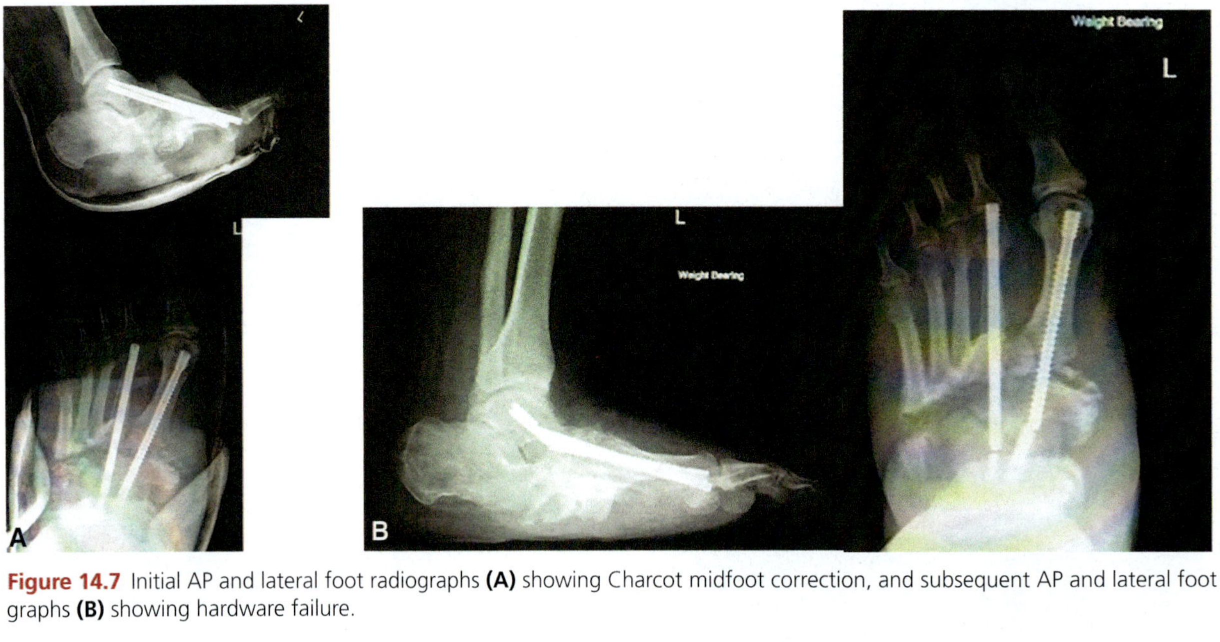

Figure 14.7 Initial AP and lateral foot radiographs **(A)** showing Charcot midfoot correction, and subsequent AP and lateral foot radiographs **(B)** showing hardware failure.

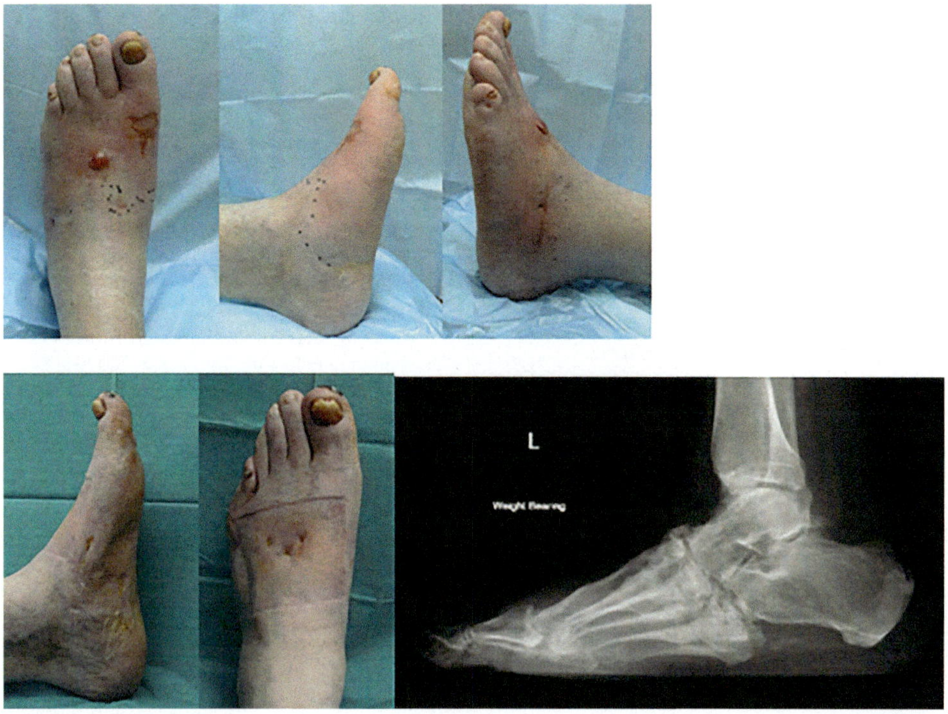

Figure 14.8 Clinical pictures showing postoperative infection (above) and postdébridement clinical pictures, and lateral foot radiograph showing eradication of infection after débridement and removal of hardware.

surrounding tissue to hold the implants in place.[35,38] Hardware failure occurs due to the high stress and pressure placed on the device during weight bearing and movement. Solid stainless steel beams may have less risk of breakage than titanium beams, as it has a higher Young modulus of elasticity.[33]

Cannulated, threaded beams facilitate reduction and fixation.[2,28,34,39-41] However, failure is a known complication of beams and bolts, so it is important to consider this risk when deciding on the best fixation technique.[30]

Infection can occur with NEMISIS. However, in cases where infection has occurred, removal of implants with copious irrigation and antibiotic loaded injectable bone graft substitute, with off-loading in TCC with Bohler iron has allowed for eradication of the infection, and maintenance of the surgical correction (Figure 14.8).[2,21,42]

Single-Stage Versus Two-Stage Procedure

Single-stage allows for a single operation and a shorter recovery time, but the compromise is a shorter foot to reduce the tension on the soft tissues. For most patients, the difference in foot length may not be a major consideration as the foot was deformed and bulky preoperatively. Two-stage procedures involve an initial period of external fixation, during which the dislocation is gradually reduced through distraction, allowing the soft tissues to lengthen and reducing the tarsometatarsal joints. The second stage procedure is then performed, in which the tarsometatarsal joints are prepared using minimally invasive burrs and fixed with intramedullary nail, beams, or bolts.[43,44] This process takes several months, and there is a risk of pin site infection with external fixation. The decision between a single-stage and two-stage procedure is based on the individual patient's needs and the surgeon's experience and expertise.

◆ OUTCOMES

The 5-year follow-up of 21 cases (19 patients) treated with NEMISIS for midfoot CN had six cases of implant failure, with three cases requiring revision. Four cases of deep infection occurred, two of which also had implant failure. Only one patient required an above-knee amputation for sepsis. There were two cases of new CN, one involving the cuboid and talus and one affecting the whole hindfoot. Although there were six deaths in this patient group, none were due to sepsis secondary to diabetic foot disease or surgery. Three patients died from cancer-related complications, two patients died from complications secondary to renal failure, and one died from respiratory complications.[45]

In summary, NEMISIS is a valuable technique for managing diabetic foot pathology. The use of minimally invasive surgical techniques and advances in implants and biologics has expanded the indications for this type of surgery. It is important to review multidisciplinary pathways to improve the escalation process for these critical procedures. The postponement of these complex reconstructions may negatively affect patient care. It is essential to complete cadaveric training and visiting fellowships to ensure that the progress made in diabetic foot surgery in the past decades is not lost.

REFERENCES

1. Sun H, Saeedi P, Karuranga S, et al. IDF diabetes atlas: global, regional and country-level diabetes prevalence estimates for 2021 and projections for 2045. *Diabetes Res Clin Pract.* 2022;183:109119.
2. Miller RJ. Neuropathic minimally invasive surgeries (NEMESIS): percutaneous diabetic foot surgery and reconstruction. *Foot Ankle Clin.* 2016;21(3):595-627. https://www.sciencedirect.com/science/article/pii/S1083751516300377
3. Apelqvist J, Bergqvist D, Eneroth M, Larsson J. The diabetic foot. Optimal prevention and treatment can halve the risk of amputation. *Lakartidningen.* 1999;96(1-2):37-41.
4. Armstrong DG, Lavery LA. Diabetic foot ulcers: prevention, diagnosis and classification. *Am Fam Physician.* 1998;57(6):1325-1328.
5. Bakker K, Dooren J. A specialized outpatient foot clinic for diabetic patients decreases the number of amputations and is cost saving. *Ned Tijdschr Geneeskd.* 1994;138(11):565-569.
6. Bus SA, van Netten JJ, Lavery LA, et al. IWGDF guidance on the prevention of foot ulcers in at-risk patients with diabetes. *Diabetes Metab Res.* 2016;32:16-24.
7. Doorgakant A, Davies MB. An approach to managing midfoot Charcot deformities. *Foot Ankle Clin.* 2020;25(2):319-335. https://www.sciencedirect.com/science/article/pii/S108375152030022X
8. Frykberg RG, Belczyk R. Epidemiology of the Charcot foot. *Clin Podiatr Med Surg.* 2008;25(1):17-28.
9. Hingorani A, LaMuraglia GM, Henke P, et al. The management of diabetic foot: a clinical practice guideline by the society for vascular surgery in collaboration with the American Podiatric Medical Association and the Society for Vascular Medicine. *J Vasc Surg.* 2016;63(2, Suppl):3S-21S. https://www.sciencedirect.com/science/article/pii/S074152141502025X
10. Pinzur MS, Evans A. Health-related quality of life in patients with Charcot foot. *Am J Orthop (Belle Mead NJ).* 2003;32(10):492-496.
11. Ragnarson Tennvall G, Apelqvist J. Prevention of diabetes-related foot ulcers and amputations: a cost-utility analysis based on Markov model simulations. *Diabetologia.* 2001;44(11):2077-2087.
12. Kennon B, Leese GP, Cochrane L, et al. Reduced incidence of lower-extremity amputations in people with diabetes in Scotland: a nationwide study. *Diabetes Care.* 2012;35(12):2588-2590.
13. Armstrong DG, Stacpoole-Shea S, Nguyen H, Harkless LB. Lengthening of the Achilles tendon in diabetic patients who are at high risk for ulceration of the foot. *J Bone Joint Surg Am.* 1999;81(4):535-538.
14. Dhawan V, Spratt KF, Pinzur MS, Baumhauer J, Rudicel S, Saltzman CL. Reliability of AOFAS diabetic foot questionnaire in Charcot arthropathy: stability, internal consistency, and measurable difference. *Foot Ankle Int.* 2005;26(9):717-731.
15. Driver VR, Fabbi M, Lavery LA, Gibbons G. The costs of diabetic foot: the economic case for the limb salvage team. *J Vasc Surg.* 2010;52(3 Suppl):17S-22S.
16. Matricali GA, Dereymaeker G, Muls E, Flour M, Mathieu C. Economic aspects of diabetic foot care in a multidisciplinary setting: a review. *Diabetes Metab Res Rev.* 2007;23(5):339-347.
17. Kroin E, Chaharbakhshi EO, Schiff A, Pinzur MS. Improvement in quality of life following operative correction of midtarsal Charcot foot deformity. *Foot Ankle Int.* 2018;39(7):808-811.
18. Hedetoft C, Rasmussen A, Fabrin J, Kølendorf K. Four-fold increase in foot ulcers in type 2 diabetic subjects without an increase in major amputations by a multidisciplinary setting. *Diabetes Res Clin Pract.* 2009;83(3):353-357.
19. Kavarthapu V. Is there a need for diabetic foot orthopaedic surgery as a sub-specialty? *J Clin Orthop Trauma.* 2021;17:72-73. https://www.sciencedirect.com/science/article/pii/S0976566221001259
20. Botezatu I, Laptoiu D. Minimally invasive surgery of diabetic foot—review of current techniques. *J Med Life.* 2016;9(3):249-254.
21. Wukich DK, Sadoskas D, Vaudreuil NJ, Fourman M. Comparison of diabetic Charcot patients with and without foot wounds. *Foot Ankle Int.* 2017;38(2):140-148.
22. Greenhagen RM, Johnson AR, Bevilacqua NJ. Gastrocnemius recession or tendo-Achilles lengthening for equinus deformity in the diabetic foot? *Clin Podiatr Med Surg.* 2012;29(3):413-424.
23. Brodsky JW. The diabetic foot. Surg. *Foot Ankle.* 2007;1281-1368.
24. Eichenholtz SN. Charcot joints. *J Bone Joint Surg.* 1962;44:1485.
25. Tiruveedhula M, Graham A, Thapar A, Dindyal S, Mulcahy M. Outcomes of tendo-Achilles lengthening and weight-bearing total contact cast for management of early midfoot Charcot neuroarthropathy. *J Clin Orthop Trauma.* 2021;17:128-138.
26. Sammarco GJ, Conti SF. Surgical treatment of neuroarthropathic foot deformity. *Foot Ankle Int.* 1998;19(2):102-109.
27. Myerson MS, Kadakia AR. 10—Surgery for the neuropathic foot and ankle. In: Myerson MS, Kadakia AR, eds. *Reconstructive Foot and Ankle Surgery: Management of Complications.* 3rd ed. Elsevier; 2019:121-140. https://www.sciencedirect.com/science/article/pii/B978032349693300010X
28. Dos Santos-Vaquinhas A, Parra G, Martínez P, Sobrón B, Cuervas-Mons M. Beaming in the Charcot foot: a case series with 12-month minimum follow-up. *The Foot.* 2021;47:101814. https://www.sciencedirect.com/science/article/pii/S0958259221000407
29. Miller R. NEMISIS minimally invasive surgical correction for midfoot Charcot arthropathy. *Foot Ankle Orthop.* 2018;3(3):2473011418S00353.
30. Miller R. NEMISIS neuropathic minimally invasive surgeries. Charcot reconstruction. Surgical technique. Pearls and pitfalls. *Foot Ankle Clin.* 2022;27(3):567-581.
31. Scott RT, DeCarbo WT, Hyer CF. Osteotomies for the management of Charcot neuroarthropathy of the foot and ankle. *Clin Podiatr Med Surg.* 2015;32(3):405-418.
32. Grant WP. Biomechanics of the Charcot foot collapse and roding the medial column of the foot as a beam to salvage the Charcot foot. 1997.
33. Sammarco VJ. Superconstructs in the treatment of Charcot foot deformity: plantar plating, locked plating, and axial screw fixation. *Foot Ankle Clin.* 2009;14(3):393-407.
34. Lamm BM, Siddiqui NA, Nair AK, LaPorta G. Intramedullary foot fixation for midfoot Charcot neuroarthropathy. *J Foot Ankle Surg.* 2012;51(4):531-536.
35. Wiewiorski M, Yasui T, Miska M, Frigg A, Valderrabano V. Solid bolt fixation of the medial column in Charcot midfoot arthropathy. *J Foot Ankle Surg.* 2013;52(1):88-94. https://www.sciencedirect.com/science/article/pii/S1067251612002086
36. Ha J, Hester T, Foley R, et al. Charcot foot reconstruction outcomes: a systematic review. *J Clin Orthop Trauma.* 2020;11(3):357-368. https://www.sciencedirect.com/science/article/pii/S0976566220301089
37. Chraim M, Krenn S, Alrabai HM, Trnka H, Bock P. Mid-term follow-up of patients with hindfoot arthrodesis with retrograde compression intramedullary nail in Charcot neuroarthropathy of the hindfoot. *Bone Joint J.* 2018;100-B(2):190-196.
38. Butt DA, Hester T, Bilal A, Edmonds M, Kavarthapu V. The medial column synthes midfoot fusion bolt is associated with unacceptable rates of failure in corrective fusion for Charcot deformity. *Bone Joint J.* 2015;97-B(6):809-813.
39. Baker JR, Glover JP, McEneaney PA. Percutaneous fixation of forefoot, midfoot, hindfoot, and ankle fracture dislocations. *Clin Podiatr Med Surg.* 2008;25(4):691-719.
40. Brandão RA, Weber JS, Larson D, et al. New fixation methods for the treatment of the diabetic foot: beaming, external fixation, and beyond. *Clin Podiatr Med Surg.* 2018;35(1):63-76.
41. Klag EA, Fisk FE, Maier LM, Zeni F. Staged percutaneous treatment of a complete Lisfranc dislocation secondary to Charcot arthropathy: a case report. *JBJS Case Connect.* 2021;11(4).
42. Biz C, Ruggieri P. Minimally invasive surgery: osteotomies for diabetic foot disease. *Foot Ankle Clin.* 2020;25(3):441-460.
43. Richter M, Mittlmeier T, Rammelt S, Agren PH, Hahn S, Eschler A. Intramedullary fixation in severe Charcot osteo-neuroarthropathy with foot deformity results in adequate correction without loss of correction—results from a multi-centre study. *Foot Ankle Surg.* 2015;21(4):269-276.
44. Lyons M, McGregor PC, Pinzur MS, Adams W, Wilkos-Prostran L. Risk reduction and perioperative complications in patients with diabetes and multiple medical comorbidities undergoing Charcot foot reconstruction. *Foot Ankle Int.* 2021;42(7):902-909.
45. Miller R. 5-year follow-up of neuropathic minimally invasive surgeries with superconstructs for mid-foot Charcot deformity. *American Foot and Ankle Society 2022 Annual Conference Presentation.*

PART

3 Midfoot/Hindfoot

15 Medializing Osteotomy

Hazibullah Waizy and Assil-Ramin Alimy

◆ INTRODUCTION

Medializing calcaneal osteotomy is an effective and frequently used technique for the restoration of hindfoot alignment and biomechanics. Calcaneal osteotomies provide correction in multiple planes, while still preserving joint and tendon function.[1] Medializing calcaneal osteotomy was first described by Gleich in 1893 for the correction of pes planovalgus deformities.[2] Gleich proposed a medial wedge resection. Dwyer popularized calcaneal osteotomy by his description of a lateral closing wedge osteotomy for the correction of cavovarus foot deformities in 1959.[3] A variation of an opening wedge calcaneal osteotomy, which provides correction through lengthening the lateral column was proposed in 1975 by Evans.[4] Koutsogiannis further popularized the medializing calcaneal osteotomy in 1971 by successfully utilizing the approach for correction of flexible pediatric flatfoot.[5] Osteotomies through the calcaneal body realign the weight-bearing forces to the structural tripod and may further redirect the pull of the Achilles tendon.[3] Medializing osteotomies are used for the correction of planovalgus deformities, whereas lateralizing osteotomies are utilized for the treatment of cavovarus deformities.

For the past 20 years, there has been growing interest and demand for minimally invasive procedures in medicine and, particularly, in orthopedic surgery. Complications with open calcaneal osteotomies through the standard lateral approach include wound dehiscence, peroneal tendon irritation, damage to the sural nerve, and delayed union, nonunion, and irritation.[6-8] Furthermore, medial neurovascular structures are at risk during medializing calcaneal osteotomies through a lateral approach.[9,10] Minimally invasive surgery (MIS) offers several advantages that may reduce the risk of these complications. MIS facilitates wound healing and avoids complications by limiting the soft-tissue dissection, decreasing postoperative pain and morbidity.[11]

◆ INDICATIONS AND CONTRAINDICATIONS

Indications for minimally invasive medializing calcaneal osteotomies (MIMCOs) include symptomatic flexible pes planovalgus deformities and failed previous conservative treatment.[5,12-14] Furthermore, MIMCO may be utilized combined with a hindfoot arthrodesis.[15] Additional soft-tissue procedure like tendon reconstructions, tendon transfers, and ligament reconstruction are frequently part of the hindfoot correction.[6,16-20]

Contraindications for the MIMCO resemble those of open surgery and include symptomatic arthritis of the subtalar, talonavicular, and calcaneocuboid joints.[12] A rigid subtalar joint with limited motion should be treated with a fusion approach.[21] Furthermore, a large dorsal displacement osteotomy for high calcaneal pitch may be considered as a contraindication for MIS and rather be performed open.[22] Further systemic risk factors that should be considered preoperatively include smoking, poor patient compliance, diabetes mellitus, inflammatory arthropathies, and medications like disease-modifying agent medications (DMARD) and glucocorticoids.[12] Moreover, local risk factors like poor vascularity, poor soft-tissue envelope at the operative site, and previous infections need to be cautiously assessed and evaluated before surgery. Although these risk factors represent a significantly higher risk with the open approach than with MIS.[1]

◆ PATIENT HISTORY AND PHYSICAL EXAMINATION

The physical examination should involve inspection, palpation, range of motion (ROM), muscle strength testing, and gait assessment. A comparison to the contralateral foot should be made. Also, the physical examination should be performed with and without weight bearing.

Inspection: The flexible flatfoot will have an arch without weight bearing, which will disappear with weight bearing.[23] The patient will be noted to overpronate. Observing the patient from the back will demonstrate the "too many toes" sign.[23,24]

Palpation: The physician should palpate various structures, including the deltoid ligament, posterior tibial tendon, lateral rearfoot, ankle joint, subtalar joint, talonavicular joint, and the calcaneocuboid joint.[4]

ROM: Examining ROM allows further differentiation regarding flexible versus rigid pes planus.[23] The Hubscher maneuver (or Jack test) is a test to determine the flexibility of a pes planovalgus in which the examiner dorsiflexes the hallux while the patient is weight bearing.[25,26] In flexible pes planovalgus, the arch of the foot increases, as opposed to rigid planovalgus in which the arch is not present with or without weight bearing.[25,26]

Muscle strength testing: The physician can evaluate muscle strength by having the patient perform a single limb heel raise.[23] The inversion against resistance may be used to evaluate the posterior tibial tendon muscle strength.[23,27]

Gait assessment: The physician may observe an antalgic gait and overpronation with ambulation.[23]

Physical examination should also focus on assessing the neurovascular status and identifying further malalignments and deformities. This is especially important as deformity may compromise postoperative results and can be corrected intraoperatively in combination with MIMCO. Additionally, the ROM of the subtalar joint must be assessed.

Workup for medializing calcaneal osteotomy consists of a thorough history and clinical examination. Complaints, medical history, previous surgeries, and risk factors, especially tobacco and alcohol, need to be further assessed and evaluated, as those can negatively influence the healing process. Understanding the patient´s expectations for activities, shoe wear, and level of pain, as well as its impact on quality of life, are fundamental for patient recovery, rehabilitation, and satisfaction.

◆ IMAGING STUDIES

Radiologic evaluation of the foot and ankle is critical in assessing the deformity.

Radiologic assessment should include weight-bearing anteroposterior, oblique, and lateral views.[28] Evaluation of the anteroposterior view should focus on the Kite angle, the talus, the first metatarsal, and the alignment of the talonavicular joint. Furthermore, the calcaneal pitch can be visualized through the lateral view of the foot.[28] Deformity may be further classified depending on the calcaneal pitch angle, where an angle between 20° and 25° may be considered normal. An angle of less than 15° is indicative of a flatfoot deformity, and an angle above 30° is indicative of a cavus deformity.[28] Moreover, the calcaneal pitch angle shows high interobserver reliability.[29] Varus or valgus deformity can be assessed and quantified through a long axial view.[28] The Saltzman view is used to assess the hindfoot axis under weight bearing.[30] If necessary, additional MRI may be utilized to assess the cartilage in the subtalar and Chopart joint in case of suspected osteoarthritis as well as evaluation of the tibialis posterior tendon in pes planovalgus and the peroneal tendons in pes cavus and also pathologies of the ligaments. Computed tomography (CT) should be obtained when a coalition is suspected.

◆ PREOPERATIVE PLANNING AND PREPARATION

SURGICAL TECHNIQUE

The MIMCO is performed with the patient under general anesthesia or sedation with a lower extremity peripheral nerve block in the supine position with a free hanging foot. The use of a bump under the ipsilateral hip allows internal rotation of the leg and simplifies access to the lateral heel.[12,22,31] Under fluoroscopic guidance, the intended osteotomy site is marked (Figure 15.1). The angle of the V-osteotomy (chevron osteotomy) lies centrally in the calcaneus on a line starting from the deepest point of the calcaneus. The osteotomy is placed ventrally at an angle of approximately 60°, whereby the osteotomy must run ventrally to the insertion of the plantar fascia.

The safe zone should be identified to minimize the risk of damage to the sural nerve.[32] A landmark line is drawn from the posterosuperior apex of the calcaneal tuberosity to the plantar fascia origin. The safe zone is defined by the area within 11 mm anterior to the defined landmark.[32] A 3- to 5-mm longitudinal lateral stab incision is made, and a curved hemostat is used to carefully expand and spread the incision down to the bone (Figure 15.2A-C).[31] The osteotomy is performed using a long (20- to 30-mm cutting surface, 10 cm length), low-speed, high torque Shannon end- and side-cutting burr (3 mm diameter) at a speed of 3,000 to 6,000 rpm.[31] Advantages of using a low-speed burr during MIMCO is to allow a more controlled osteotomy to minimize soft-tissue contact and irritation.

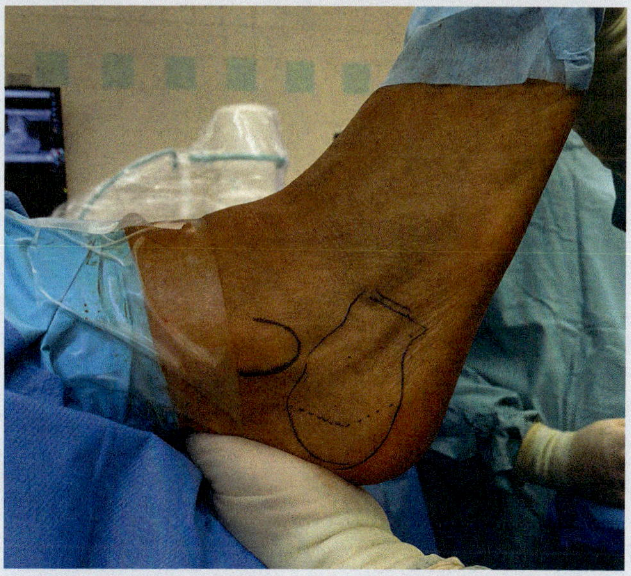

Figure 15.1 The planned osteotomy level is drawn under image intensifier control. A straight or chevron osteotomy may be performed. The chevron osteotomy is made with an angle of ~60°, whereby the osteotomy must run plantar ventrally to the insertion of the plantar fascia. At the same time, the planned screw position can be marked. Lengthening of the calcaneus is challenging due to the soft-tissue tension. If a significant shift is desired, a neutral osteotomy or, in the case of pes cavus, a slight shortening and dorsalization of the calcaneal tuberosity is preferred.

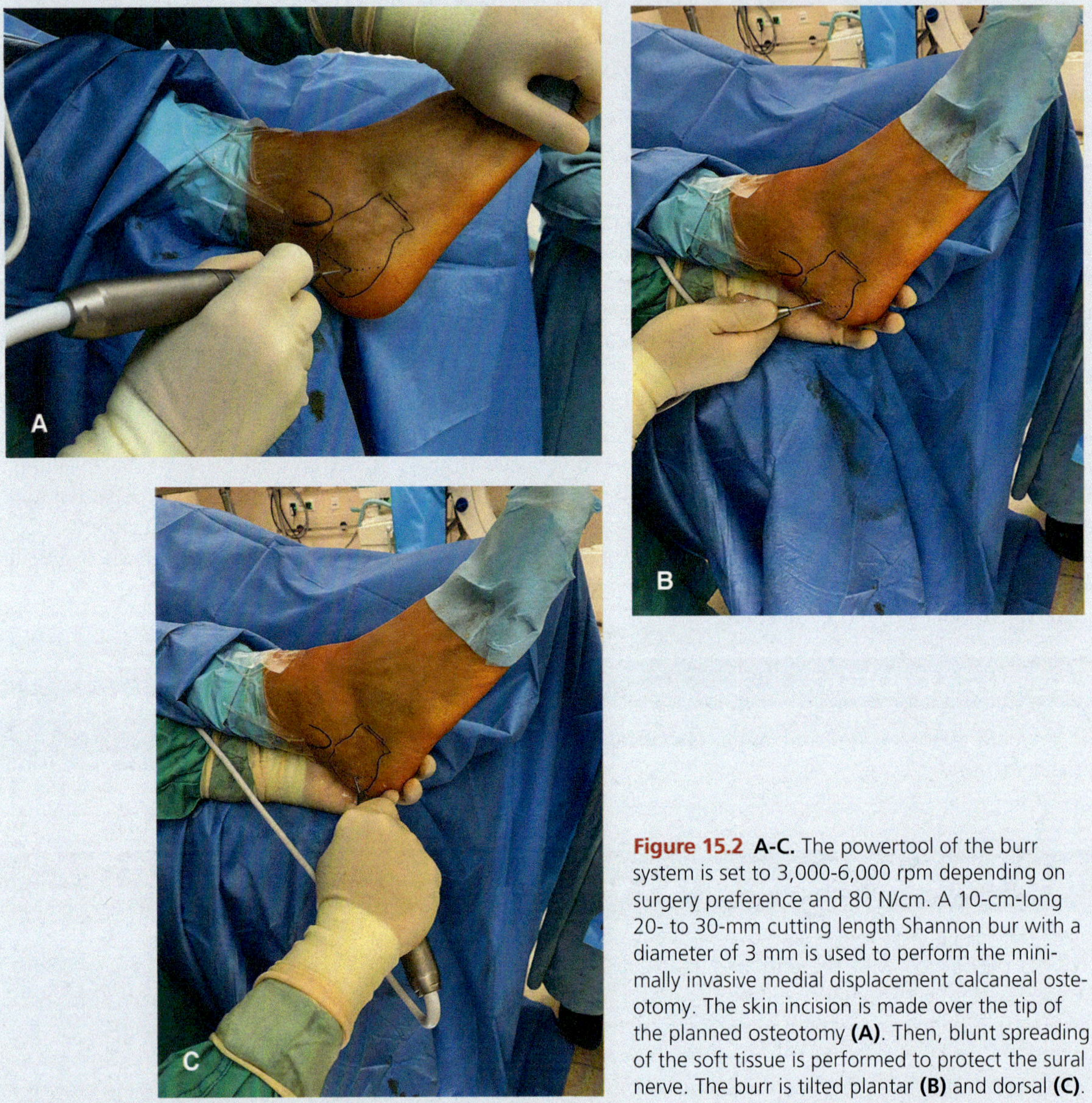

Figure 15.2 A-C. The powertool of the burr system is set to 3,000-6,000 rpm depending on surgery preference and 80 N/cm. A 10-cm-long 20- to 30-mm cutting length Shannon bur with a diameter of 3 mm is used to perform the minimally invasive medial displacement calcaneal osteotomy. The skin incision is made over the tip of the planned osteotomy **(A)**. Then, blunt spreading of the soft tissue is performed to protect the sural nerve. The burr is tilted plantar **(B)** and dorsal **(C)**.

To prevent thermal injury to the tissues the use of a tourniquet is discouraged, and continuous bulb syringe irrigation of the burr with saline is imperative.[31] The calcaneal tubercle can be lengthened, shortened, plantarized, or even dorsalized by tilting the burr.[33] A lengthening could be achieved by aiming the tip of the burr distally. Tilting to dorsal would result in shortening. The kerf of the Shannon burr is at least 3.0 mm. This should be taken into account when planning the osteotomy level. Experience has shown that tension in the soft tissues complicates lengthening of the calcaneus. To achieve a significant shift, a neutral osteotomy or, in the case of pes cavus, a slight shortening and dorsalization are recommended.

A straight transverse or chevron-shaped osteotomy may be performed. The chevron-shaped technique provides greater stability, but their correction capacity is limited. Especially, plantarization or dorsalization is limited with the chevron osteotomy. First, the osteotomy of the dorsal leg of the osteotomy is performed. The burr is retracted so that the cutting portion is fully within the bone starting from the lateral cortex. This minimizes the risk of soft-tissue injury. The burr is guided dorsally in a curve with continuous cooling. The osteotomy levels previously drawn on the skin facilitate orientation, which is followed by the plantar leg of the chevron osteotomy. The center of rotation of the burr lies strictly in the plane of the skin incision. Once the osteotomy is complete, the calcaneal tubercle can be moved medially or laterally. If the osteotomy is not complete, bony bridges can be felt and cut with the tip of the Shannon burr. Displacement of the calcaneal tubercle medial or lateral is possible to a greater extent after a minimally invasive osteotomy than with an open displacement osteotomy of the calcaneus. A displacement of more than 50% of the width of the calcaneus is possible medially or laterally. The calcaneal tuberosity can be levered into the desired position with an elevator or clamp placed in the osteotomy gap (Figure 15.3). In addition to pure displacement, rotation of the calcaneal

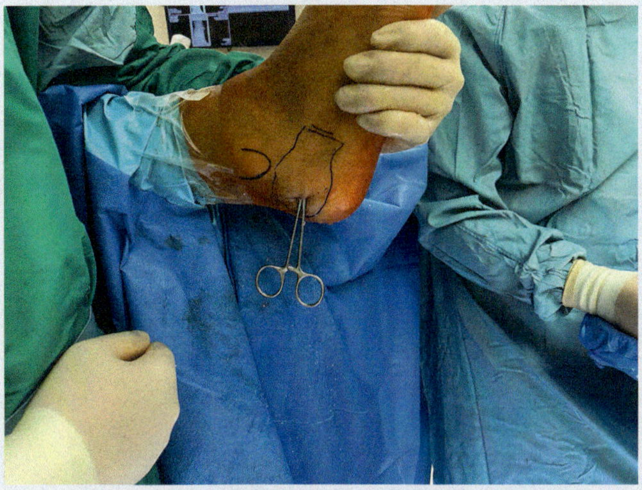

Figure 15.3 The calcaneal tuberosity can be levered into the desired position with a clamp placed in the osteotomy gap.

tuberosity is also possible. The insertion of the Achilles tendon can be shifted further by rotating the tuber fragment, but the risk of overcorrection also increases. Once the clinically desired correction of the hindfoot has been achieved, one to two K-wires are inserted via a stab incision on the calcaneal tubercle according to the skin markings. Skin incisions in the area of the weight-bearing surface of the calcaneus should be avoided. The chevron osteotomy can be fixed in a rotation-stable manner with a screw. In the case of significant translation, additional stability can be achieved with a second screw. The translation must be taken into account when inserting the wire. The correction achieved and the position of the K-wire can be documented with a calcaneal axial image (Figure 15.4A and B). An overcorrection can also be detected. In addition, the documentation is carried out in the second level (calcaneus laterally) (Figure 15.4C). Once the desired correction has been achieved and the wires are in the correct position, the length of the required screws is determined via the stab incision and the osteosynthesis is carried out. The cannulated screws are predominantly self-drilling and self-tapping. Therefore, a 15-mm deep drill hole and head milling are sufficient to perforate the hard cortex. Whenever screws with heads are used, it is recommended to countersink the screw head to bone level. Finally, axial and lateral calcaneal fluoroscopy views are obtained to check tuberosity and screw position (Figure 15.5A and B). During the osteotomy, the lateral portal, in particular, should be diligently irrigated in order to avoid long-term irritation from bone paste in the soft tissue. The dressing is made with a nonadhesive wound dressing, compresses, cotton pads, and an elastocompressive bandage. A short leg splint is placed in a neutral position.

Pitfalls

- Skin and bone thermal injury due to insufficient irrigation of the burr
- Overcorrection
- Nonunion
- Injury to tendons, nerves, or vessels

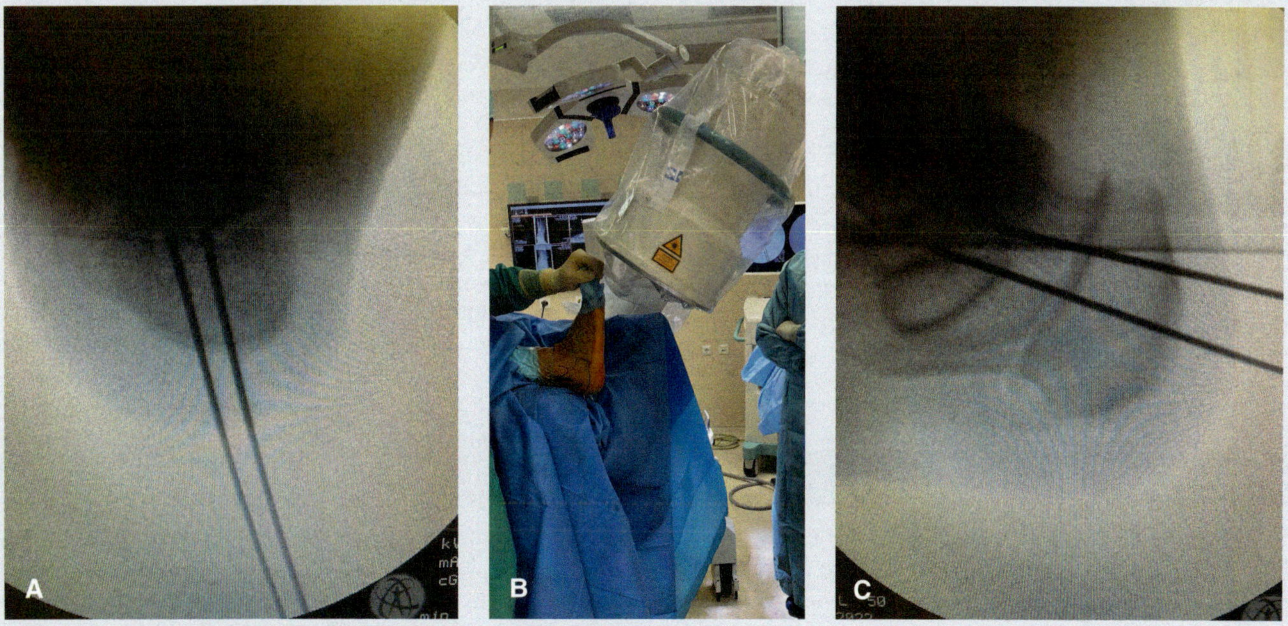

Figure 15.4 The correction achieved and the position of the K-wire can be documented with a calcaneal axial view **(A, B)**. In addition, the documentation is carried out in the calcaneus lateral view **(C)**.

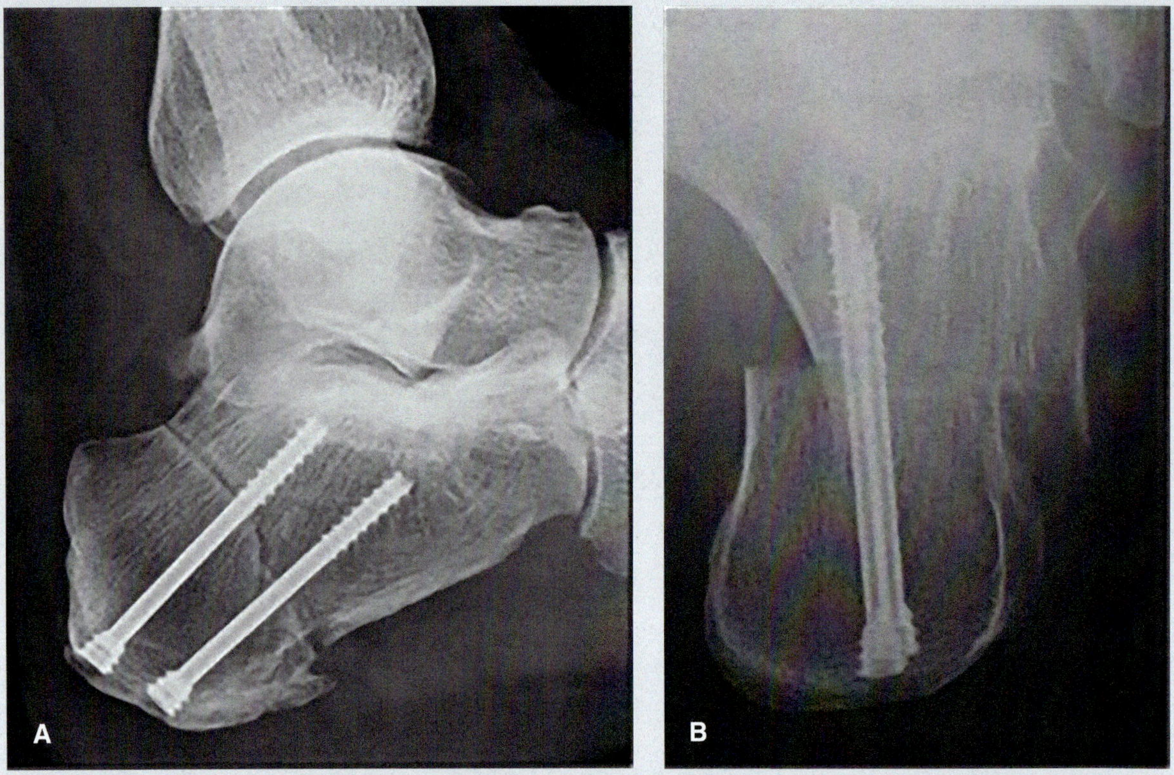

Figure 15.5 **A.** Lateral view of the calcaneus showing two headless compression screws placed across the minimally invasive medial displacement calcaneal osteotomy. **B.** Harris axial view of the calcaneus showing two headless compression screws placed across the minimally invasive medial displacement calcaneal osteotomy with the desired correction.

◆ POSTOPERATIVE MANAGEMENT

The patient is placed in a splint for the first 2 weeks followed by a short cam walker boot for the following 4 weeks. The patient may use a below-knee scooter, with 2 weeks non-weight bearing followed by partial weight bearing of 20 kg for an additional 4 weeks.[31]

Sutures may be removed after 10 to 14 days. Postoperative radiographs are obtained, and weight bearing as tolerated is initiated at 6 weeks postoperatively. In the midterm, insoles may be necessary to support the hindfoot. In addition, stretching of the dorsal muscle chain is recommended. Thromboembolic prophylaxis should be implemented according to standard guidelines.

◆ OUTCOMES

Limited literature exists reporting on MIMCO outcomes. However, several studies support the safety and efficacy of MIS for MIMCO. Kheir et al. retrospectively reviewed the outcomes of MIMCO in a case series of 30 patients.[34] Radiological and clinical union was observed in all patients, and no complications regarding wound infection or neurovascular injury were described. Kendal et al. conducted a retrospective cohort study that evaluated and compared open and MIS calcaneal osteotomies.[35] The MIS osteotomies were associated with a statistically significant reduction in postoperative complications compared to the open osteotomy group. Complications included delayed wound healing, wound infection, damage to the sural nerve, and implant removal for hardware irritation. Wound complications with open calcaneal osteotomy may be as high as 10%.[36,37] Waizy et al. compared MIS and open calcaneal osteotomies in 60 patients and found similar improvements in the Foot and Ankle Outcome Score (FAOS).[31] Furthermore, they observed a statistically significant shorter operative time among patients following MIS, which is a major advantage for MIS as longer durations of surgery are associated with increased morbidity and higher rates of complications.[36,38] Additionally, they observed no neurovascular injuries in MIS but reported sural neuropathy in 9% of patients following open surgery. Proposed disadvantages of MIS include increased radiation exposure.[29] However, Waizy et al. described no statistically significant difference between MIS and open calcaneal osteotomies regarding fluoroscopy time and radiation dose, with a tendency toward shorter fluoroscopy time and radiation dose in the MIS group.[31]

Overall, MIMCO provides a safe and effective correction. Results demonstrate comparable outcomes to open calcaneal osteotomies. Future research should focus on implementing prospective comparative studies with the use of validated outcome measures to provide an evidence-based foundation. However, existing data support the application of MIMCO.

References

1. Trnka H-J, Easley ME, Myerson MS. The role of calcaneal osteotomies for correction of adult flatfoot. *Clin Orthop Relat Res.* 1999;365:50-64.
2. Gleich A. Beitrag zur operativen plattfussbehandlung. *Arch Klin Chir.* 1893;46(1):358-362.
3. Dwyer F. Osteotomy of the calcaneum for pes cavus. *J Bone Joint Surg Br.* 1959;41(1):80-86.
4. Evans D. Calcaneo-valgus deformity. *J Bone Joint Surg Br.* 1975;57(3):270-278.
5. Koutsogiannis E. Treatment of mobile flat foot by displacement osteotomy of the calcaneus. *J Bone Joint Surg Br.* 1971;53(1):96-100.
6. Weinfeld SB. Medial slide calcaneal osteotomy: technique, patient selection, and results. *Foot Ankle Clin.* 2001;6(1):89-94.
7. Ray R, Jameson S, Kumar S, eds. Complications of calcaneal osteotomy. *Orthopaedic Proceedings*. The British Editorial Society of Bone & Joint Surgery; 2010.
8. Abbasian A, Zaidi R, Guha A, Goldberg A, Cullen N, Singh D. Comparison of three different fixation methods of calcaneal osteotomies. *Foot Ankle Int.* 2013;34(3):420-425.
9. Greene DL, Thompson MC, Gesink DS, Graves SC. Anatomic study of the medial neurovascular structures in relation to calcaneal osteotomy. *Foot Ankle Int.* 2001;22(7):569-571.
10. Haugsdal J, Dawson J, Phisitkul P. Nerve injury and pain after operative repair of calcaneal fractures: a literature review. *Iowa Orthop J.* 2013;33:202-207.
11. Jowett CR, Rodda D, Amin A, Bradshaw A, Bedi HS. Minimally invasive calcaneal osteotomy: a cadaveric and clinical evaluation. *Foot Ankle Surg.* 2016;22(4):244-247.
12. Sherman TI, Guyton GP. Minimal incision/minimally invasive medializing displacement calcaneal osteotomy. *Foot Ankle Int.* 2018;39(1):119-128.
13. Parks RM, Mirmiran R. Posterior calcaneal displacement osteotomy with lateral wall reduction. *J Foot Ankle Surg.* 2002;41(2):135-137.
14. Torosian CM, Dias LS. Surgical treatment of severe hindfoot valgus by medial displacement osteotomy of the os calcis in children with myelomeningocele. *J Pediatr Orthop.* 2000;20(2):226-229.
15. Johnson JE, Yu J. Arthrodesis techniques in the management of stage II and III acquired adult flatfoot deformity. *Instr Course Lect.* 2006;55:531-542.
16. D'Souza NA, Kinchelow T, Lin S. Posterior tibial tendon dysfunction: tendon transfers, osteotomies, and lateral column lengthening. *Curr Opin Orthop.* 2002;13(2):81-88.
17. Guyton GP, Jeng C, Krieger LE, Mann RA. Flexor digitorum longus transfer and medial displacement calcaneal osteotomy for posterior tibial tendon dysfunction: a middle-term clinical follow-up. *Foot Ankle Int.* 2001;22(8):627-632.
18. Myerson MS, Corrigan J, Thompson F, Schon LC. Tendon transfer combined with calcaneal osteotomy for treatment of posterior tibial tendon insufficiency: a radiological investigation. *Foot Ankle Int.* 1995;16(11):712-718.
19. Myerson MS, Corrigan J. *Treatment of Posterior Tibial Tendon Dysfunction with Flexor Digitorum Longus Tendon Transfer and Calcaneal Osteotomy.* SLACK Incorporated; 1996:383-388.
20. Mann R, Guyton G. Medial displacement osteotomy of the calcaneus and flexor digitorum longus transfer. *The Foot and Ankle.* Lippincott Williams and Wilkins; 2002:369-385.
21. Greenfield S, Cohen B. Calcaneal osteotomies: pearls and pitfalls. *Foot Ankle Clin.* 2017;22(3):563-571.
22. Guyton GP. Minimally invasive osteotomies of the calcaneus. *Foot Ankle Clin.* 2016;21(3):551-566.
23. Raj MA, Tafti D, Kiel J. Pes planus. *StatPearls [Internet].* StatPearls Publishing; 2021.
24. Knapp PW, Constant D. Posterior tibial tendon dysfunction. 2019.
25. Nowacki RM, Air ME, Rietveld A. Hyperpronation in dancers incidence and relation to calcaneal angle. *J Dance Med Sci.* 2012;16(3):126-132.
26. Cass AD, Camasta CA. A review of tarsal coalition and pes planovalgus: clinical examination, diagnostic imaging, and surgical planning. *J Foot Ankle Surg.* 2010;49(3):274-293.
27. Kohls-Gatzoulis J, Angel JC, Singh D, Haddad F, Livingstone J, Berry G. Tibialis posterior dysfunction: a common and treatable cause of adult acquired flatfoot. *BMJ.* 2004;329(7478):1328-1333.
28. DiDomenico LA, Anain JM, LaCivita MD. Percutaneous calcaneal displacement osteotomy. *Minimally Invasive Surgery of the Foot and Ankle.* Springer; 2010:231-244.
29. Sensiba PR, Coffey MJ, Williams NE, Mariscalco M, Laughlin RT. Inter- and intraobserver reliability in the radiographic evaluation of adult flatfoot deformity. *Foot Ankle Int.* 2010;31(2):141-145.
30. Springfeld R. Arthrodesen und Korrekturarthrodesen des subtalaren Gelenkkomplexes: Indikationen, operative Fusionstechniken bei Funktionsstörungen des Rückfußes. *Fuß Sprunggelenk.* 2011;9(4):176-191.
31. Waizy H, Jowett C, Andric V. Minimally invasive versus open calcaneal osteotomies—comparing the intraoperative parameters. *Foot (Ed inb).* 2018;37:113-118.
32. Talusan PG, Cata E, Tan EW, Parks BG, Guyton GP. Safe zone for neural structures in medial displacement calcaneal osteotomy: a cadaveric and radiographic investigation. *Foot Ankle Int.* 2015;36(12):1493-1498.
33. Walther M, Kriegelstein S, Altenberger S, Röser A. Die perkutane Kalkaneusverschiebeosteotomie. *Oper Orthop Traumatol.* 2016;28(4):309-320.
34. Kheir E, Borse V, Sharpe J, Lavalette D, Farndon M. Medial displacement calcaneal osteotomy using minimally invasive technique. *Foot Ankle Int.* 2015;36(3):248-252.
35. Kendal AR, Khalid A, Ball T, Rogers M, Cooke P, Sharp R. Complications of minimally invasive calcaneal osteotomy versus open osteotomy. *Foot Ankle Int.* 2015;36(6):685-690.
36. Eastwood DM, Atkins RM. Lateral approaches to the heel A comparison of two incisions for the fixation of calcaneal fractures. *The Foot.* 1992;2(3):143-147.
37. Freeman BJC, Duff S, Allen PE, Nicholson HD, Atkins RM. The extended lateral approach to the hindfoot. *J Bone Joint Surg Br.* 1998;80-B(1):139-143.
38. Iverson RE; Facilities ATFoPSiO-BS. Patient safety in office-based surgery. *Plast Reconstr Surg.* 2002;110(5):1337-1342.

16 Percutaneous Dwyer and Lateral Displacement Calcaneal Osteotomy

Jonathan R. M. Kaplan

◆ INTRODUCTION

The calcaneal osteotomy has a long-standing history of use in various disorders of the foot and ankle. While traditionally performed through a 4- to 6-cm incision, advancements in minimally invasive technique and technology have allowed the calcaneal osteotomy to be performed through 1- to 2-mm "keyhole" incisions. Through these minimally invasive techniques, excellent correction is achieved while minimizing soft-tissue disruption.

Both the lateral displacement calcaneal osteotomy and the Dwyer lateral closing wedge osteotomy can be used to correct a hindfoot varus deformity.[1] The author prefers to perform a combination of the Dwyer and lateral closing wedge osteotomy in order to achieve sufficient correction. Additionally, if needed, proximal translation of the calcaneus can also be performed in order to achieve three-dimensional correction of the deformity when needed.

◆ INDICATIONS AND CONTRAINDICATIONS

The primary indication for the lateral displacement calcaneal osteotomy is to correct a hindfoot varus deformity. This includes primarily correction of the cavovarus foot or subtle hindfoot varus. Other indications may include treatment of Mueller-Weiss syndrome in which there is hindfoot varus with a compensatory flatfoot[2] (Figure 16.1). Additionally, this calcaneal osteotomy can be considered as part of the treatment algorithm in patients undergoing surgery for a fifth metatarsal fracture, peroneal tendon pathology, or ankle instability with associated hindfoot varus. Furthermore, the minimally invasive calcaneal osteotomy is beneficial for preserving the soft tissues. Examples include relatively close adjacent incisions such as a concomitant lateral ligament reconstruction incision (Figure 16.2), patients at risk for infection (tobacco use, diabetes, corticosteroid usage), or nearby prior surgical scars.

Contraindications to a lateral displacement calcaneal osteotomy include neutral hindfoot alignment or hindfoot valgus. Additionally, it should be avoided in patients with active infection in the hindfoot. Lastly, in patients with a rigid hindfoot deformity, consideration should be made for arthrodesis-type procedures to correct the deformity instead of periarticular osteotomies; however, this is a relative contraindication as a calcaneal osteotomy can be performed in addition to a hindfoot arthrodesis procedure if needing to achieve additional correction.

◆ PATIENT HISTORY AND PHYSICAL EXAMINATION

A thorough history and physical examination is critical to determine the need for a lateral displacement calcaneal osteotomy. On the history, patients with hindfoot varus may report an array of symptoms related to lateral ankle and foot overload. Patients may occasionally develop pain and callosities along the lateral column of the foot; however, more often patients will present with symptoms related to other pathology that are related to having a hindfoot varus alignment. This includes pain or weakness related to peroneal tendon pathology, recurrent ankle sprains or ankle instability, symptoms related to hindfoot or midfoot arthritis, or even fifth metatarsal stress fracture symptoms due to their alignment and chronic lateral foot overload.

The physical examination should include assessment of the patient in both the standing and seated position. The author prefers to first start with having the patient stand facing away from the examiner to best evaluate the hindfoot alignment. Additionally, Coleman block testing can be performed while the patient is standing so as to assess for a forefoot-driven hindfoot varus. If the hindfoot corrects into physiologic valgus, the deformity is flexible and secondary to plantarflexion of the first ray. In this case, a first metatarsal osteotomy is better indicated for correction rather than a lateral displacement calcaneal osteotomy. With the patient in a seated position, the hindfoot deformity should be assessed to determine if it is passively correctable. If the deformity is not passively correctable, an arthrodesis-type procedure would be more likely indicated than a calcaneal osteotomy. Finally, thorough examination of the foot and ankle should

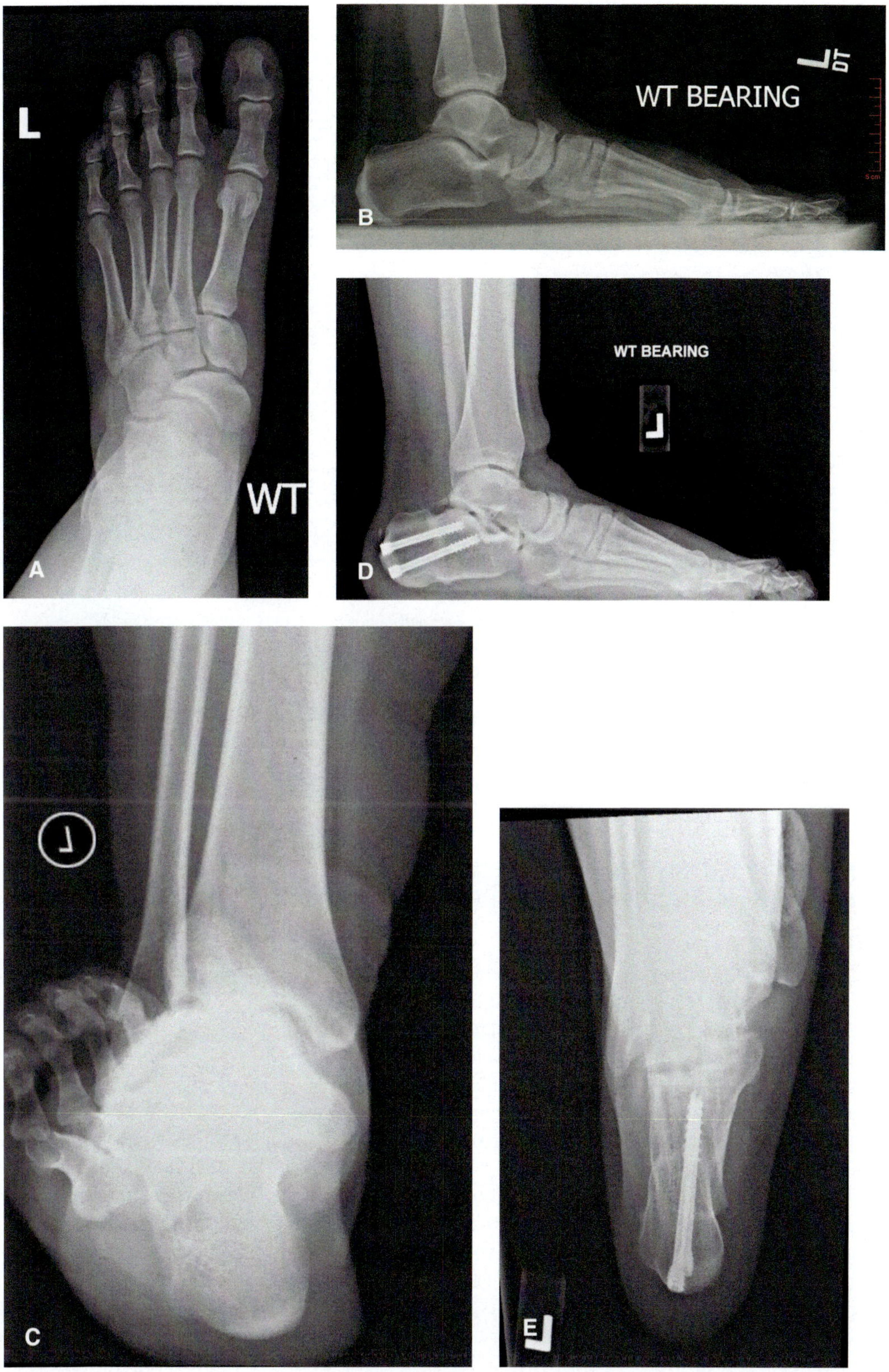

Figure 16.1 **A.** AP foot radiograph of a patient with Mueller-Weiss syndrome with comma-shaped dysplastic navicular. **B.** Lateral foot radiograph of a patient with Mueller-Weiss syndrome with flatfoot appearance including decreased calcaneal pitch as well as dysplastic navicular. **C.** Hindfoot alignment radiograph of a patient with Mueller-Weiss syndrome showing hindfoot varus. **D.** Postoperative lateral foot radiograph of a patient with Mueller-Weiss syndrome with healed calcaneal osteotomy. **E.** Postoperative hindfoot alignment radiograph of a patient with Mueller-Weiss syndrome with laterally translated calcaneal osteotomy.

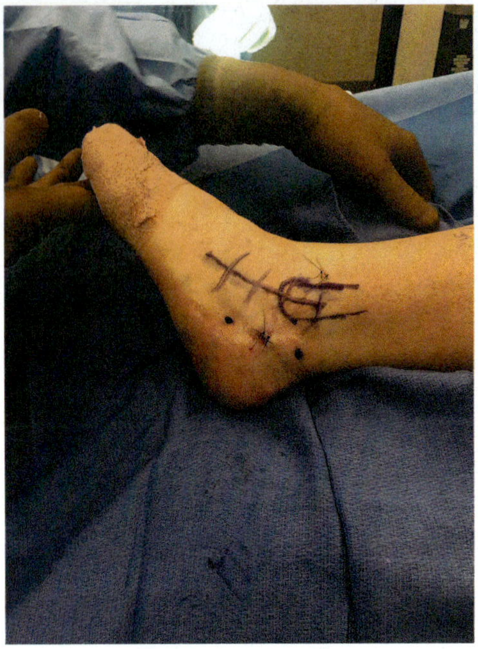

Figure 16.2 Intraoperative image showing planned incision for lateral ligament reconstruction (*full line*) and adjacent completed calcaneal osteotomy (*dotted line*).

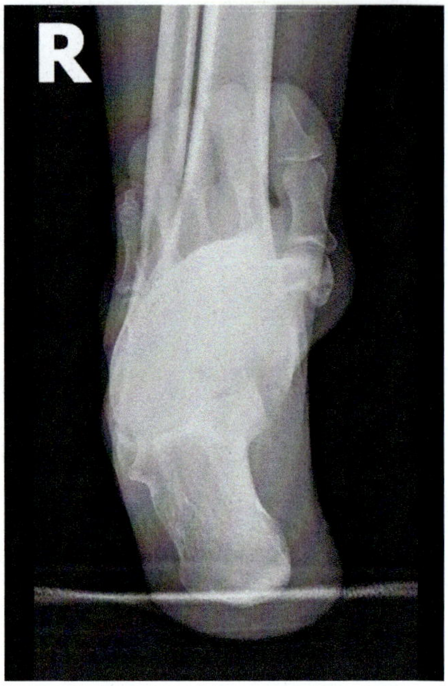

Figure 16.3 Hindfoot alignment radiograph showing hindfoot varus.

be completed including soft-tissue evaluation, strength and sensory testing, palpation of pulses, range of motion of the ankle and hindfoot joints, as well as diagnosis-specific examination.

◆ IMAGING STUDIES

Radiographs

Weight-bearing radiographs should be obtained if possible as they are better indicators of true alignment compared to non–weight-bearing radiographs. Three views of the ankle, including anteroposterior (AP), oblique, and lateral, and three views of the foot, including AP, oblique, and lateral, should be obtained. Additionally, a Saltzman hindfoot alignment view should be obtained to allow for better assessment of the extend of hindfoot varus deformity[3] (Figure 16.3).

Pertinent findings on the AP and oblique ankle radiographs would include any presence of ankle arthritis as well as potential varus or compensatory valgus deformity of the ankle. On the lateral radiographs of the foot and ankle, there may be evidence of increased calcaneal pitch, metatarsal stacking, increased sinus tarsi visualization, and posterior appearance of the fibula due to a cavovarus deformity, as well as potential hindfoot arthritis across the triple joint complex. The AP and oblique radiographs of the foot may show associated adduction deformity across the transverse tarsal joint and/or metatarsus adductus, or midfoot arthritis across the tarsometatarsal joints. Furthermore, specific pathologic abnormalities should be considered on the radiographs such as the presence of Mueller-Weiss syndrome with talonavicular arthritis and avascular changes to the navicular associated with hindfoot varus and compensatory flattening of the arch.

MRI

Magnetic resonance imaging is often not needed for the assessment of hindfoot varus; however, it is valuable for assessing pathology associated with hindfoot varus deformities. MRI of the ankle is valuable in assessing for the presence of any osteochondral defects, lateral ligament integrity, peroneal tendon pathology, or early arthritic changes with bone marrow edema of the ankle or hindfoot joints.

CT

Computed tomography has multiple benefits in the setting of assessment of hindfoot varus and associated pathology with this deformity. While non–weight-bearing CT scans are limited in assessing true deformity, the ongoing advancements in weight-bearing CT scans provides a more three-dimensional assessment of the hindfoot deformity.[4,5] An additional benefit to weight-bearing CT scans include decreased radiation compared to more traditional CT scans. Specific pathology seen on CT scans includes the presence of arthritis of the ankle, hindfoot, or midfoot joints assessment for fifth metatarsal fractures, and while not as accurate as MRI, in cases in which a patient is unable to obtain an MRI (ie, pacemakers), a CT scan may at least allow for a degree of evaluation of peroneal tendon pathology.

SURGICAL TECHNIQUE

The patient can be positioned supine or semilateral depending on what other associated procedures need to be completed. In the case of supine positioning, the author elects to use a large C-arm to allow for ease of imaging without having to move the operative extremity. However, in the semilateral positioning, the author elects to use a mini C-arm for ease of imaging. In cases for an isolated lateral displacement and lateral closing wedge osteotomy, the author elects to perform the procedure in the semilateral position.

The landmarks are first triangulated using fluoroscopy, including the entry point for the osteotomy using a radiopaque marker such as a freer elevator. The entry point should take into account the safe zone for the calcaneal osteotomy as described by Talusan and colleagues in order to minimize risk to the sural nerve.[6] They defined the landmark line as a line drawn from the posterior superior apex of the calcaneal tuberosity to the origin of the plantar fascia, and based on cadaveric assessment, they determined the save zone to be with the area 11.2 ± 2.7 mm anterior to this landmark line. Once the entry point is determined with fluoroscopy, a surgical marker is used to mark out the skin incision. Additionally, the proximal and distal exit points on the calcaneus are triangulated with fluoroscopy and marked out with surgical mark to allow for a visualizable trajectory on the skin during burring (Figure 16.4).

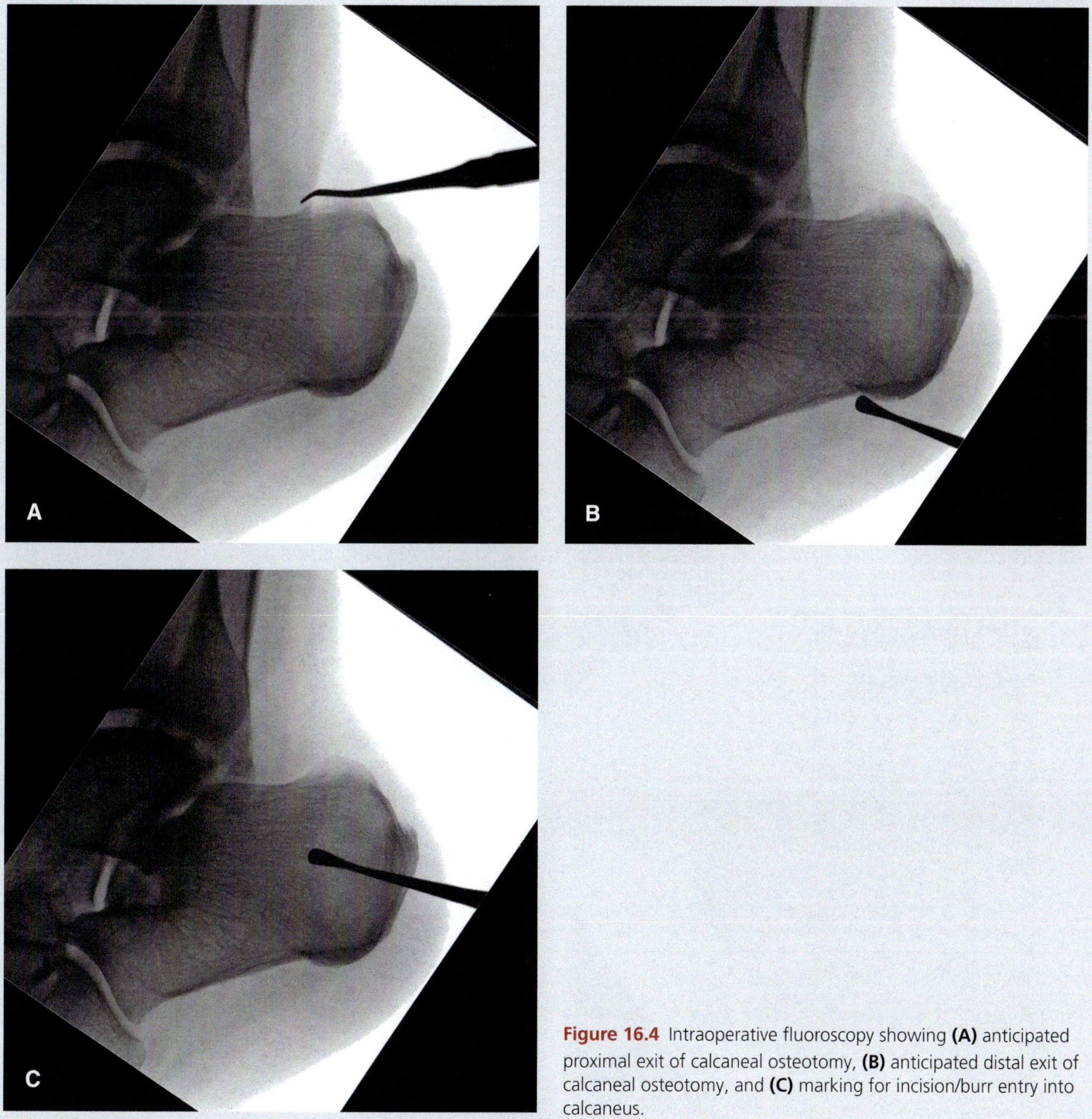

Figure 16.4 Intraoperative fluoroscopy showing **(A)** anticipated proximal exit of calcaneal osteotomy, **(B)** anticipated distal exit of calcaneal osteotomy, and **(C)** marking for incision/burr entry into calcaneus.

Once the trajectory is marked out, a skin incision is made measuring approximately 1 to 2 mm with a Beaver blade through the skin only. A blunt snap is then used to spread the soft tissues down to the bone to protect the adjacent structures. A freer elevator can then be used to gently elevate the adjacent periosteal tissue. At this point, the 3 × 20 mm or 3 × 30 mm Shannon burr is entered into the calcaneus. The author prefers to disconnect the handpiece at this point and confirm with fluoroscopy the entry point as well as visualize the trajectory for the osteotomy prior to proceeding with the osteotomy. The osteotomy is then completed in quadrants including the lateral proximal, medial proximal, lateral distal, and medial distal quadrants. The osteotomy can be completed in a linear or chevron shape depending on surgeon's preference; however, the author prefers to perform a linear osteotomy due to ease and excellent healing potential regardless of technique. While burring, it is critical to ensure copious irrigation whether through the burr system tubing or with an assistant using continuous bulb irrigation. Chilled saline is beneficial here as the cooling aspect of the saline theoretically prevents soft-tissue burns as well as bony necrosis at the osteotomy site. Once the lateral and medial aspects of the osteotomy is completed, the burr is then brought back to midline, and approximately 50% depth and the lateral proximal and lateral distal quadrants are again burred to allow for additional lateral closing wedge correction. Upon completion of the osteotomy, the burr is removed and manual testing of the osteotomy site is beneficial to ensure a complete osteotomy is achieved. The calcaneal tuber should be able to be translated medially or laterally by manual testing, and if this is not achievable, then there is likely an incomplete osteotomy. In this case, the burr can be used to sweep the cortices without running the burr or alternatively a tool such as a freer elevator can be used to feel for any residual uncut cortices.

Once the osteotomy is confirmed to be completed, the surgeon can proceed with reduction and fixation. The author prefers to use a sayre elevator to achieve reduction; however, other tools can be used such as a large hemostat or peon elevator. The reduction tool is placed through the wound and into the calcaneal tuber while it is levered against the lateral skin edges of the adjacent calcaneal body (Figure 16.5). Additionally, to aide in reduction, a small bump can be placed under only the calcaneal tuber thus providing additional lateral force to the tuber. A fluoroscopic calcaneal view should be obtained to confirm sufficient correction including lateral translation as well as closure of the lateral closing wedge with good bony contact prior to pinning and fixation. Once reduction is achieved, the author elects to place two Kirschner wires (K-wires) across the osteotomy site to achieve provisional fixation. Two wires are used in case one wire is inadvertently removed during drilling for screw fixation in order to prevent loss of reduction and alignment of the osteotomy site. Fluoroscopy is used to confirm K-wire placement on lateral and calcaneal views. Once confirmed, one or two large partially threaded cannulated screws can be placed depending on surgeon's preference (Figure 16.6).

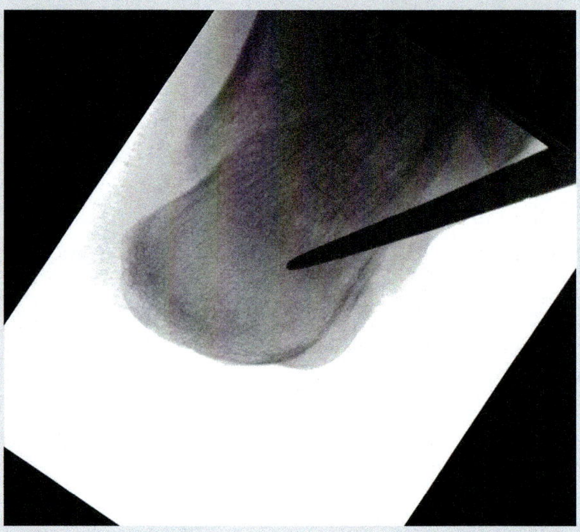

Figure 16.5 Intraoperative fluoroscopy showing lateral translation with use of Sayre elevator.

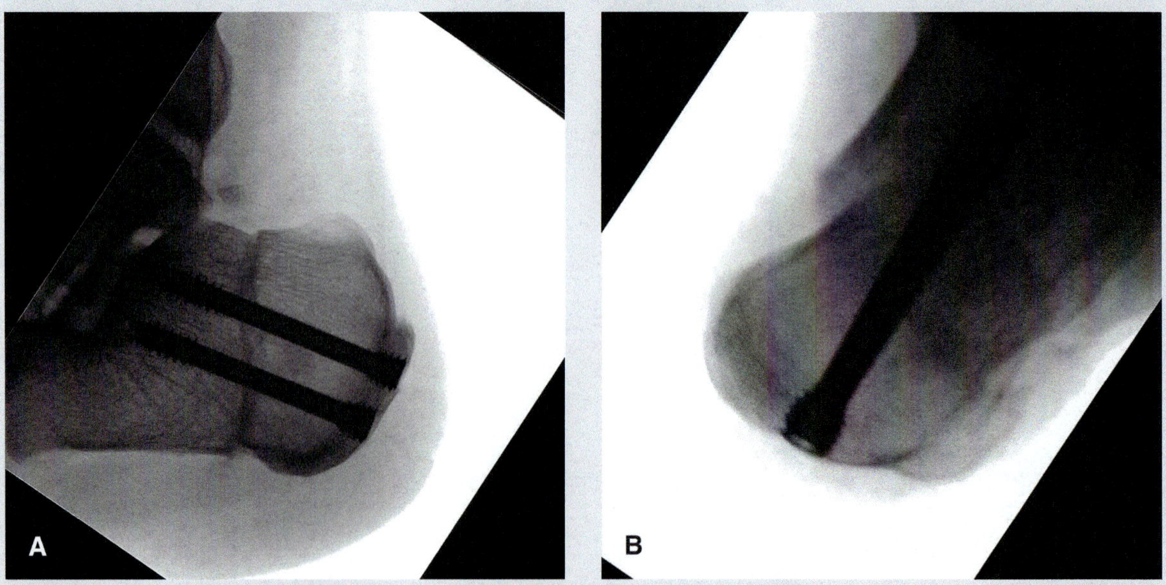

Figure 16.6 Final fixation for calcaneal osteotomy including **(A)** lateral view and **(B)** calcaneal view to confirm screw placement.

In cases of osteoporotic bone or compromised bone health, the author elects to place one partially threaded cannulated screw to achieve compression across the osteotomy site and a second fully threaded cannulated screw to avoid loss of fixation in the postoperative period. Final fluoroscopic views are obtained to confirm placement of all hardware as well as maintenance of reduction and alignment of the osteotomy site.

Upon completion of the procedure, the wound is irrigated copiously using normal saline to remove any residual debris. The author prefers to close the incision with a 4-0 absorbable subcutaneous stich as well as a 3-0 nylon in simple interrupted fashion for the skin layer; however, this is simply surgeon's preference. Associated ancillary procedures are then completed.

◆ POSTOPERATIVE MANAGEMENT

Options for dressings and splint are often dependent on associated ancillary procedure as well as surgeon's preference; however, even in cases of an isolated calcaneal osteotomy, the author prefers to use a Robert-Jones short leg splint in order to protect the osteotomy and the incision sites.

The specific postoperative protocol will often depend on associated ancillary procedures. In cases of isolated calcaneal osteotomies, the author prefers to keep the patient non–weight bearing in the splint for 2 weeks. At the first postoperative visit, the patient is transitioned to a tall controlled ankle motion boot and instructed on range of motion exercises; however, they are kept non–weight bearing until 4 weeks postoperatively. At that point, they are allowed to progress weight bearing as tolerated in the boot. The patient is transitioned out of the boot at the 6-week postoperative visit based on clinical and radiographic healing.

◆ OUTCOMES

The traditional open approach for calcaneal osteotomies allows for good correction of a hindfoot deformity; however, it is associated with wound complications in 5% to 10% of cases and sural nerve injury in 7% to 25% of patients.[7,8] When comparing all calcaneal osteotomies in an open versus percutaneous approach, there have been lower rates of wound complications and sural nerve injuries in the percutaneous group compared to the open group.

Kendal and colleagues compared 50 open calcaneal osteotomies to 31 minimally invasive calcaneal osteotomies to assess safety and compare complications between these two techniques.[9] The majority of these patients underwent medial displacement calcaneal osteotomies; however, there were 9 patients in the minimally invasive group and 18 patients in the open group who were treated for hindfoot varus. The results showed a similar amount of calcaneal shift achieved and rate of union of the osteotomy with significantly fewer complications in the minimally invasive group (6%) compared to the open group (28%) for all calcaneal osteotomies. This includes a lower rate of wound complications (6% vs 28%) and sural neuropathy (0% vs 6%). However, this study did not specifically compare the complications with lateral displacement calcaneal osteotomies.

More recently, Gutteck and colleagues in 2019 reported on their experience in 122 patients undergoing a calcaneal osteotomy for a hindfoot alignment procedure.[10] This included 58 patients in the open group and 64 patients in the minimally invasive group, with hindfoot varus accounting for 16 patients in the open group and 12 patients in the minimally invasive group. In all patients, the authors found that the minimally invasive group had a significantly lower risk of wound healing issues, shorter hospitalization, and lower rate of sural nerve injury while maintaining equal radiographic parameters, AOFAS scores, and overall healing rate of the osteotomy. However, again, there was no specific subset analysis looking exclusively at lateral displacement/closing wedge osteotomies.

Ultimately, while there are limited studies looking exclusively at the outcomes related to minimally invasive lateral displacement/closing wedge osteotomies, given that multiple studies have shown similar efficacy to open procedures while decreasing wound complications and sural nerve injury, the author of this chapter believes that the percutaneous lateral displacement/closing wedge osteotomy is a good option for surgical correction of hindfoot varus in isolation or in combination with associated ancillary procedures.

References

1. Dwyer FC. Osteotomy of the calcaneus for pes cavus. *J Bone Joint Surg Br*. 1959;41-B(1):80-86.
2. Li S, Myerson MS, Monteagudo M, Maceira E. Efficacy of calcaneus osteotomy for treatment of symptomatic Mueller-Weiss disease. *Foot Ankle Int*. 2017;38(3):261-269.
3. Saltzman CL, el-Khoury GY. The hindfoot alignment view. *Foot Ankle Int*. 1995;16(9):572-576.
4. Lintz F, Jepsen M, de Cesar Netto C, Bernasconi A, Ruiz M, Siegler S. Distance mapping of the foot and ankle joints using weightbearing CT: the cavovarus configuration. *Foot Ankle Surg*. 2021;27(4):412-420.
5. An T, Haupt E, Michalski M, Salo J, Pfeffer G. Cavovarus with a twist: midfoot coronal and axial plane rotational deformity in Charcot-Marie-Tooth Disease. *Foot Ankle Int*. 2022;43(5):676-682.
6. Talusan PG, Cata E, Tan EW, Parks BG, Guyton GP. Safe zone for neural structures in medial displacement calcaneal osteotomy: a cadaveric and radiographic investigation. *Foot Ankle Int*. 2015;36(12):1493-1498.
7. Catanzariti AR, Lee MS, Mendicino RW. Posterior calcaneal displacement osteotomy for adult acquired flatfoot. *J Foot Ankle Surg*. 2000;39:2-14.
8. Wacker JT, Hennessy MS, Saxby TS. Calcaneal osteotomy and transfer of the tendon of flexor digitorum longus for stage-II dysfunction of tibialis posterior: three to five year results. *J Bone Joint Surg Br*. 2002;84:54-58.
9. Kendal AR, Khalid A, Ball T, Rogers M, Cooke P, Shapr R. Complications of minimally invasive calcaneal osteotomy versus open osteotomy. *Foot Ankle Int*. 2015;36(6):685-690.
10. Gutteck N, Zeh A, Wohlrab D, Delank KS. Comparative results of percutaneous calcaneal osteotomy in correction of hindfoot deformities. *Foot Ankle Int*. 2019;40(3):276-281.

17 Percutaneous Zadek Osteotomy to Treat Insertional Achilles Tendinopathy

Taylor L. Paskey and Ettore Vulcano

◆ INSERTIONAL ACHILLES TENDINOPATHY

Insertional Achilles tendinopathy (IAT) is the chronic degeneration of the Achilles tendon at its insertion at the midportion of the posterior aspect of the calcaneus. Hallmarks of this disease include ossification of the entheseal fibrocartilage leading to bone spurs and tendon tears with associated pain at the insertion site. IAT is a chronic degenerative condition in the absence of underlying inflammation and is commonly observed in active individuals as well as overweight females in their 40s and in individuals over age 60.[1] Since running can apply 4 to 6 times the force of body weight on the Achilles tendon, IAT has been noted to end careers for up to 5% of professional athletes.[2]

The changes within the Achilles insertion that result from this disease include a loss of parallel collagen fibers due to disorganization from fatty infiltration, intratendinous degeneration, and the proliferation of capillaries. Clinically, patients often present with pain at the prominent posterior heel bump and Achilles/gastrocnemius tightness. Pain is exacerbated by physical activity and after walking following a period of rest (ie, with the first steps in the morning). Radiographically, posterior calcaneus spurs will typically be observed on lateral hindfoot radiographs, although the spurs themselves are not the cause of the pain but rather a manifestation of the chronic tendon degeneration. More advanced imaging (magnetic resonance imaging or ultrasonography) may be necessary in cases where the clinician is uncertain whether the diagnosis is an IAT or a true Haglund deformity, the latter causing inflammation of the tendon in the absence of tendinopathy.

Risk Factors for Achilles Tendinopathy

Risk factors for Achilles tendinopathy can be extrinsic, intrinsic, or systemic. Some of the most important intrinsic risk factors are related to biomechanical abnormalities such as limb length discrepancies, varus deformity of the forefoot, pes cavus, or limited mobility of the subtalar joint. Relevant systemic conditions include those related to age and body mass index, inflammatory arthropathies, endocrine abnormalities, and adverse medication effects. Of the extrinsic factors described, excessive mechanical overload or errors in training practices are the most cited. Examples of this include changes in training schedule, duration of training, and varying inclinations while training.[3-6] Athletes who perform repetitive push-off activities, such as in basketball and soccer, are at most risk for this disease process.[7]

◆ TREATMENT OPTIONS FOR INSERTIONAL ACHILLES TENDINOPATHY

The first approach to treat IAT consists of physical therapy to stretch and eccentrically strengthen the tendon, with the addition of icing, open-back shoes, and a heel lift to mitigate the pain. Extracorporeal shock wave therapy, night splinting, open-back shoes, and platelet-rich plasma have also been described.[2,8]

Operative Management

Traditionally, IAT has been surgically managed with open débridement, calcaneus exostectomy, detachment, and reinsertion of the tendon in patients failing 3 months of nonoperative management. However, this normally requires up to 6 weeks of immobilization and non–weight bearing and is associated with postoperative complications such as wound infection and dehiscence, sural nerve injury, tendon rupture, and ankle stiffness.[7,9] In more recent years, a growing body of literature has emerged supporting the use of a purely bony approach (Zadek osteotomy [ZO]) to the disease to change the biomechanics of the Achilles, ultimately leading to its healing.[7,9-13]

Zadek Osteotomy

The calcaneal dorsal closing wedge osteotomy was first described by Zadek in 1939 for the treatment of Achilles bursitis.[7,13-15] The purpose of this technique for IAT is to decrease the zone of impingement between the superior angle of the calcaneal tuberosity and the anterior portion of the Achilles tendon. As a result of the ZO, the calcaneus is shortened, the tendon is translated anteriorly, the Fowler-Philip angle is lowered, and the distal insertion point of the Achilles is elevated. These alterations lead to less friction and compression of the retrocalcaneal bursa, less irritation of the tendon by the calcaneal prominence, and decreased tightness of the gastroc-soleus muscles.[7,9-13]

Percutaneous Zadek Osteotomy

The open ZO demonstrated good clinical results for IAT, but due to the risks of postoperative complications associated with the large L-shaped lateral incision, the technique was never particularly popular.[13,16,17] This has led to the development of minimally invasive techniques to reduce wound complications.[13,18] As suggested by several studies, the use of keyhole incisions (2-3 mm) is associated with less postoperative pain, fewer soft-tissue complications, and faster healing.[7,10,17,19,20]

◆ INDICATIONS AND CONTRAINDICATIONS

Any patient with a diagnosis of IAT who has failed 3 months of nonoperative treatment is a candidate for the procedure.

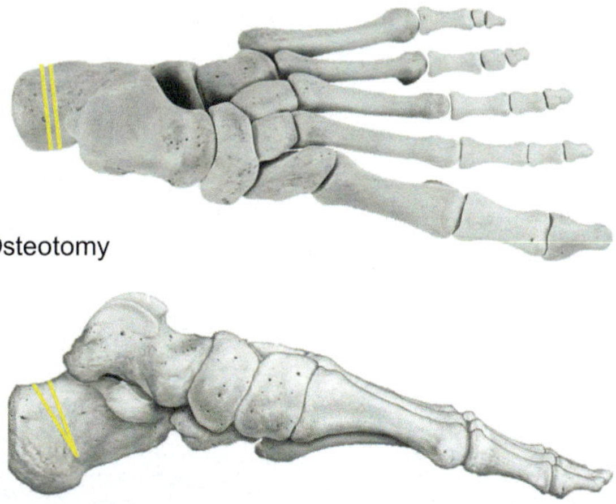

Figure 17.1 The image demonstrates the anatomy and orientation of the Zadek osteotomy. The goal is to remove 8 to 10 mm of a dorsal wedge.

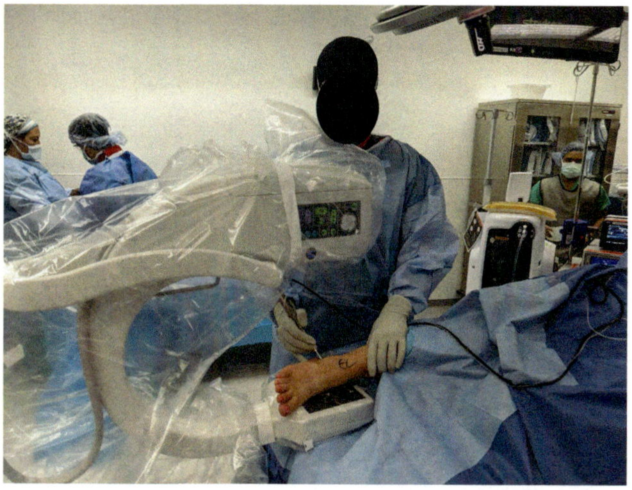

Figure 17.2 The photo illustrates patient, surgeon, and C-arm positioning. The lateral position of the patient is preferred by the senior author.

◆ PREOPERATIVE PLANNING AND PREPARATION

The osteotomy is planned at the posterior tuberosity of the calcaneus, taking care to avoid the subtalar joint. The dorsal closing wedge osteotomy should remove 8 to 10 mm of dorsal bone, and the apex of the wedge should be 5 to 10 mm proximal to the plantar cortex of the calcaneus (Figure 17.1). Violating the plantar hinge of the osteotomy might increase the risk of nonunion.

Room Setup

- The authors routinely place the patient in a lateral position supine (surgical side facing the ceiling) with the surgical foot at the edge of the table. The mini C-arm is positioned at the end of the bed, and the surgical foot should rest directly on it (Figure 17.2).
- The power box should be set at 6,000 rpm but may be increased to 7,000 rpm in patients with harder bone.
- The use of a tourniquet is **highly discouraged** as the intraosseous bleeding may help cool down the burr during the procedure, thus reducing the risk of heat necrosis.
- Saline irrigation of the burr throughout the procedure is also crucial to reduce the risk of thermal injury to the soft tissues. This may be in the form of automated irrigation systems provided by several manufacturers distributing minimally invasive surgery instrumentation or manually by the surgical assistant with the use of a bulb syringe.

SURGICAL TECHNIQUE

- If right-handed, the surgeon will stand at the left side of the patient for a left foot or at the right side of the patient for a right foot.
- The first step is to mark the osteotomy on the lateral aspect of the hindfoot under fluoroscopic guidance (Figure 17.3). The three marks to be made are the anterior and posterior limbs of the osteotomy as well as the apex/plantar hinge of the wedge.
- A superficial skin incision of 3 mm is made in correspondence of the apex of the osteotomy.
- Use mosquito clamps to bluntly dissect the soft tissues until down on bone.
- While the mosquito clamps are keeping the soft tissues retracted, advance a 3 × 30 mm Shannon or cutting burr directly across the calcaneus (Figure 17.4).
- With the tip of the burr feel the far cortex and poke through it without plunging all the way in the medial hindfoot soft tissues.
- Slightly retract the burr and start making the osteotomy (either the anterior or the posterior limb of the wedge).
- The senior author's preference is to burr through the near cancellous bone first, then through the far cancellous, and then making poke holes at the far cortex. Lastly, the burr will be used to "connect" the poke holes. One way to

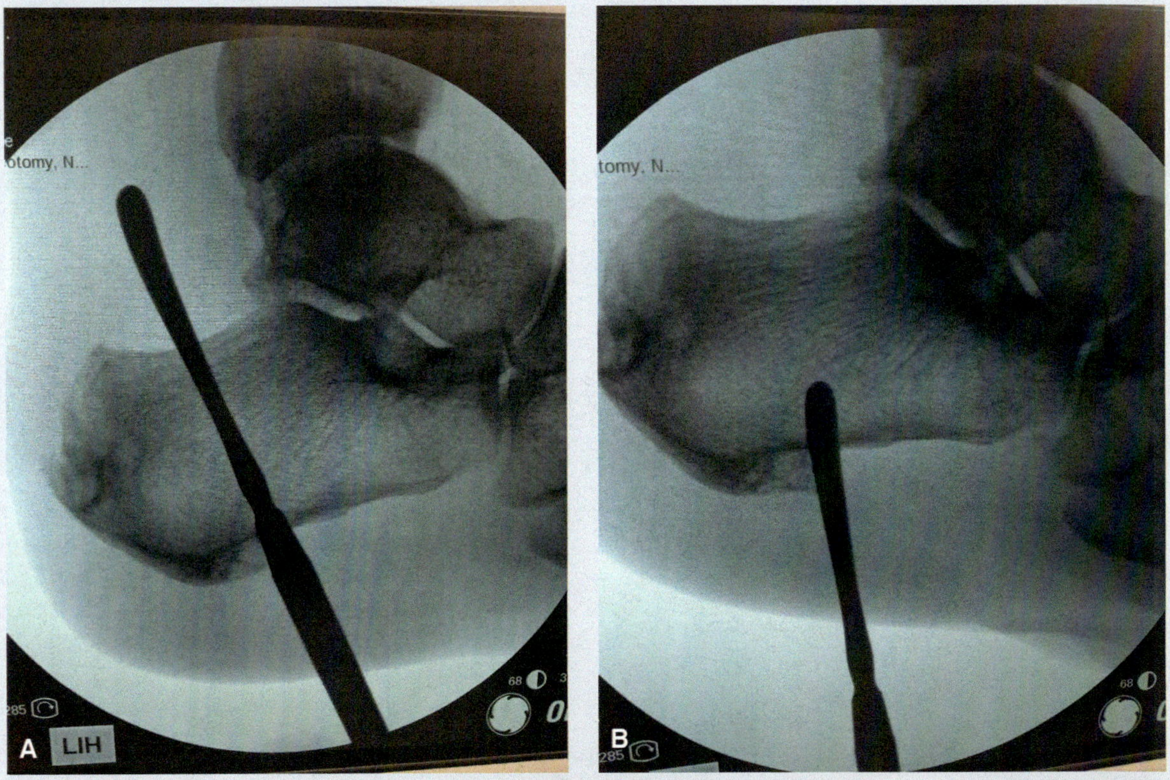

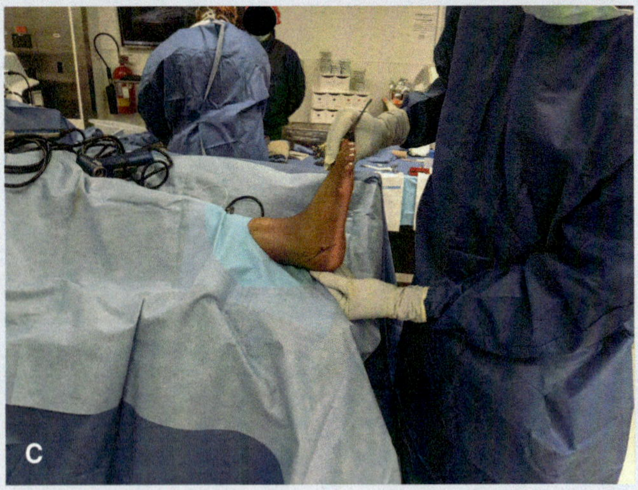

Figure 17.3 **A.** The photo shows the outline of the osteotomy marked under fluoroscopic guidance. **B.** The photo shows the hinge outline of the osteotomy marked under fluoroscopic guidance. **C.** The photo demonstrates the planned osteotomy.

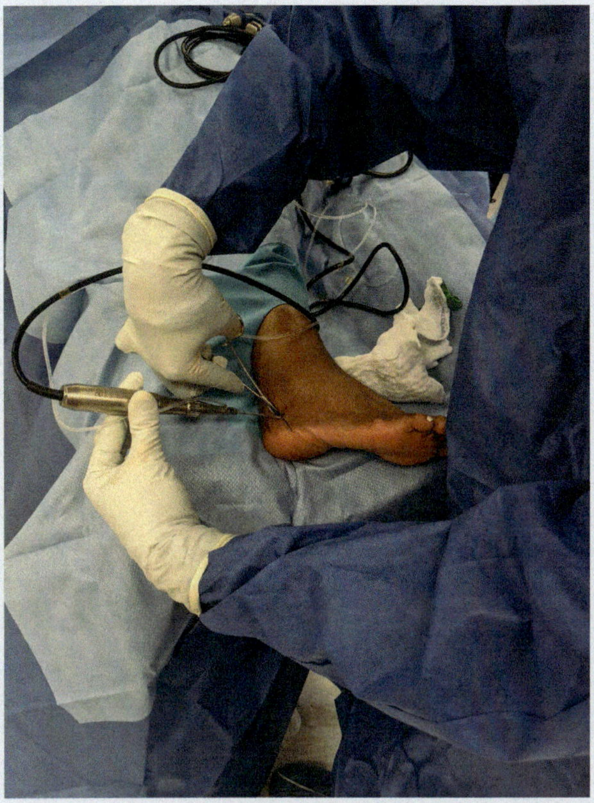

Figure 17.4 The photo demonstrated blunt dissection and retraction of the soft tissues to allow passage of the 3 × 30 mm Shannon burr.

assess if the osteotomy is fully completed is by inserting a freer elevator in the osteotomy and palpate for any bone bridges that might need to be burred down.

- Once the first limb of the osteotomy is completed, there are two possible ways to continue the procedure.
    - Using the same technique, perform the osteotomy along the other remaining leg of the wedge. Then, change the burr to a 3- or 4-mm wedge burr and resect the wedge of bone between the two limbs of the osteotomy. Using this technique might result in overresection especially for less experienced surgeons. Therefore, frequent use of fluoroscopy is recommended to monitor the progress of the osteotomy.
    - Use the same 3 × 30 mm Shannon burr, or convert to a 3- to 4-mm wedge burr, to start shaving bone on either side of the osteotomy. Under fluoroscopic guidance, monitor the amount of bone resected. Make sure to evenly remove bone across the calcaneus, thus avoiding varus or valgus deformities of the hindfoot.
- There is no need to irrigate the osteotomy site as the bone paste will be automatically extruded through the skin incision upon reduction of the osteotomy. Any remaining bone paste will act as bone graft and is very unlikely to cause heterotopic ossification.
- Once the wedge resection is complete, the surgeon can reduce the osteotomy by hyperdorsiflexing the ankle (Figure 17.5). This is actually a fun part of the case to observe under live fluoroscopy. At this point, the surgeon

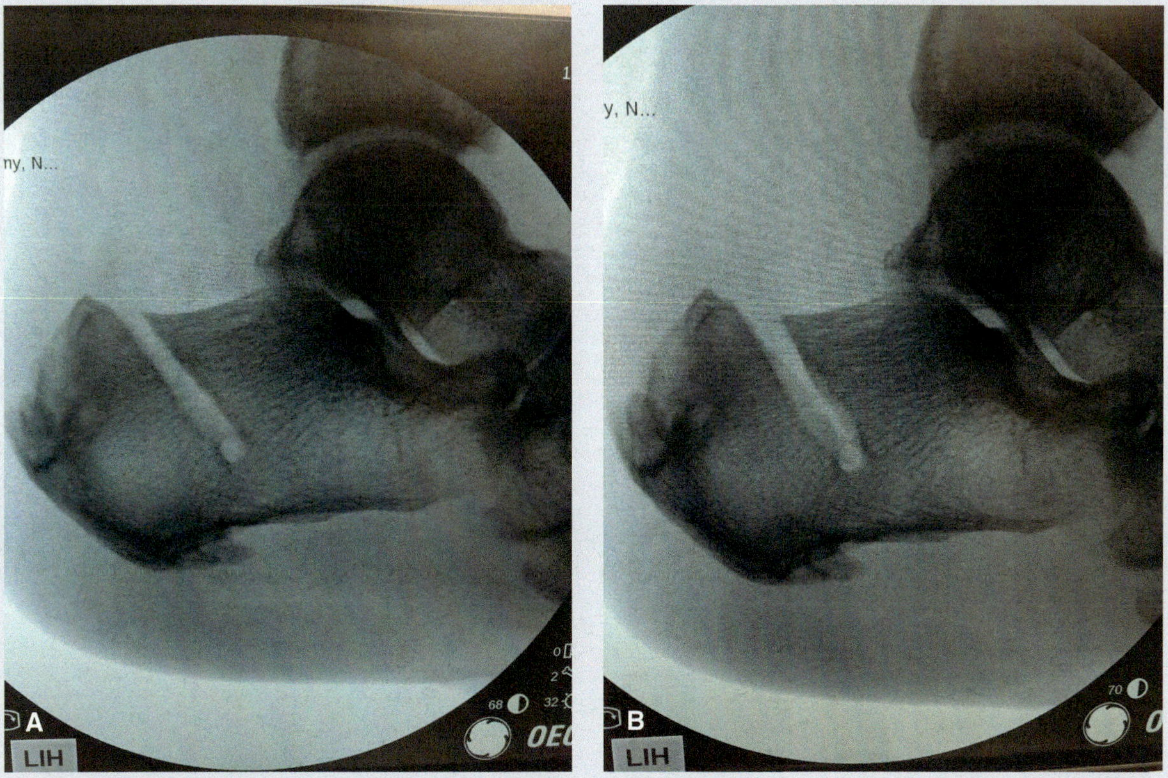

Figure 17.5 **A.** The fluoroscopic image demonstrates the main osteotomy limb. **B.** The fluoroscopic image demonstrates the osteotomy site following shaving of the dorsal wedge prior to being closed. **C.** The fluoroscopic image demonstrates the osteotomy closed by hyperdorsiflexing the ankle.

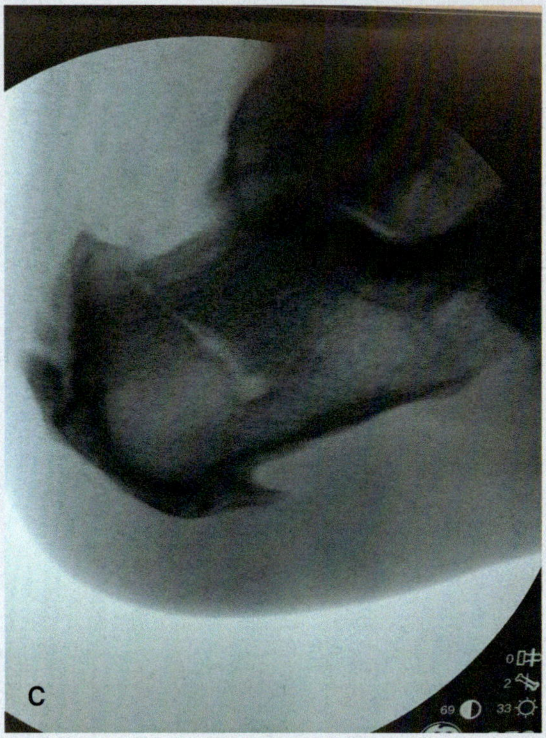

Figure 17.5 *(Continued)*

will note an improved ankle dorsiflexion (to about 20°). If the dorsiflexion feels "tight," it might be advisable to reintroduce the burr and remove more bone from the osteotomy. In the senior author's experience, it is extremely rare to have to excise more than 10 mm of dorsal wedge; hence, caution is recommended if considering added resection.

- The osteotomy is stabilized with one or two 5- to 7-mm headless compression screws driven across the calcaneus (Figure 17.6). If the plantar cortex is fractured or violated, the authors recommend to drive one of the screws along the inferior portion of the bone to stabilize the hinge.
- The skin is closed with the surgeon's sutures of choice, and soft dressings are applied to the lower extremity (Figure 17.7).

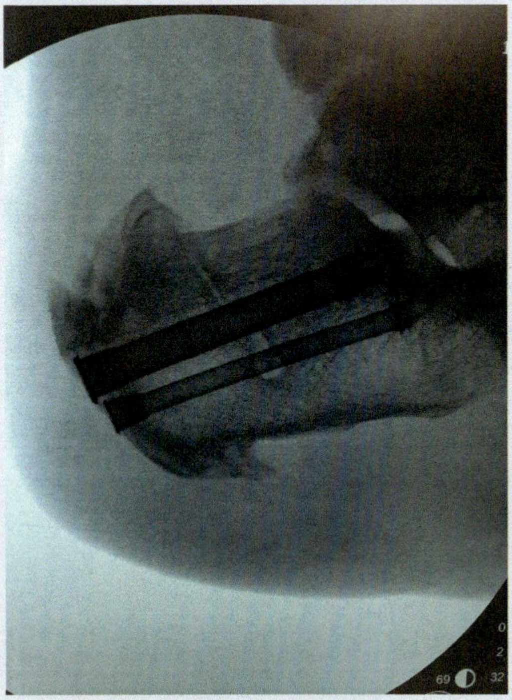

Figure 17.6 The image demonstrates stabilization of the osteotomy site by means of headless compression screws.

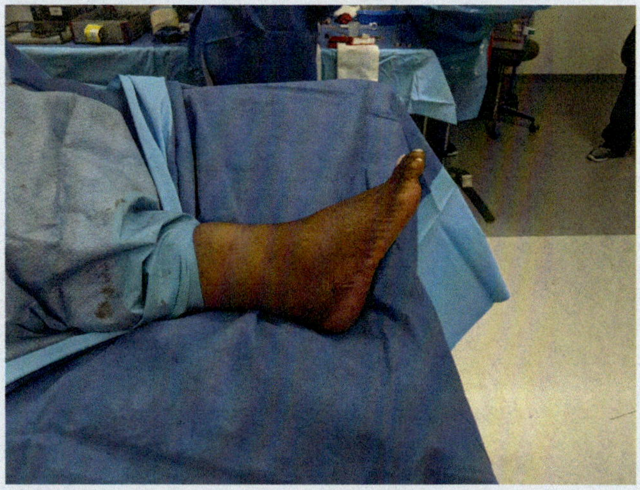

Figure 17.7 The photo shows closure of the wound with a single stitch.

PEARLS AND PITFALLS

- In the setting of a flatfoot, the osteotomy should be more obliquely oriented to minimize a decrease in the calcaneal pitch. Conversely, in cavus feet, the osteotomy can be made more vertical to slightly reduce the calcaneal pitch.
- Occasionally, when the osteotomy is reduced, existing (and particularly prominent) plantar heel spurs might rotate more plantar causing pain. It is advisable to consent the patient for a possible plantar spur exostectomy should this occur.
- Do not keep the burr activated for more than 5 seconds. This might lead to thermal injury to the tissues. Stop the power, allow a few seconds to cool down without removing the burr from its position, and resume the procedure.
- While making the osteotomy, use a gentle sawing motion of the hand to facilitate penetration of the burr into the bone.
- Remember to use a rotational hand movement while making the osteotomy. Imagine the hinge of the burr to be at the skin incision. Ignoring this will cause a widening of the skin incision.

POSTOPERATIVE MANAGEMENT

- Patients are allowed full weight bearing in a controlled ankle motion boot.
- Low-impact activities such as walking, stationary bike, elliptical, upper and several lower body weight-lifting, etc., are allowed in the surgical sandal.
- Early ankle range of motion is encouraged.
- Deep vein thrombosis chemoprophylaxis is not routinely recommended.
- Dressings and stiches are removed 2 weeks postoperatively. At that point, patients are allowed to bathe the surgical foot and can wear socks.

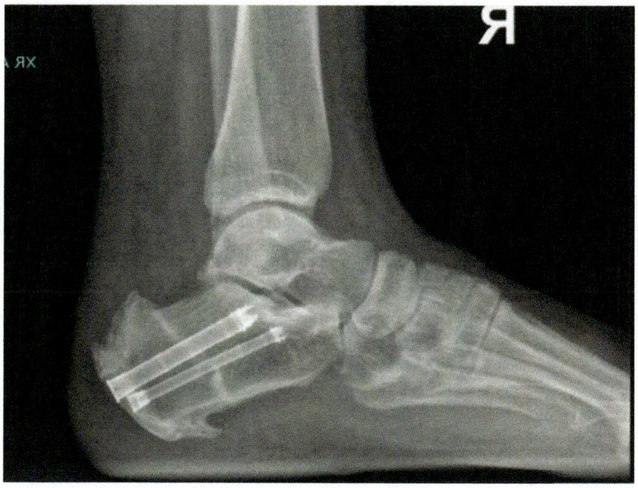

Figure 17.8 The lateral view radiograph of the foot demonstrates a healed osteotomy 3 months following the procedure.

- Two weeks postoperatively, three-view weight-bearing radiographs of the foot or ankle are obtained to confirm there is no displacement of the osteotomy.
- Six weeks postoperatively, new radiographs are obtained. Patients are allowed to wear comfortable shoes, avoiding impact activities. Physical therapy for ankle range of motion, proprioception, and strengthening is also recommended.
- Three months postoperatively, new radiographs are obtained. At this time, most patients will show signs of bone healing (Figure 17.8). Most patients will already report full resolution of the preoperative symptoms but will report lateral and medial heel discomfort. This is normal and resolves around 4 months after surgery.
- At 3 months, if comfortable, patients are allowed to return to any shoe and to any activity as tolerated.
- Remind the patient that postoperative swelling will resolve around 4 months postoperatively.
- Patients should be followed every 3 months in their first year, with or without radiographs depending on symptoms and bone healing at the previous visits.

OUTCOMES

The senior author reported on the experience with 26 patients who underwent percutaneous ZO for IAT. The study found a significant improvement in patient-reported outcomes measured by the Foot Function Index as well as the visual analog scale. The patient satisfaction rate at final follow-up was high at 92%.[13]

In terms of postoperative complications, the open lateral approach for the ZO has been reported to have a high rate of wound complications (5%-25%) across multiple studies.[9,13,21,22] In the cohort of patients who underwent open ZO in the study by Georgiannos et al., the complication rate was 10.9%, with four cases (6.3%) of superficial wound infection.[7] One systematic review demonstrated a wound infection rate of up to 13% in patients undergoing the open ZO, while Paavola et al. found wound-related complications in 4.7% of a cohort of 432 patients undergoing the open ZO.[23,24] Kendal et al. also demonstrated that of 81 patients who underwent calcaneal osteotomy (50 patients in the open group and 31 patients in the percutaneous group), there was a significantly lower risk of wound complications in the percutaneous group (6.45%) compared to the open group (28%). There was also a significantly lower rate of wound infections in the percutaneous group compared to those receiving the open osteotomy (3% vs 20%). In the senior author's study on percutaneous ZO, there were 0 cases of superficial or deep wound infections or wound dehiscence.[13] In terms of neurovascular injuries, the percutaneous approach was found to have a decreased risk of nerve injury (0%) compared to the open approach.[13] In fact, there reported sural nerve injury with open ZO has been reported in 1.6% to 25% of the studied population There is an approximately 7% to 25% risk of nerve injury in the open approach, with complications mostly affecting the sural nerve.[7,9,25,26]

Nonunion is rare in the setting of the ZO, and there has been no significant difference between the incidence of nonunion in the percutaneous approach and the traditional open approach.[9,13,25] In the senior author's percutaneous ZO study, there was one nonunion in 26 patients, which likely resulted from a technical error in violating the plantar hinge at the apex of the osteotomy. This violation created translation of the posterior calcaneal process and failure of the hardware.[13]

◆ CONCLUSION

IAT is a chronic degeneration of the Achilles tendon at its insertion on the calcaneus, plaguing a significant proportion of the population, including recreational and professional athletes. The relatively low success rates of nonoperative treatment often lead patients to seek surgical options to address their condition. The reported data on percutaneous ZO suggest that said technique can be safely and effectively utilized as an alternative to open débridement or open ZO to reduce postoperative pain, reduce soft-tissue complications, and expedite recovery.

References

1. Kader D, Saxena A, Movin T, Maffulli N. Achilles tendinopathy: some aspects of basic science and clinical management. *Br J Sports Med.* 2002;36(4):239-249.
2. Li HY, Hua YH. Achilles tendinopathy: current concepts about the basic science and clinical treatments. *Biomed Res Int.* 2016;2016:6492597.
3. Järvinen TA, Kannus P, Paavola M, Järvinen TL, Józsa L, Järvinen M. Achilles tendon injuries. *Curr Opin Rheumatol.* 2001;13(2):150-155.
4. Krishna Sayana M, Maffulli N. Insertional Achilles tendinopathy. *Foot Ankle Clin.* 2005;10(2):309-320.
5. Holmes GB, Lin J. Etiologic factors associated with symptomatic Achilles tendinopathy. *Foot Ankle Int.* 2006;27(11):952-959.
6. Myerson MS, McGarvey W. Disorders of the Achilles tendon insertion and Achilles tendinitis. *Instr Course Lect.* 1999;48:211-218.
7. Georgiannos D, Lampridis V, Vasiliadis A, Bisbinas I. Treatment of insertional Achilles pathology with dorsal wedge calcaneal osteotomy in athletes. *Foot Ankle Int.* 2017;38(4):381-387.
8. Chimenti RL, Cychosz CC, Hall MM, Phisitkul P. Current concepts review update: insertional Achilles tendinopathy. *Foot Ankle Int.* 2017;38(10):1160-1169.
9. Kendal AR, Khalid A, Ball T, Rogers M, Cooke P, Sharp R. Complications of minimally invasive calcaneal osteotomy versus open osteotomy. *Foot Ankle Int.* 2015;36(6):685-690.
10. Vernois J, Redfern D, Ferraz L, Laborde J. Minimally invasive surgery osteotomy of the hindfoot. *Clin Podiatr Med Surg.* 2015;32(3):419-434.
11. Georgiannos D, Kitridis D, Bisbinas I. Dorsal closing wedge calcaneal osteotomy for the treatment of insertional Achilles tendinopathy: a technical tip to optimize its results and reduce complications. *Foot Ankle Surg.* 2018;24(2):115-118.
12. Boffeli TJ, Peterson MC. The Keck and Kelly wedge calcaneal osteotomy for Haglund's deformity: a technique for reproducible results. *J Foot Ankle Surg.* 2012;51(3):398-401.
13. Nordio A, Chan JJ, Guzman JZ, Hasija R, Vulcano E. Percutaneous Zadek osteotomy for the treatment of insertional Achilles tendinopathy. *Foot Ankle Surg.* 2020;26(7):818-821.
14. Zadek I. An operation for the cure of achillobursitis. *Am J Surg.* 1939;43:542-546.
15. Keck SW, Kelly PJ. Bursitis of the posterior part of the heel; evaluation of surgical treatment of eighteen patients. *J Bone Joint Surg Am.* 1965;47:267-273.
16. Miller AE, Vogel TA. Haglund's deformity and the Keck and Kelly osteotomy: a retrospective analysis. *J Foot Surg.* 1989;28(1):23-29.
17. Maynou C, Mestdagh H, Dubois HH, Petroff E, Elise S. L'Ostéotomie calcanéenne est-elle justifiée dans la maladie de Haglund? [Is calcaneal osteotomy justified in Haglund's disease?]. *Rev Chir Orthop Reparatrice Appar Mot.* 1998;84(8):734-738.
18. Group W. M. *Annual Report 2017.* 2017.
19. Syed TA, Perera A. A proposed staging classification for minimally invasive management of Haglund's syndrome with percutaneous and endoscopic surgery. *Foot Ankle Clin.* 2016;21(3):641-664.
20. Maffulli N, Longo UG, Marinozzi A, Denaro V. Hallux valgus: effectiveness and safety of minimally invasive surgery. A systematic review. *Br Med Bull.* 2011;97:149-167.
21. Catanzariti AR, Lee MS, Mendicino RW. Posterior calcaneal displacement osteotomy for adult acquired flatfoot. *J Foot Ankle Surg.* 2000;39(1):2-14.
22. Folk JW, Starr AJ, Early JS. Early wound complications of operative treatment of calcaneus fractures: analysis of 190 fractures. *J Orthop Trauma.* 1999;13(5):369-372.
23. Kearney R, Costa ML. Insertional Achilles tendinopathy management: a systematic review. *Foot Ankle Int.* 2010;31(8):689-694.
24. Paavola M, Orava S, Leppilahti J, Kannus P, Järvinen M. Chronic Achilles tendon overuse injury: complications after surgical treatment. An analysis of 432 consecutive patients. *Am J Sports Med.* 2000;28(1):77-82.
25. Gutteck N, Zeh A, Wohlrab D, Delank KS. Comparative results of percutaneous calcaneal osteotomy in correction of hindfoot deformities. *Foot Ankle Int.* 2019;40(3):276-281.
26. Talusan PG, Cata E, Tan EW, Parks BG, Guyton GP. Safe zone for neural structures in medial displacement calcaneal osteotomy: a cadaveric and radiographic investigation. *Foot Ankle Int.* 2015;36(12):1493-1498.

18 Percutaneous Haglund Resection

Ettore Vulcano

◆ INTRODUCTION

In 1928, the Swedish orthopedic surgeon, Patrick Haglund,[1] described a condition involving a painful osseous prominence of the posterolateral corner of the calcaneus, large posterior callus, and retrocalcaneal bursitis. In the absence of Achilles tendinopathy, a Haglund deformity can be addressed by performing an exostectomy of the calcaneus. Open and endoscopic techniques have been described for this. The complication rate for open surgery in one study is 12.3% (range, 0%-53%).[2] The complications reported included transient paresthesia around the wound (4.3%), superficial infection (3%), incision site tenderness (0.8%), delayed wound healing (0.6%), heel numbness (0.6%), extensive hematoma (0.6%), Achilles tendon rupture (0.4%), complex regional pain syndrome (0.2%), hypertrophic scar (0.2%), sural nerve neuropathy (0.2%), and deep vein thrombosis (0.2%).[2] Endoscopic techniques, on the other hand, have demonstrated a significantly lower complication rates of 5.3% (range, 0%-18%).[2] Such complications include superficial wound infection (1.8%), sural nerve neuropathy (0.9%), delayed wound healing (0.6%), heel numbness (0.6%), portal site tenderness (0.6%), deep vein thrombosis (0.3%), Achilles tendon rupture (0.3%), and complex regional pain syndrome (0.3%).[2] Endoscopic resection of the Haglund deformity is technically difficult, deterring less experienced surgeons or those who do not routinely employ arthroscopic techniques in their practice. For such reason, the use a fully percutaneous technique might be of interest to surgeons less willing to use an arthroscope but nonetheless eager to perform the procedure through a keyhole incision that should minimize soft-tissue complications.

◆ INDICATIONS

Indications for percutaneous Haglund resection in patients who have failed at least 3 months of nonoperative treatments (ie, oral anti-inflammatories, activity modification, and physical therapy) include the following:

1. Painful posterior bony impingement with posterior facet edema on MRI
2. Minimal or no Achilles tendinopathy

◆ PATIENT HISTORY AND PHYSICAL EXAMINATION

The diagnosis of Haglund syndrome is generally straightforward with obvious posterior heel pain, swelling, and redness. Tenderness is reported at the posterolateral "bump," the retrocalcaneal burse anterior to the Achilles tendon. Of note, posteromedial bumps are more suggestive of an insertional Achilles tendinopathy instead of a true Haglund syndrome. Most patients are young adults, physically active, who complain of pain when walking or exercising. The pain dissipates with rest and often improves with the use of heels or a small heel lift.

◆ IMAGING STUDIES

Weight-bearing radiographs including three views of the foot and ankle should be obtained in all patients. The radiographs will demonstrate a prominent Haglund deformity (Figure 18.1) and, in most cases, the lack of intratendinous insertional Achilles calcifications. An MRI is useful in differentiating an insertional tendinopathy of the Achilles versus a true Haglund's. The latter will present with edema of the exostosis and Achilles bursitis, without signs of Achilles degeneration or tearing.

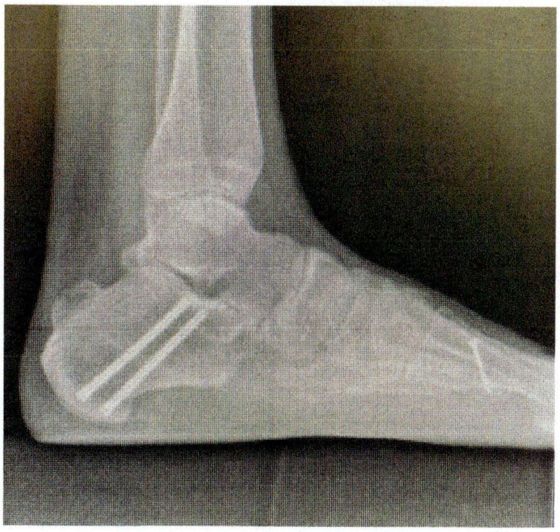

Figure 18.1 The lateral radiograph demonstrates a prominent Haglund deformity.

SURGICAL TECHNIQUE

Once the chosen nerve block has been performed (the senior author prefers an ankle or a popliteal block), the patient is placed in a lateral position with the surgical side facing the ceiling (Figure 18.2). The mini C-arm is positioned at the end of the surgical table allowing for the foot to rest on the image intensifier while the surgeon stands at either side of the bed. The power box should be set to 6,000 rpm, and irrigation should be available throughout the entire case. The use of the tourniquet is strongly discouraged to prevent thermal injury to the tissues.

Upon prepping and draping of the surgical site, the entry point for the exostectomy is identified under fluoroscopic visualization. Ideally, the portal is at the base of the Haglund's, roughly midway (Figure 18.3). A 3-mm skin incision is made at this level, and the subcutaneous tissues are bluntly dissected with a mosquito clamp. A 3-mm wedge burr is advanced into the wound, aiming for the apex of the Haglund deformity (Figure 18.4). Under repeated fluoroscopic visualization, the burr is activated and a gentle sweeping motion is applied to resect the bony prominence gradually (Figure 18.5). The senior author's preference is to start shaving from medial to lateral.

Once the deformity is resected (Figure 18.6), the wound is copiously irrigated with an 18-gauge blunt needle and a 50-mL syringe. A small bone rasp can also be used to help remove any debris.

The wound is closed with the suture of preference (Figure 18.7), followed by application of sterile dressings and a surgical boot.

Postoperatively, patients are allowed immediate weight-bearing in the surgical boot and are encouraged to work on ankle range of motion as soon as possible. Two weeks after surgery, patients are allowed to transition into comfortable shoes and may return to activities as tolerated.

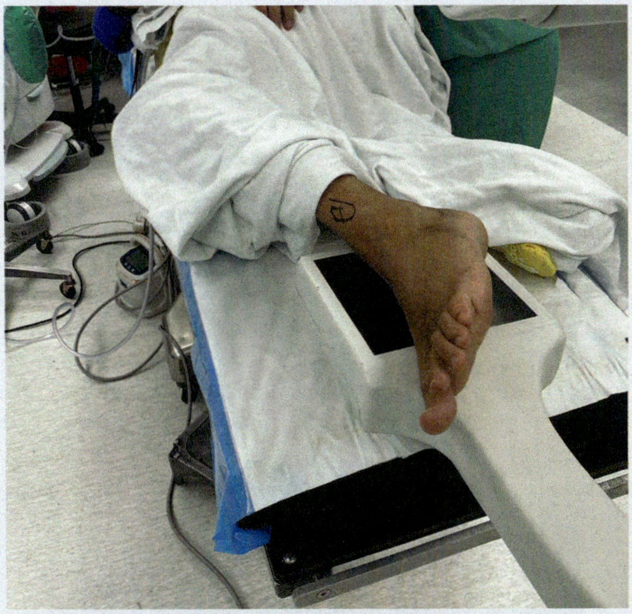

Figure 18.2 The patient is positioned in the lateral position, allowing the foot to rest on the C-arm.

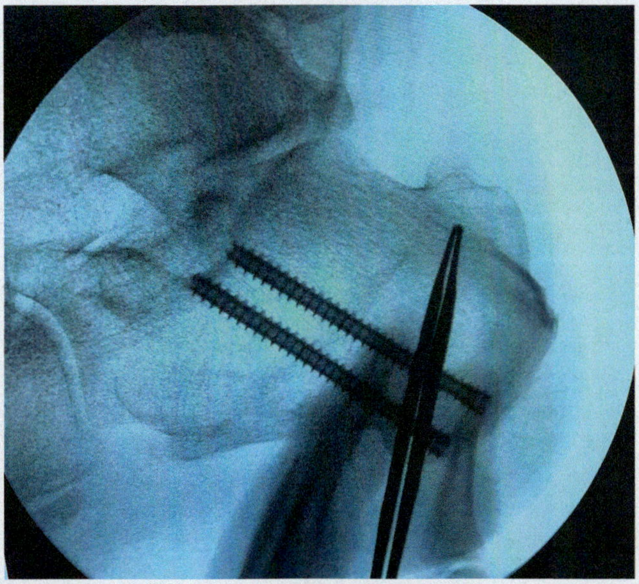

Figure 18.3 The entry point is identified under fluoroscopy. This is at the midline of the base of the Haglund bump.

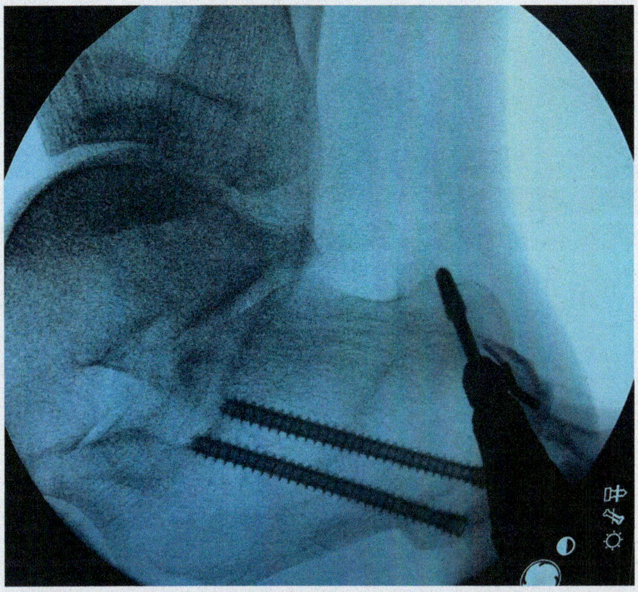

Figure 18.4 The 3-mm wedge burr is advanced to reach the apex of the deformity.

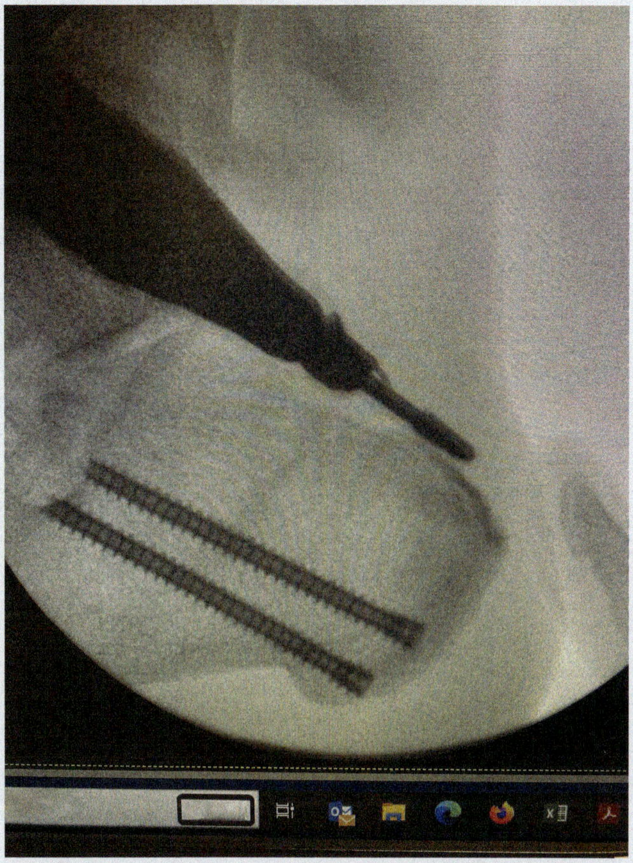

Figure 18.5 The deformity is gradually resected from medial to lateral and from anterior to posterior.

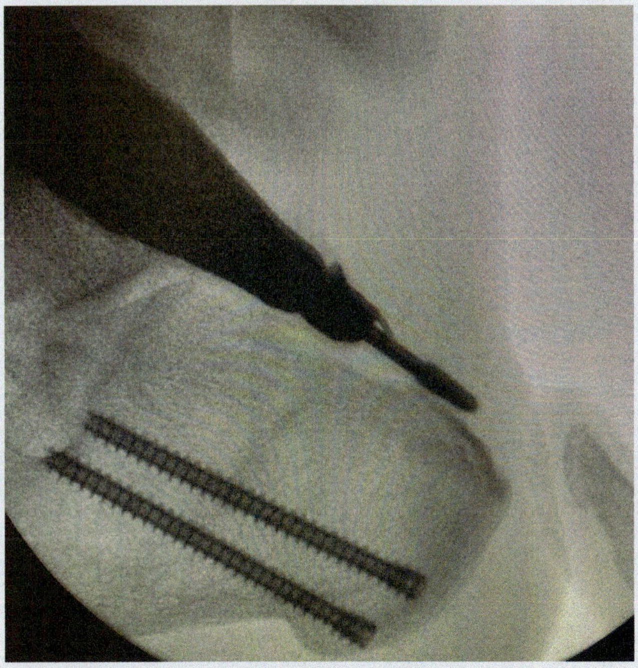

Figure 18.6 The fluoroscopic image demonstrates satisfactory resection of the Haglund deformity.

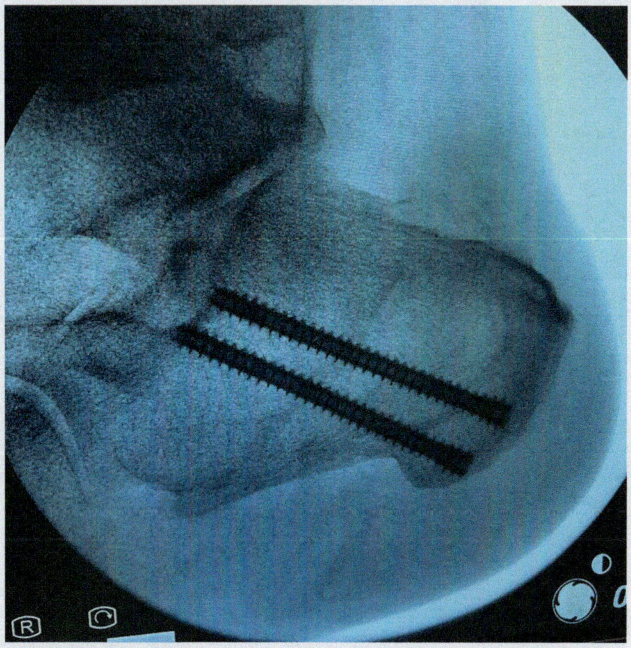

Figure 18.7 A single suture is given to close the wound.

PEARLS AND PITFALLS

- While shaving the exostosis, it is important to remember that the burr should hinge/rotate at the level of the skin incision, avoiding any left-right translation of the hand, which will result in lacerating the wound.
- Always ensure that the irrigation system of the burr is functioning throughout the case or that an assistant is constantly dripping saline on the burr during the procedure. This is important to prevent thermal injury to the soft tissues. For the same reason, a tourniquet should not be used as it would prevent the cooling effect caused by bleeding.
- The exostectomy can be performed with either a 3- or 4-mm wedge burr.
- The surgeon should be cautious not to apply too much pressure when shaving the most posterior aspect of the Haglund's so as to avoid "falling" into the Achilles tendon. Performing this step of the procedure under fluoroscopy may also be helpful in preventing such injury.

References

1. Haglund P. Beitrag zur Klinik der Achilles tendon. *Zeitschr Orthop Chir*. 1928;49:49-58.
2. Yuen WLP, Tan PT, Kon KKC. Surgical treatment of Haglund's deformity: a systematic review and meta-analysis. *Cureus*. 2022;14(7):e27500.

19 Arthroscopic and Percutaneous Triple Arthrodesis

Alastair Younger and Andrea Veljkovic

◆ INTRODUCTION

Arthroscopic triple arthrodesis is an alternative to the open procedure, avoiding the risks of wound complications and periarticular dissection. Reports to date are case reports for arthroscopic triple arthrodesis. The principles used for arthroscopic ankle fusion can be followed. The main challenges are getting appropriate portal placement. Arthroscopy and percutaneous techniques are used to remove the cartilage from all three joints. Subsequent screw fixation is used to immobilize the three joints in a neutral position to achieve fusion in the corrected position. Potential benefits of arthroscopic triple arthrodesis are the reduction of wound complications, maintenance of bone blood supply, better cartilage débridement, reduction of bleeding, and assessment of other pathology arthroscopically. Challenges include the steep learning curve, the potential for nerve injury, and correct placement of fixation. To assist in successful surgery, the surgeon should be capable and well trained in the open surgery, as well as arthroscopic and percutaneous techniques. These skills can be obtained through cadaver labs as well as attempting arthroscopy in open cases with consent of the patient. Much of the guidance is through palpation. To assist in the initial débridement and creation of a joint space, a percutaneous Shannon burr can be used to remove osteophytes and get initial cartilage removal within the joint under C-arm control and palpation. This creates a much bigger space for the insertion of the arthroscope. The procedure can also be hybrid arthroscopic and open, with, for example, the subtalar fusion done arthroscopic and the talonavicular fusion done open. For example, this may be determined by prior incisions.

◆ INDICATIONS AND CONTRAINDICATIONS

Indications

- End-stage talonavicular arthritis (Figure 19.1)
- Planovalgus foot deformity
- Congenital conditions
- Charcot arthropathy without major bone loss
- Posttraumatic arthritis of the triple joint complex
- Old scars compromising an open procedure

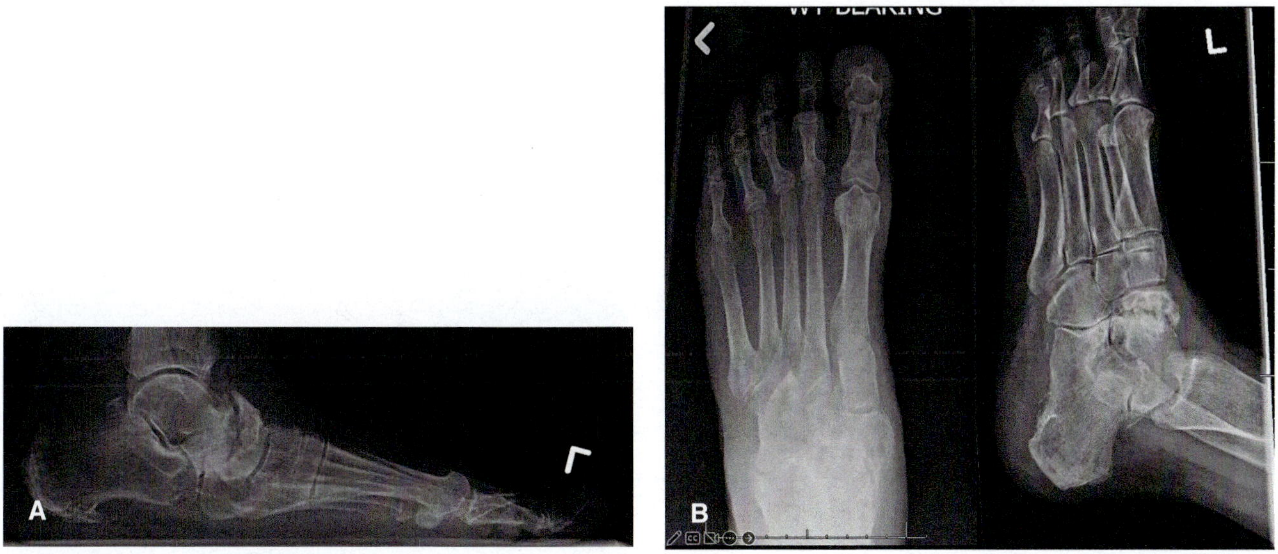

Figure 19.1 **A, B.** AP and lateral view of a patient with talonavicular arthritis amenable to arthroscopic fusion to preserve the blood supply to the bones.

- Patients at risk of wound healing complications
- Staged surgery such as a triple arthrodesis prior to a total ankle arthroplasty
- Mueller-Weiss disease in combination with a navicular-cuneiform fusion

Contraindications

- Major bone loss
- Major deformity, particularly cavus, requiring major bone resection
- Infection (relative contraindication)

◆ EQUIPMENT

A larger arthroscope allows better fluid flow and a wider field of visualization. A 2.9 scope has an approximately 5-mm cannula. This can fit into the joint in most cases. Arthroscopic shavers, such as a 3.5- or 5-mm resector, plus a cutting burr with an auger shaft for debris removal are invaluable. Pump or gravity irrigation can be used. Bone graft if used should be injectable so that it can be placed through the portals. A 2 × 12 mm Shannon burr with the appropriate handpiece and power supply can assist in the early joint débridement and removal of osteophytes. Screw fixation should ideally be nonvariable pitch full thread 6- to 7-mm cannulated screws for the subtalar joint. The talonavicular joint and calcaneocuboid joints can be transfixed by full thread screws in a diameter range between 3.5 and 5 mm in size. Headless screws are helpful in avoiding hardware irritation and removal. Intraoperative imaging can be achieved with a mini or large C-arm. The author prefers the small C-arm.

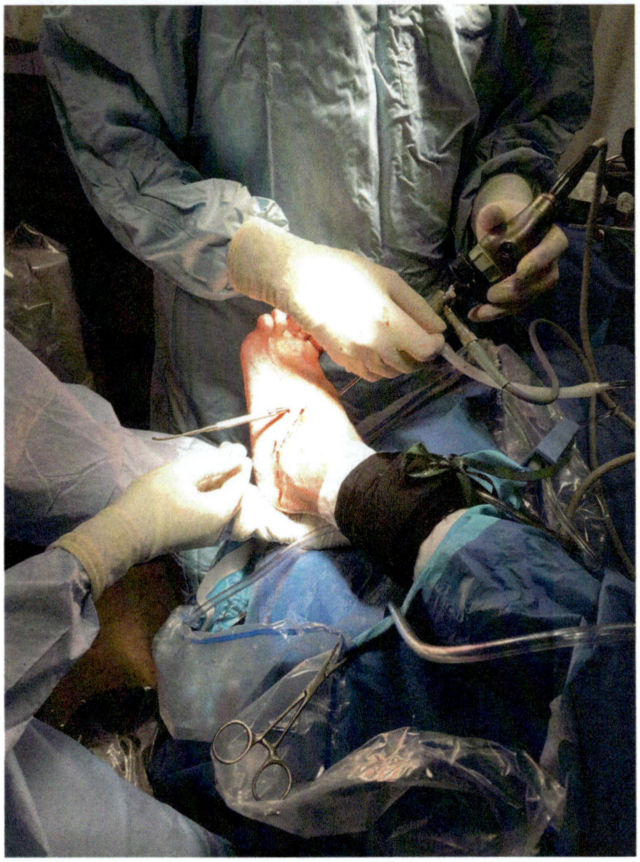

Figure 19.2 Positioning in the operating room with a calf tourniquet, regional block, and internal rotation of the hip to allow access to the lateral border of the foot.

◆ POSITIONING AND OPERATING ROOM ORGANIZATION

The procedure is done supine with the hip internally rotated (Figure 19.2). A beanbag can allow correct positioning with the foot being 10° to 20° internally rotated on the operating room table.

The procedure can be done under nerve block with a sterile calf tourniquet or with a spinal or general with a thigh tourniquet. The arthroscopy tower is placed on the opposite side of the bed toward the patient's head. The C-arm is placed at the base of the bed. It is best to release all three joints using a blunt elevator first, then débride all three joints working from back to front, and then transfix all joints with screw fixation in the order of subtalar joint, talonavicular joint, and calcaneocuboid joint.

◆ PORTAL PLACEMENT

Subtalar Joint

The subtalar joint can be approached safely through the sinus tarsi as described by Walter and Winson[1] (Figure 19.3). The first portal is placed just lateral to the talar neck. The top of the calcaneus is palpated, and the anterior side of the posterior facet is identified. Two more portals are required, one posterior to the peroneal tendons and proximal to the posterior facet joint line, and one next to the Achilles tendon and about a centimeter more proximal to this (Figure 19.4). This last portal will allow access to the medial side of the posterior facet for cartilage removal.[2]

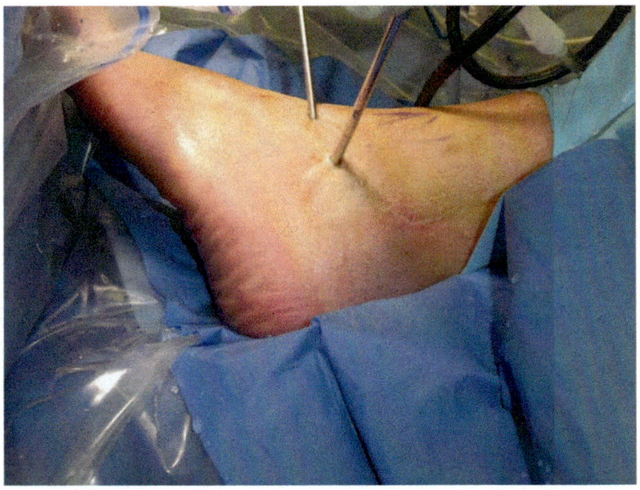

Figure 19.3 Demonstration of the portals used for anterior subtalar arthroscopy.

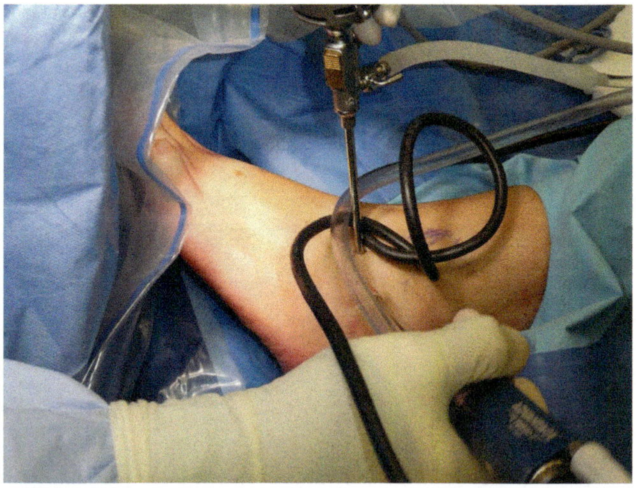

Figure 19.4 The direct lateral portals for subtalar arthroscopy.

The Shannon burr can be placed into the sinus tarsi portal to allow osteophyte and cartilage removal. Care should be taken to avoid the sural nerve laterally and the tibial nerve medially.[3]

Calcaneocuboid Joint

The calcaneocuboid joint lies immediately under and lateral to the talonavicular joint. The lateral portal for the talonavicular joint can also be used for the calcaneocuboid joint (Figure 19.5). The other two portals can be placed direct lateral and dorsal lateral. Initial débridement can be done with the Shannon burr using the two dorsal portals to remove osteophytes and dorsal cartilage. Care is taken not to damage the saphenous nerve.

Talonavicular Joint

The easiest access to the talonavicular joint is lateral and just above the calcaneus and the cuboid (Figure 19.6). Portals can also be placed each side of the neurovascular bundle on the dorsal side of the foot and an additional portal placed over the medial side of the joint proximal to the tuberosity of the navicular.[4] Nerves at risk based on a cadaver study include the superficial and deep peroneal nerve, particularly with the dorsal medial portal. Care is taken not to damage the deep branch of the peroneal nerve, which is dorsal and central to the talonavicular joint and closely opposed to it, and to avoid the saphenous nerve medially.

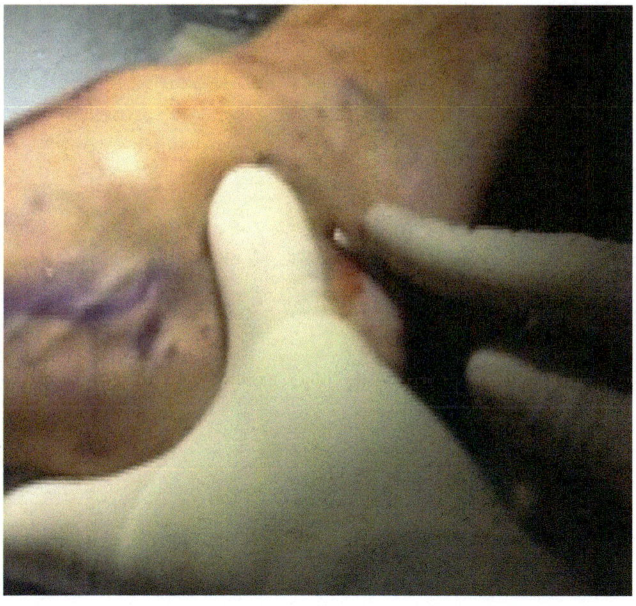

Figure 19.5 The calcaneocuboid portals. The instrument is in the lower portal; the upper portal is above the surgeon's left hand.

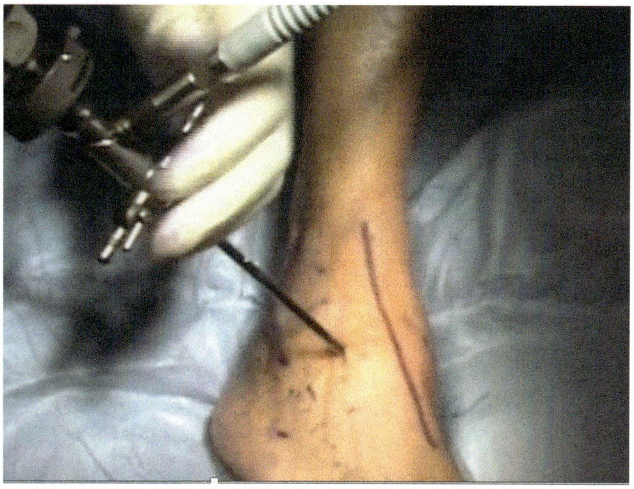

Figure 19.6 The arthroscope in the lateral portal to the talonavicular joint.

◆ SUBTALAR DÉBRIDEMENT

The initial débridement is performed using the Shannon burr. To correctly release and identify the joint, a blunt instrument is used to palpate the joint through the portal. The nondominant hand is placed medially palpating the medial and posterior joint line. The Shannon burr is then placed to remove the osteophytes and anterior lateral cartilage from the talus and calcaneus. C-arm views can be used to assess the correct placement if there is concern. Palpation will also determine if both joint lines are moving at the time of débridement confirming correct placement.

The 2.9 scope is then placed in the talar neck portal with the shaver in the sinus tarsi portal. The debris is washed out and the joint visualized. With this combination, the anterior half of the subtalar joint can be débrided of cartilage. A combination of the shaver and the burr is used.

Once the anterior cartilage has been removed, the arthroscope is switched to the sinus tarsi portal and the joint penetrated with a blunt instrument from the peroneal portal. The instrument is visualized via the arthroscope and the portal expanded to allow the insertion of the burr. Sequential posterior cartilage removal is then performed (Figure 19.7).

The medial side of the joint is débrided with the arthroscope placed either in the sinus tarsi or the peroneal portal with the burr placed from the Achilles tendon portal. The initial dissection is blunt and penetration of the joint confirmed. This portal is closest to the tibial nerve, so care is

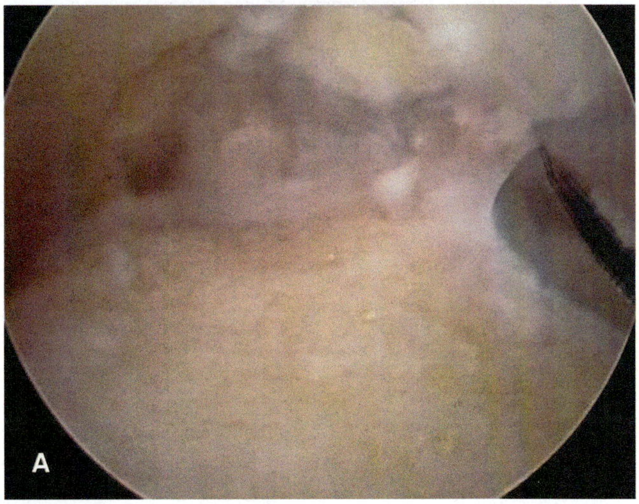

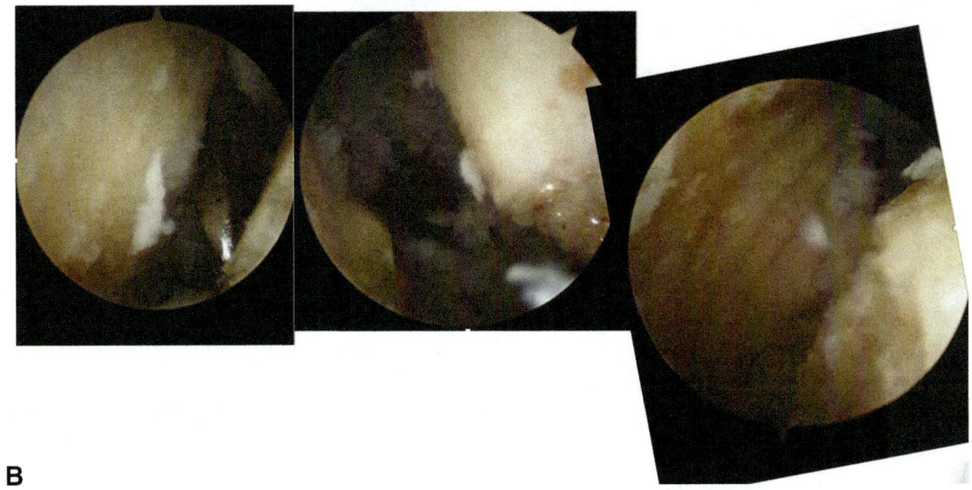

Figure 19.7 **A.** The débridement of the subtalar joint and **(B)** the débridement of the talonavicular joint.

taken to stay medial, and no shaver is used within the joint without direct visualization through the arthroscope of the entire working end of the instrument. The burr is used to remove the remainder of the cartilage.

Complete cartilage removal through the arthroscope should be confirmed. All cartilage debris should be removed from the joint as cartilage can act as a biological and physiological barrier to bone healing.

Talonavicular Joint

The dorsal side of the talonavicular joint cannot be approached using the Shannon burr as this may damage the neurovascular bundle. The talonavicular joint is the hardest joint to débride, and in early cases, the surgeon may need to consider converting to open. Sometimes the joint space can be tighter than expected.

The initial portal is placed laterally in the soft spot palpated between the talus, navicular, calcaneus, and cuboid. A portal is made and the joint palpated with a blunt elevator. Confirmation is achieved using C-arm and palpation. The 2 × 12 mm Shannon burr can be used for initial cartilage removal with care being taken not to penetrate the subchondral bone. This, however, will create space for the arthroscope and shaver in tighter joints.

The lateral portal can then be used to access the dorsal lateral and dorsal medial portals each side of the neurovascular bundle by going from inside to outside.

A shaver can be placed from dorsal lateral with the arthroscope placed lateral. After removal of debris the burr can be used to sequentially remove cartilage moving medial. The dorsal medial portal is used next. The direct medial portal is required for removal of the plantar and most medial cartilage. Again, complete cartilage removal is required.

Calcaneocuboid Joint

Initial débridement can be achieved from the dorsal lateral portal. An incision is made and the joint palpated with a blunt instrument. The Shannon burr is used to remove the dorsal osteophytes and cartilage. The arthroscope can be placed in this portal and the shaver in the more medial portal used for the lateral talonavicular joint.

Sequential cartilage removal can then be performed from dorsal to plantar in the calcaneocuboid joint. Once the dorsal half of the joint has been débrided, the arthroscope is then switched to the dorsal lateral portal, and the shaver is inserted via the lateral portal to the plantar side of the joint to remove the remainder of the cartilage. Complete cartilage removal should be performed to the medial side of the joint.

◆ SCREW FIXATION

Joint reduction and screw fixation is performed in the subtalar joint first, the talonavicular joint second, and the calcaneocuboid joint third.

Subtalar Joint

Three screws are placed from the tuberosity into the body or neck of the talus. Care is taken to ensure that the wires or drill bits do not penetrate the ankle joint. The joint is reduced into about 5° of hindfoot valgus and checked (Figure 19.8).

After confirmation of position on an anterior-posterior view of the ankle and foot, a calcaneal axial view and lateral view of the hindfoot three screws are placed. The first can be partially threaded and the second two fully thread. Arthroscopic fusion preserves the subchondral bone, which has excellent strength so screw fixation can be achieved at this level. Two screws are required to immobilize the joint to all forces, and a third is beneficial as an insurance screw. 6.5- to 7-mm cannulated screws or 4.5 solid screws can be used. Single screw fixation results in a higher nonunion rate.[5]

Dr. Lui has also published an earlier technical note on the procedure.[6]

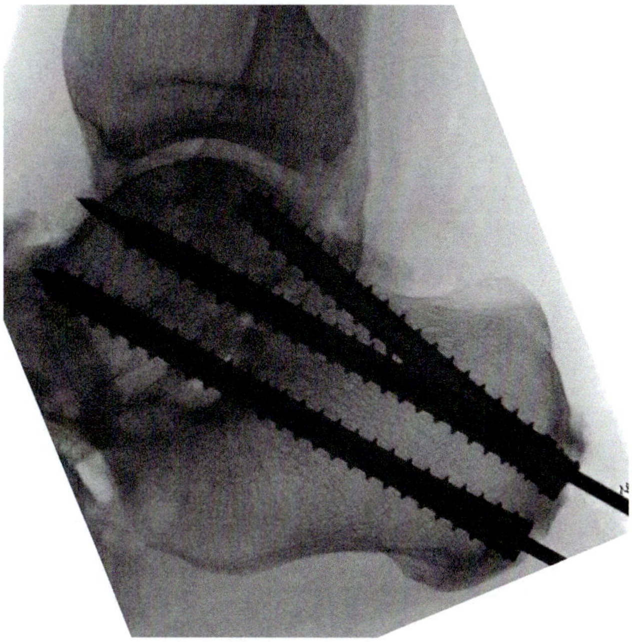

Figure 19.8 Subtalar screw placement. Views are also checked on an AP ankle, a calcaneal axial, and an AP of the foot to ensure that all screws are in bone. Penetration of the ankle joint with a wire should be avoided.

Talonavicular Joint

Reduction is achieved initially using the guidewire from the cannulated screw set. Typically, the navicular will need to be brought plantar and medial to correct forefoot varus and adduction. This can be checked against the tibial axis and the forefoot rotation confirmed. The author prefers the 4-mm fully threaded screws for this application as they have appropriate thread diameter, are headless, and nonvariable pitch. Fixation can be achieved percutaneously from the medial side and from the dorsal medial and dorsal lateral side (Figure 19.9). Care is taken to avoid the neurovascular bundle. The screws should avoid penetration of the navicular cuneiform joint.

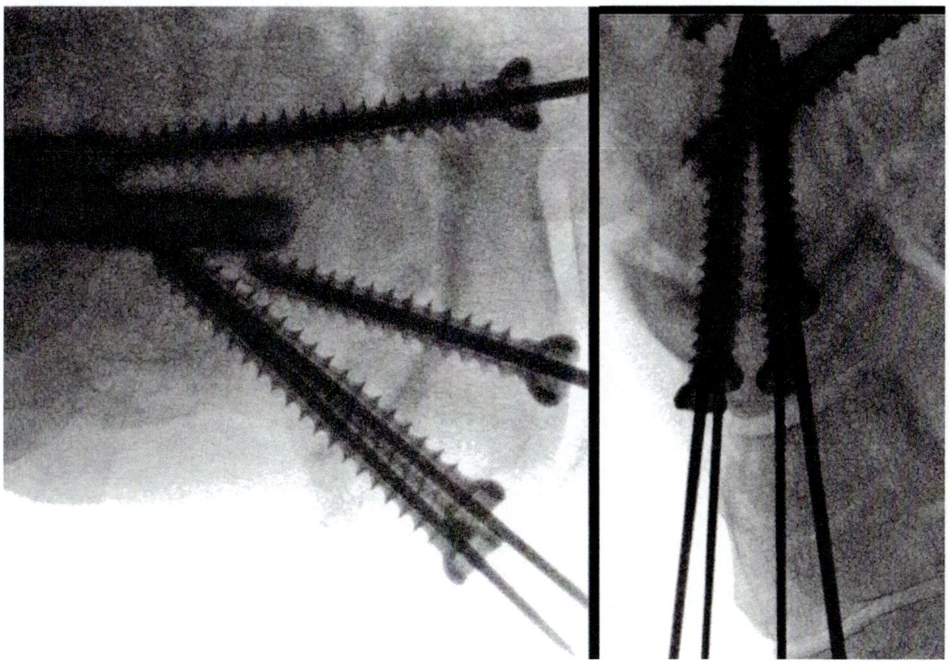

Figure 19.9 Placement of the talonavicular joint screws.

◆ CALCANEOCUBOID JOINT FIXATION

The calcaneocuboid joint typically needs to be reduced into dorsiflexion as the forefoot is often in varus. Initial fixation is performed percutaneously from the anterior process of the calcaneus to the cuboid. The 4- or 3-mm fully threaded, noncompression screws can be used. Additional screws can be placed from the anterior process of the calcaneus to the cuboid and from the cuboid into the medial calcaneus.

◆ BONE GRAFT SUBSTITUTE

Bone graft can be placed from the portals prior to screw fixation or after screw fixation. Injectable formats are preferable. Bone graft or substitute is indicated for patients with nonunion risk such as smokers, the older adults, or patients with diabetes.

At the end of the procedure, the portals are closed with nylon, and the patient placed in a below the knee plaster slab. Elevation is encouraged.

◆ POSTOPERATIVE MANAGEMENT

Patients can undergo the procedure as a day care or short inpatient stay. Arthroscopy can shorten the admission rate and duration of admission.

Patients are kept non-weight bearing for 6 weeks. They are seen at 2 weeks for suture removal and 6 weeks for radiograph and remobilization.

◆ CASES

Enclosed are images of a number of cases and utilization of arthroscopic triple arthrodesis to assist in the treatment of hindfoot arthritis.

In Figure 19.10, a patient is illustrated with combined ankle and subtalar plus talonavicular posttraumatic arthritis. The patient needed to be treated in an outpatient setting. An arthroscopic triple arthrodesis was performed first to reduce the wound risk and to preserve blood supply to bone (Figure 19.11). At 4 weeks, a laterally placed total ankle arthroplasty was performed. The patient was seen back 5 years after surgery and doing well, and had the lateral fibular plate removed.

In Figure 19.12, another case of staged total ankle and triple arthrodesis can be seen, illustrating the screw configuration. In this case, a fibular nail was used for the fibular osteotomy.

In Figure 19.13, postoperative views of an isolated triple arthrodesis performed arthroscopically can be seen.

In Figure 19.14, a similar case is shown demonstrating the incisions and the minimal swelling of the foot.

In Figure 19.15, in a case of Mueller-Weiss disease, a combined arthroscopic triple and NC fusion was performed with successful fusion and correction of foot shape.

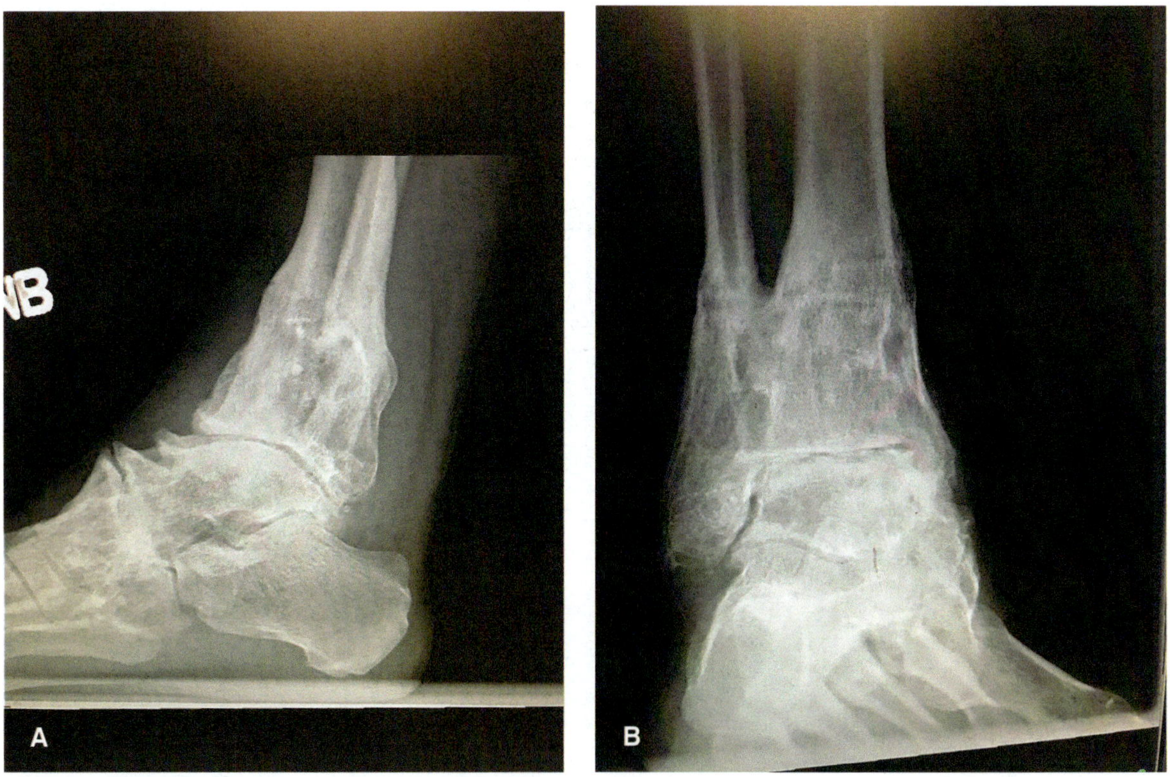

Figure 19.10 A, B. A case of ankle and subtalar arthritis.

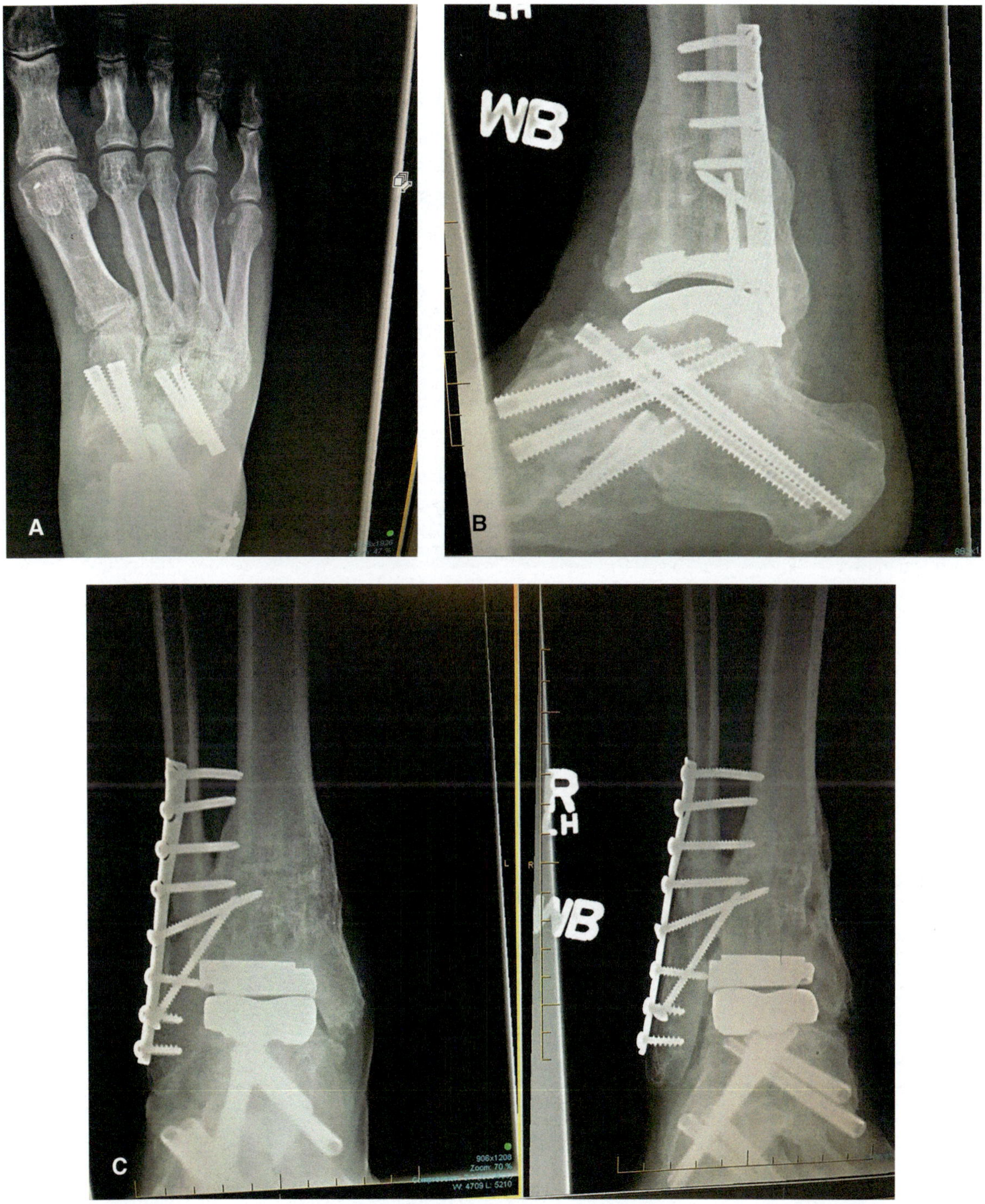

Figure 19.11 **A-C.** The case at 10 weeks post two stage surgery. The first stage was an arthroscopic triple arthrodesis.

◆ OUTCOMES

Subtalar arthroscopic fusion has been reviewed. Fusion rates of 96% are recorded, and hardware issues remain the primary reason for reoperation. Nerve injury rates were in the 4% range. Infection rates may be lower with arthroscopic subtalar fusion.[7]

A randomized prospective study of open versus arthroscopic subtalar fusion demonstrated shorter recovery times and similar union rates and complication rates between two groups of 28 patients.[7]

Most of the outcomes reported are case reports for triple arthrodesis[8] and for club foot.[9]

One paper reported on a case series of six patients treated for Mueller-Weiss disease with arthroscopic triple arthrodesis.[10]

Li and Lui report on a three portal technique for flatfoot deformity.[11]

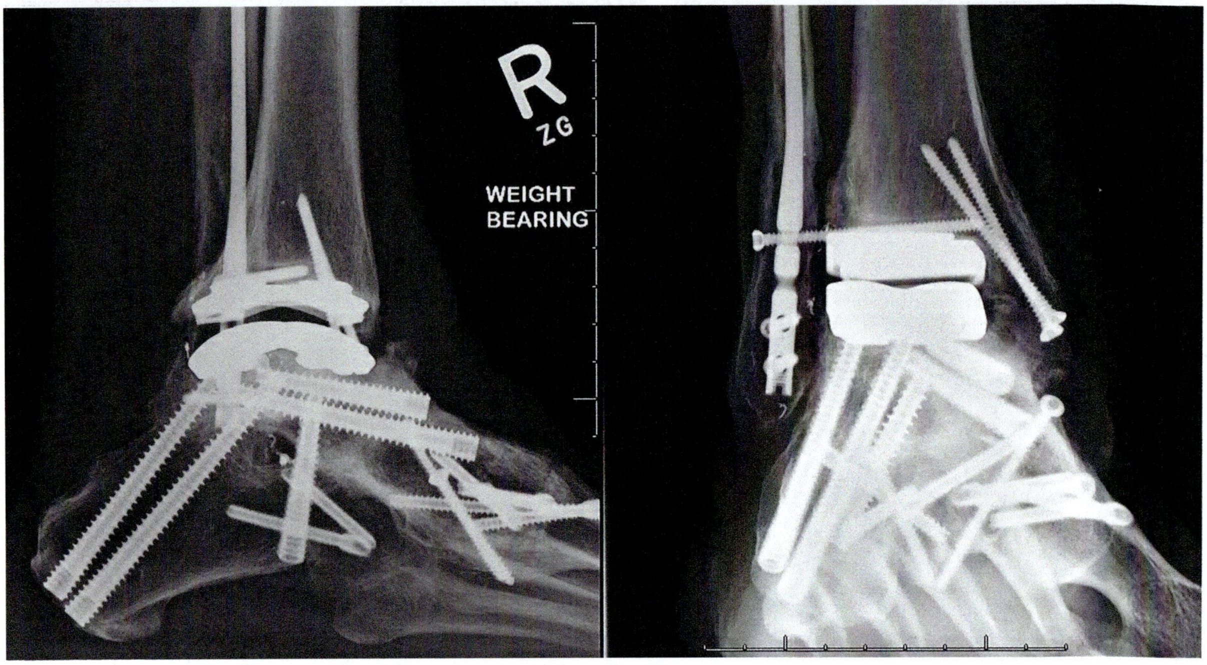

Figure 19.12 Another case of staged triple arthrodesis and total ankle arthroplasty.

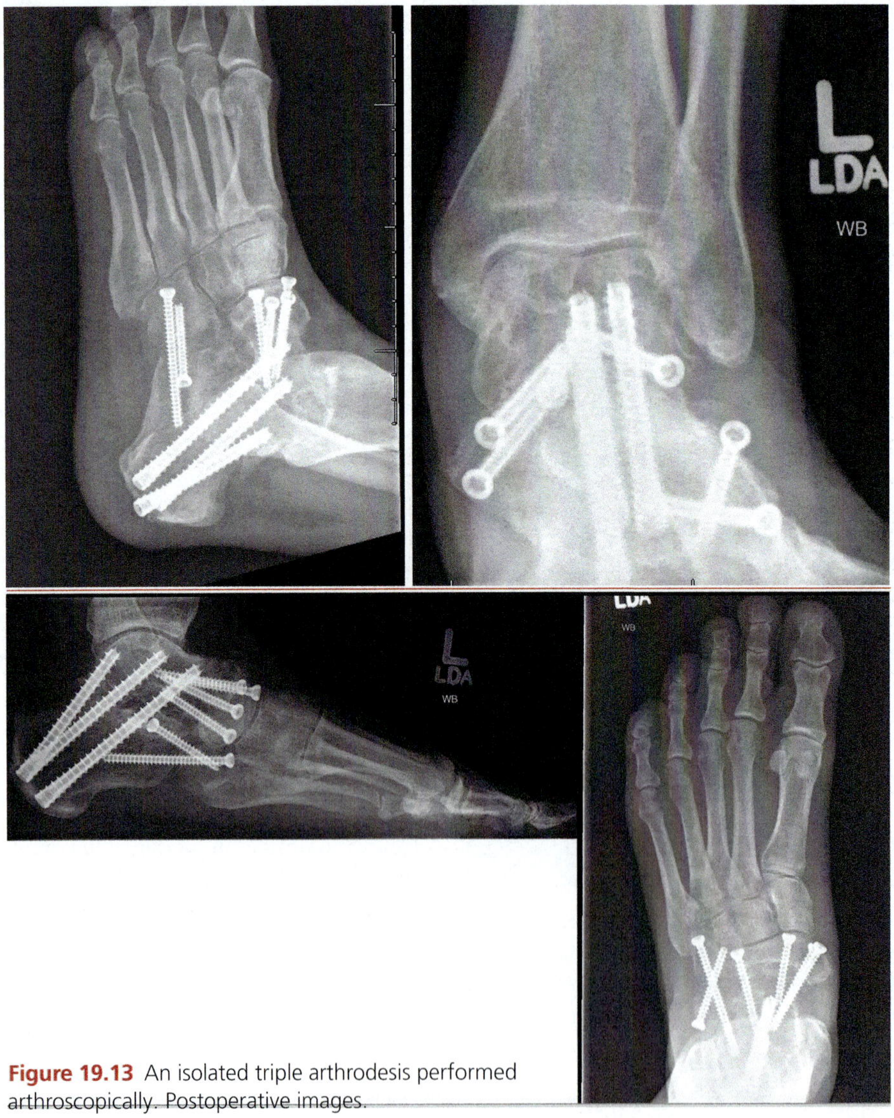

Figure 19.13 An isolated triple arthrodesis performed arthroscopically. Postoperative images.

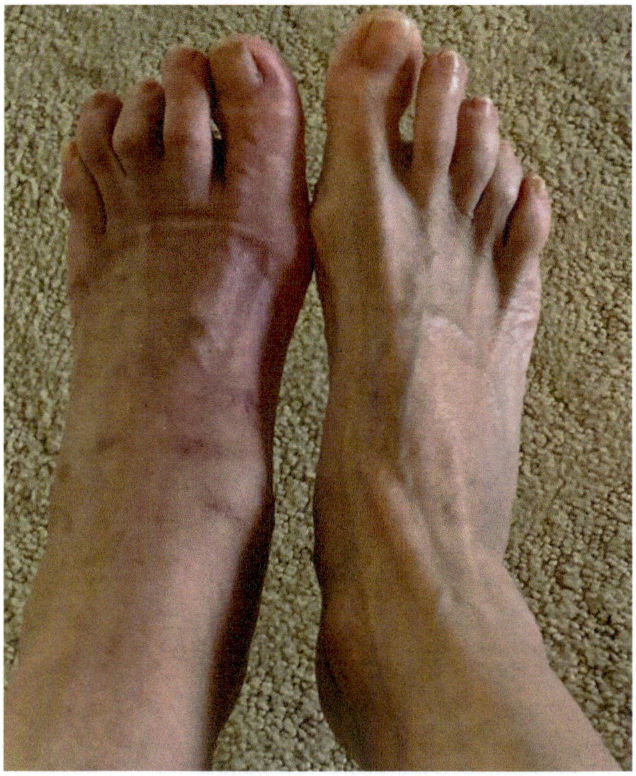

Figure 19.14 Clinical picture of a postoperative foot.

References

1. Walter R, Parsons S, Winson I. Arthroscopic subtalar, double, and triple fusion. *Foot Ankle Clin.* 2016;21(3):681-693.
2. Perera A, Kandhari VK, Portal-Banker T, Guillod S. Lateral hind-foot endoscopic anterolateral/posterolateral (LEAP) subtalar arthrodesis: an effective minimally invasive technique to achieve subtalar fusion and deformity correction. *Arthrosc Tech.* 2021;10(2):e423-e429.
3. Hughes AM, Gosling O, McKenzie J, Amirfeyz R, Winson IG. Arthroscopic triple fusion joint preparation using two lateral portals: a cadaveric study to evaluate efficacy and safety. *Foot Ankle Surg.* 2014;20(2):135-139.
4. Lui TH, Chan LK. Safety and efficacy of talonavicular arthroscopy in arthroscopic triple arthrodesis. A cadaveric study. *Knee Surg Sports Traumatol Arthrosc.* 2010;18(5):607-611.
5. Vila-Rico J, Bravo-Gimenez B, Jimenez-Diaz V, Mellado-Romero MA, Ojeda-Thies C. Arthroscopic subtalar arthrodesis: does the type of fixation modify outcomes? *J Foot Ankle Surg.* 2018;57(4):726-731.
6. Lui TH. Arthroscopic triple arthrodesis in management of chronic flatfoot deformity. *Arthrosc Tech.* 2017;6(3):e871-e877.
7. Oshba H, Shaaban RHA, Abdelrahman I, Gougoulias N. Arthroscopic subtalar joint arthrodesis: topical review. *Foot Ankle Int.* 2022;43(1):131-145.
8. Nakasa T, Ikuta Y, Kanemitsu M, Adachi N. Arthroscopic triple arthrodesis for the patient with rheumatoid arthritis; a case report. *Mod Rheumatol Case Rep.* 2021;5(1):29-35.
9. Lui TH. Case report: correction of neglected club foot deformity by arthroscopic assisted triple arthrodesis. *Arch Orthop Trauma Surg.* 2010;130(8):1007-1011.
10. Lui TH. Arthroscopic triple arthrodesis in patients with Muller Weiss disease. *Foot Ankle Surg.* 2009;15(3):119-122.
11. Li HM, Lui TH. Correction of severe flatfoot deformity by 3-portal arthroscopic triple arthrodesis. *Arthrosc Tech.* 2020;9(1):e103-e109.

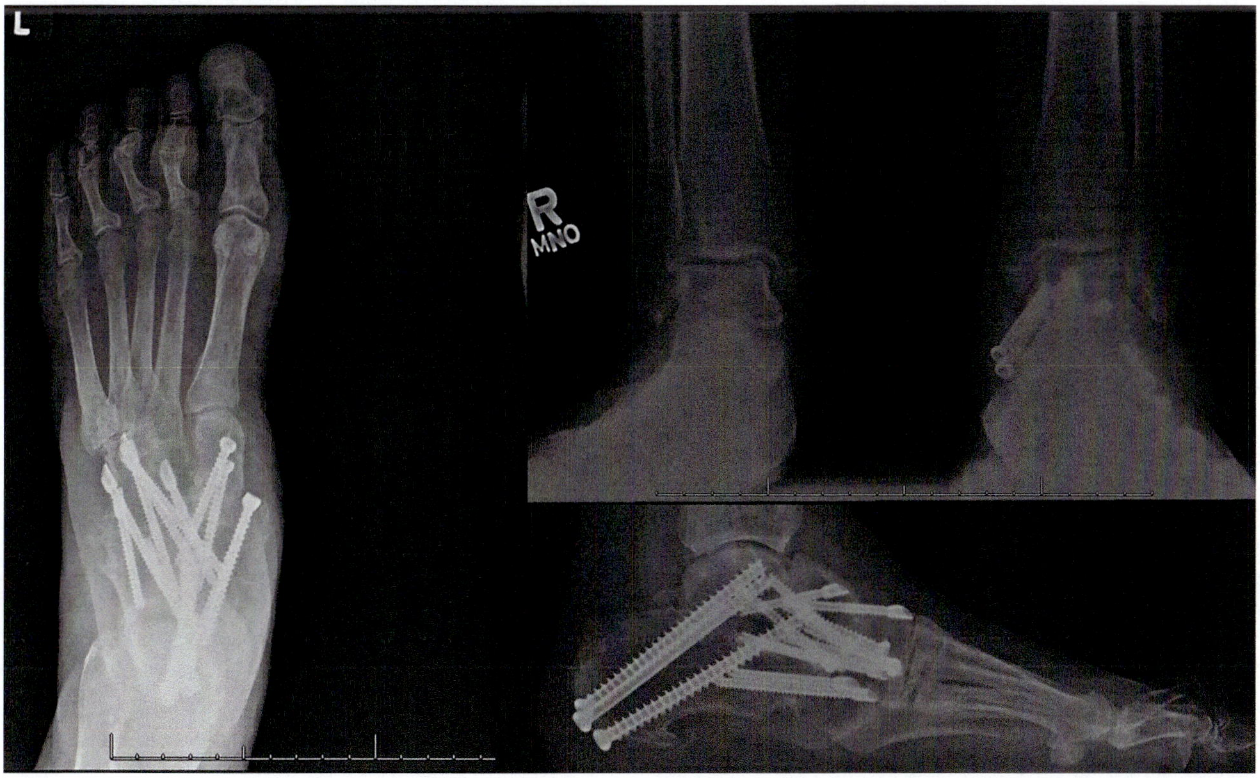

Figure 19.15 Postoperative views of a combined arthroscopic triple and navicular-cuneiform fusion performed for Mueller-Weiss disease.

20 Triple Arthrodesis: A Fully Percutaneous Approach

Ettore Vulcano

◆ PREPARATION

Room Setup

The author routinely places the patient supine with the surgical foot at the edge of the table with a bump under the ipsilateral hip so as for the ankle to be facing "straight up." The contralateral leg is frog-legged to avoid interference with the mini C-arm and/or the operator. The power box and the scrub technician are always at the left side of the patient, whereas the mini C-arm is always at the right side of the patient, regardless of surgical site laterality (Figure 20.1). The power box should be set at 6,000 rpm. The use of a tourniquet is highly discouraged as the intraosseous bleeding may help cool down the burr during the procedure, thus reducing the risk of heat necrosis.

Saline irrigation of the burr throughout the procedure is also crucial to reduce the risk of thermal injury to the soft tissues. This may be in the form of automated irrigation systems provided by several manufacturers distributing minimally invasive surgery instrumentation or manually by the surgical assistant with the use of a bulb syringe.

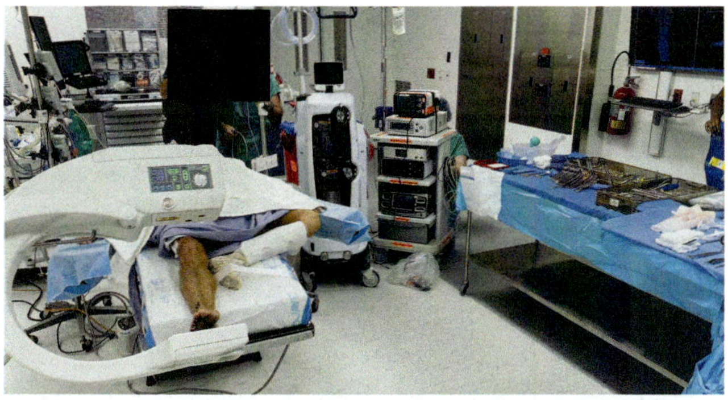

Figure 20.1 Room setup. The contralateral side is frog-legged, and fluoroscopy is positioned to the right side of the patient regardless of surgical laterality.

SURGICAL TECHNIQUE

The surgeon will stand at the end of the bed and may move to the side of the patient as needed. A bump under the ipsilateral hip is recommended to internally rotate the foot, facilitating access to the subtalar and calcaneocuboid joints. By the time the talonavicular joint is addressed, the surgeon may opt to remove the bump as needed.

Subtalar Joint Approach

The author has transitioned from using a dual-portal approach (posterolateral and sinus tarsi) to a single-portal approach (posterolateral) as no technical advantage was perceived and to avoid injuring the sinus tarsi artery. Under fluoroscopic guidance, the posterolateral aspect of the subtalar joint is identified and a 3-mm incision is made between just posterior to the peroneal tendons. The subcutaneous tissues are dissected bluntly with a mosquito clamp. A freer elevator is advanced into the joint to "get a feel" of the joint anatomy and orientation (Figure 20.2).

Next, under fluoroscopy, the 3 × 30 cutting burr is advanced into the joint and débridement is begun (Figure 20.3). The author prefers to work from distal to proximal, tackling the talar surface first and the calcaneal cartilage next. After the débridement is completed, the joint surfaces are palpated with a curette to feel for any remaining areas of cartilage that can be removed with the curette itself (Figure 20.4). Next, a small bone rasp and a pituitary rongeur are used to remove debris from the joint and to further assist with cartilage débridement (Figure 20.5). Prior to preparing the joint with a 2-mm wire (Figure 20.6), the joint is flushed copiously with a 50-mL syringe and an 18-gauge blunt needle.

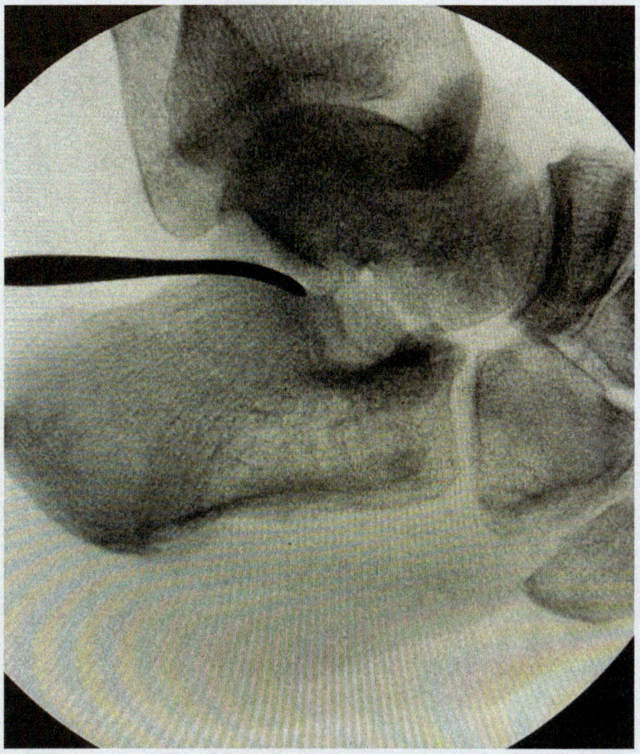

Figure 20.2 Upon making the incision, a freer elevator is advanced into the subtalar joint to appreciate the anatomy and joint orientation.

Calcaneocuboid Joint Approach

A single 3-mm stab incision is made at the lateral aspect of the midline calcaneocuboid joint. A freer elevator is advanced to feel the joint. A 2 × 12 cutting burr is advanced into the joint and the débridement is performed. The author prefers to work from medial to lateral, addressing the cuboid first and the calcaneus next. The débridement and preparation of the joint (curette, rasp, irrigation, 2-mm drill holes) is then completed as described for the subtalar joint.

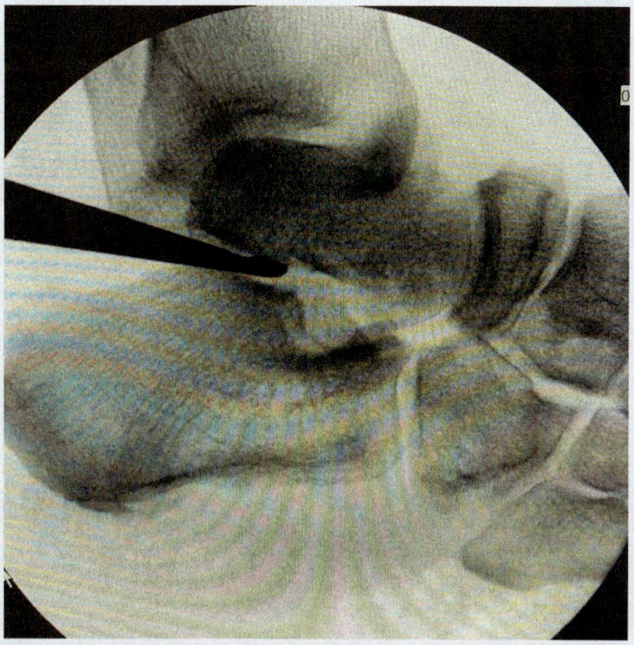

Figure 20.4 The joint is palpated with a curette to feel for remaining cartilage areas and to further help with débridement.

Talonavicular Joint Approach

The surgeon utilizes two 2-mm portals: one straight medial and one dorsolateral (between the anterior tibial and extensor hallucis longus tendons). Once the subcutaneous tissues are dissected with a mosquito clamp, a freer elevator is advanced into the joint to feel the anatomy and orientation (Figure 20.7). A 2 × 12 mm cutting burr is advanced

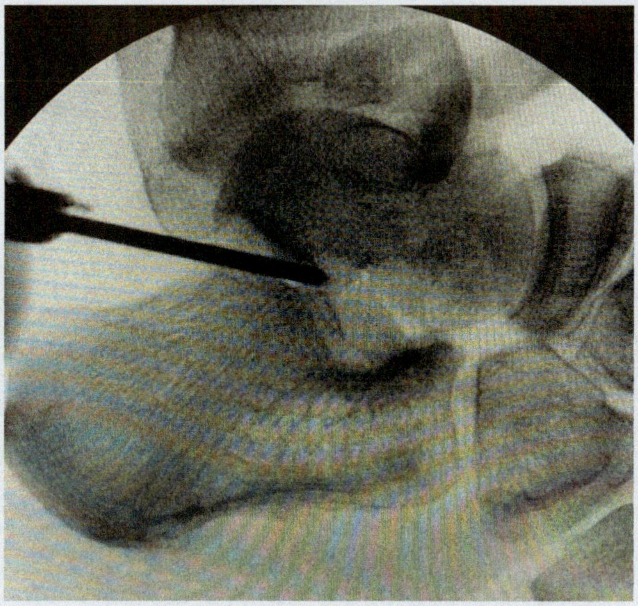

Figure 20.3 A 3 × 30 mm cutting burr is advanced into the subtalar joint to perform the débridement.

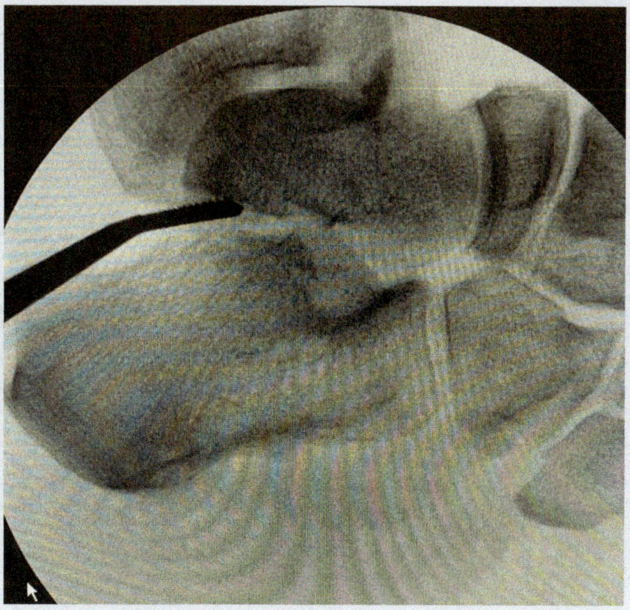

Figure 20.5 A small bone rasp is utilized to remove part of the debris and to further assist with joint débridement.

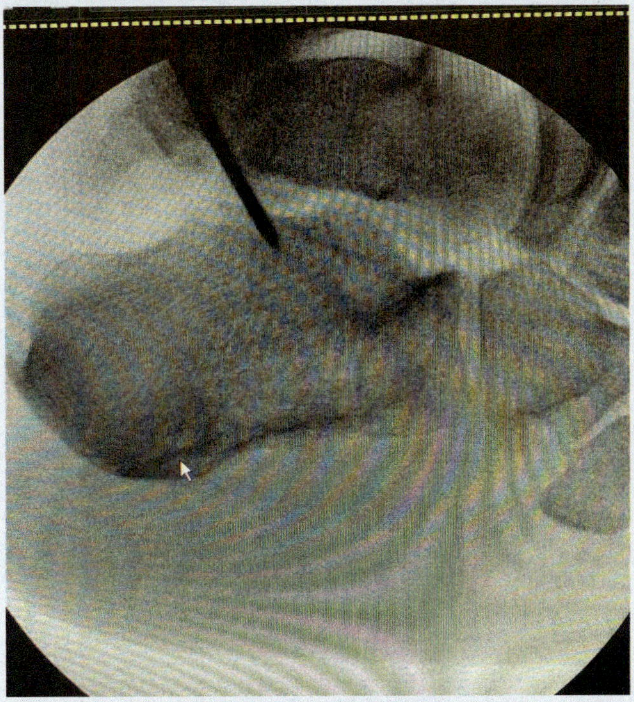

Figure 20.6 A 2-mm wire is used to fenestrate the joint.

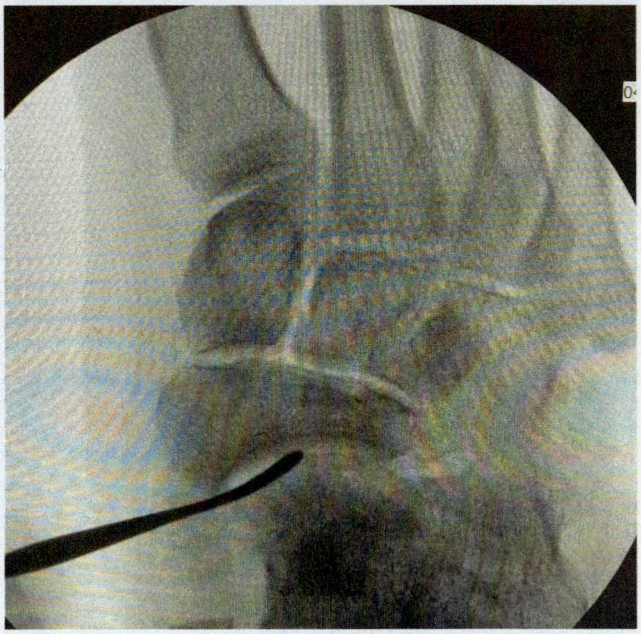

Figure 20.7 The talonavicular joint is explored with a freer to understand its anatomy prior to joint débridement.

through the medial portal (Figure 20.8A), and the débridement is performed from lateral to medial, addressing the navicular surface first and the talar head next. Caution needs to be taken when débriding the notoriously soft talar head so as to avoid notching the bone. Next, the burr is introduced through the dorsolateral portal, and the joint is débrided from plantar to dorsal (Figure 20.8B). The débridement is completed by means of a curved curette (facilitates reaching around the talus), small bone rasp, and irrigation of the joint (Figure 20.9). The latter is then prepped by drilling multiple 2-mm holes (Figure 20.10).

Bone Grafting and Fixation

Prior to adding bone graft, all joints are irrigated with a 50-mL syringe and 18-gauge blunt needle. Bone graft is morselized, and a straight mosquito clamp is used to advance the bone into the joints. Then, all portals are closed with the surgeon's suture of choice.

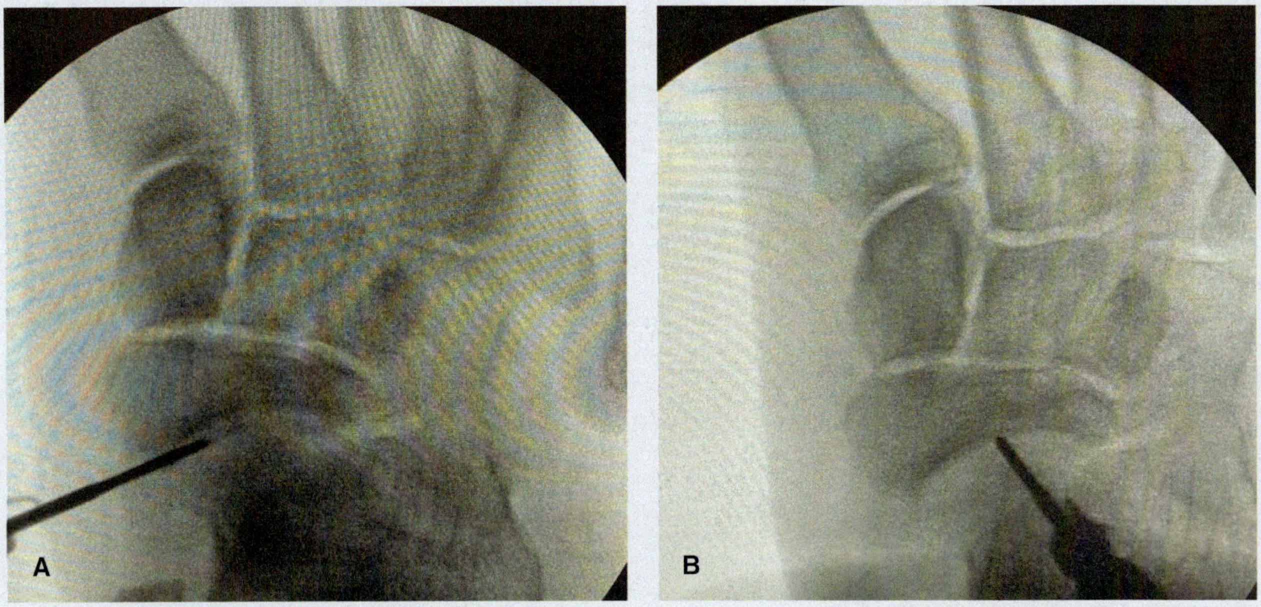

Figure 20.8 With the use of a 2 × 12 mm cutting burr, the joint is débrided through the medial **(A)** and lateral (**B**, dorsolateral) portals.

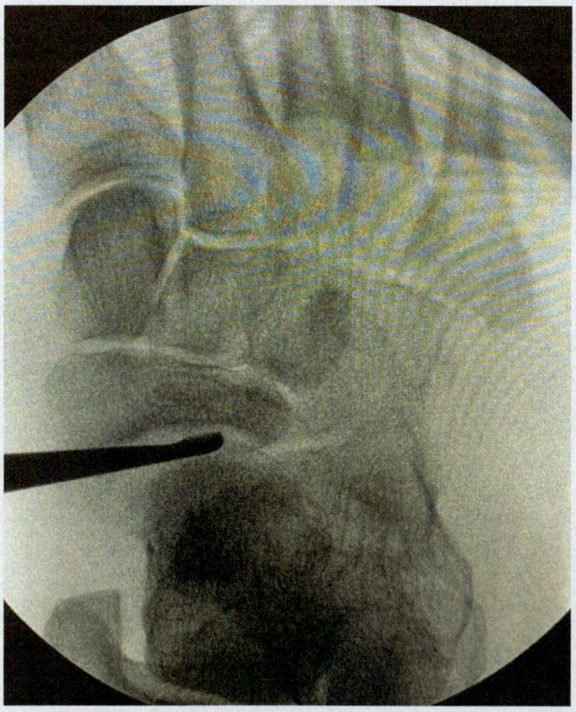

Figure 20.9 A curette is used to palpate the joint for any remaining cartilage.

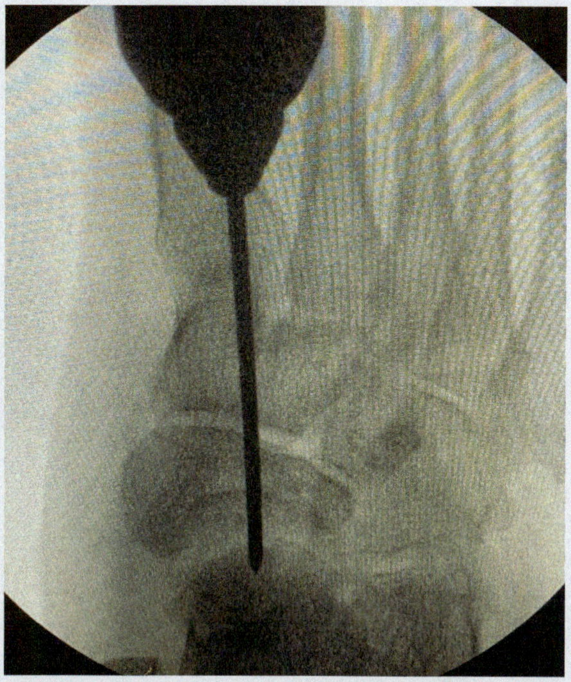

Figure 20.10 The joint surfaces are fenestrated with a 2-mm wire or the 2-mm burr.

The author always starts by stabilizing the talonavicular joint as it is the one that tends to stiffen up the most when the calcaneocuboid or subtalar joints are pinned first. Three wires are advanced across the talonavicular joint from distal to proximal. Once the position is confirmed, the skin is incised, the wires are measured and overdrilled, and three 4-mm fully threaded screws are advanced across the joint.

Next, the calcaneocuboid or subtalar joints can be addressed in any order. The calcaneocuboid joint can be stabilized with a 7-mm headless compression screw inserted from the calcaneus posterior tuberosity to the cuboid, with two 4-mm crossed screws, or with a single 4- to 5-mm screw across the anterior process-cuboid. The subtalar joint is stabilized with two or three 5- to 7-mm headless compression screws in any orientation.

Lastly, all wounds are closed with sutures, and a well-padded splint is applied to the surgical leg.

PEARLS AND PITFALLS

- Do not keep the burr activated for more than 8 to 10 seconds. This might lead to thermal injury to the tissues. Stop the power, allow a few seconds to cool down without removing the burr from its position, and resume the procedure.
- While débriding the joint, exert sufficient pressure to remove the cartilage but not excessive to cause toughing of the burr into the bone. Until a good tactile feedback is developed by the surgeon, frequent use of fluoroscopy is helpful in preventing such complications.
- Remember to use a rotational hand movement while débriding the joint. Imagine the hinge of the burr to be at the skin incision. Ignoring this will cause a widening of the skin incision.
- At the calcaneocuboid joint and at the navicular surface, a 3-mm wedge burr might be useful to complete the débridement in patients with advanced arthritis and particularly hard subchondral bone.

POSTOPERATIVE MANAGEMENT

Patients are kept non–weight bearing for 6 weeks. Two weeks postoperatively, the splint is removed and exchanged for a controlled ankle motion boot. Deep vein thrombosis chemoprophylaxis consists of aspirin 81 mg daily for low-risk patients or rivaroxaban 10 mg daily for high-risk patients. At 2 weeks postoperatively, patients are allowed to bathe the surgical foot and can wear socks. Two weeks postoperatively, three-view weight-beating radiographs of the foot are obtained to confirm alignment. Six weeks postoperatively, new radiographs are obtained. Patients are allowed to start weight bearing as tolerated in the surgical boot.

Three months postoperatively, patients are allowed comfortable shoes, and a CT scan is ordered to confirm bone healing. Remind the patient that postoperative swelling will resolve around 4 months postoperatively (Figure 20.11).

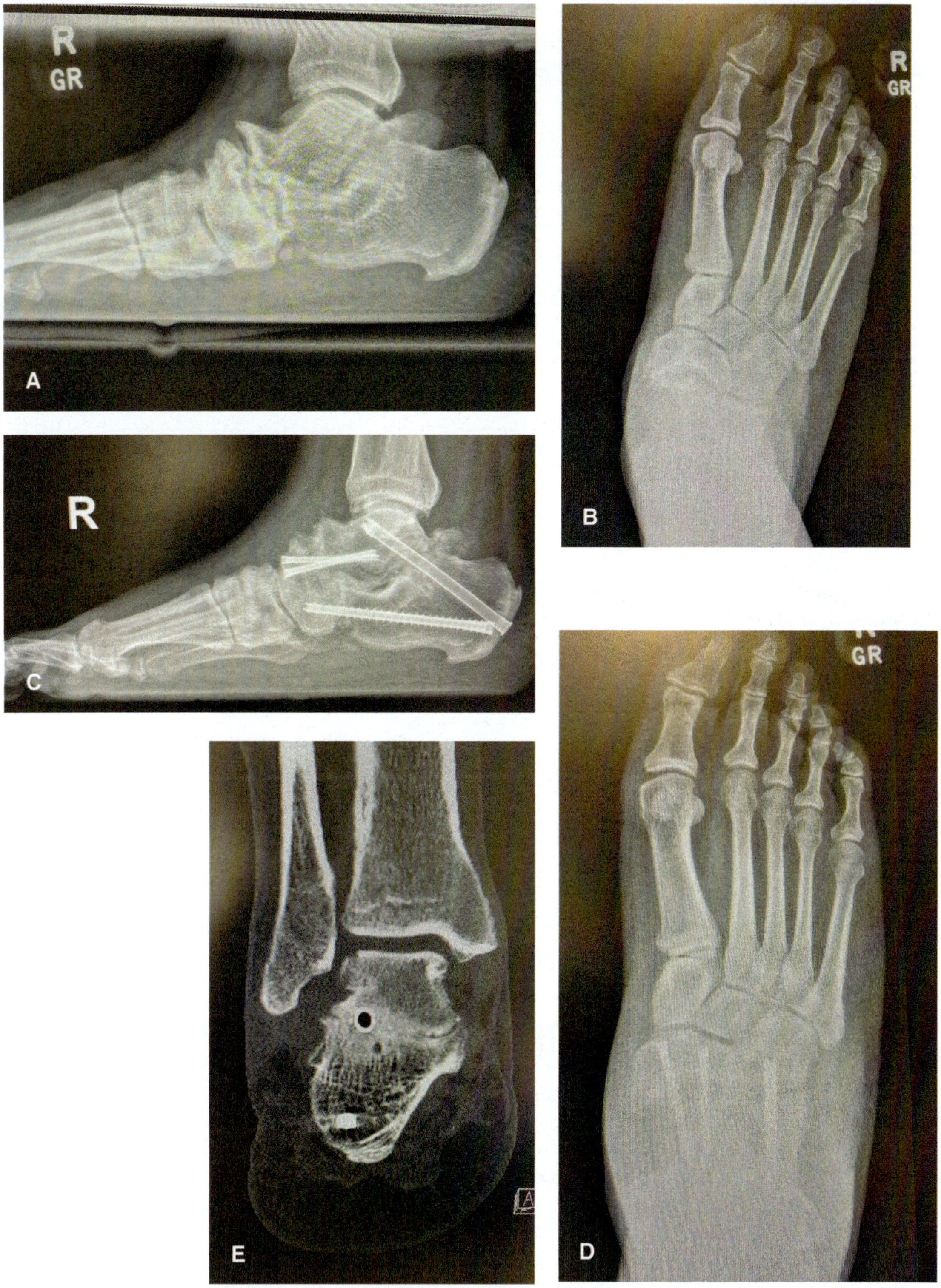

Figure 20.11 Preoperative lateral **(A)** and anteroposterior **(B)** radiographs of a 78-year old healthy female with a right rigid flatfoot deformity; 8-week postoperative lateral **(C)** and anteroposterior **(D)** radiographs of the same foot; coronal, sagittal, and axial CT images obtained 3 months postoperatively confirming fusion at the subtalar **(E)**, talonavicular **(F)**, and calcaneocuboid **(G)** joints. The image **(H)** demonstrates the healed portals used to perform the percutaneous triple arthrodesis.

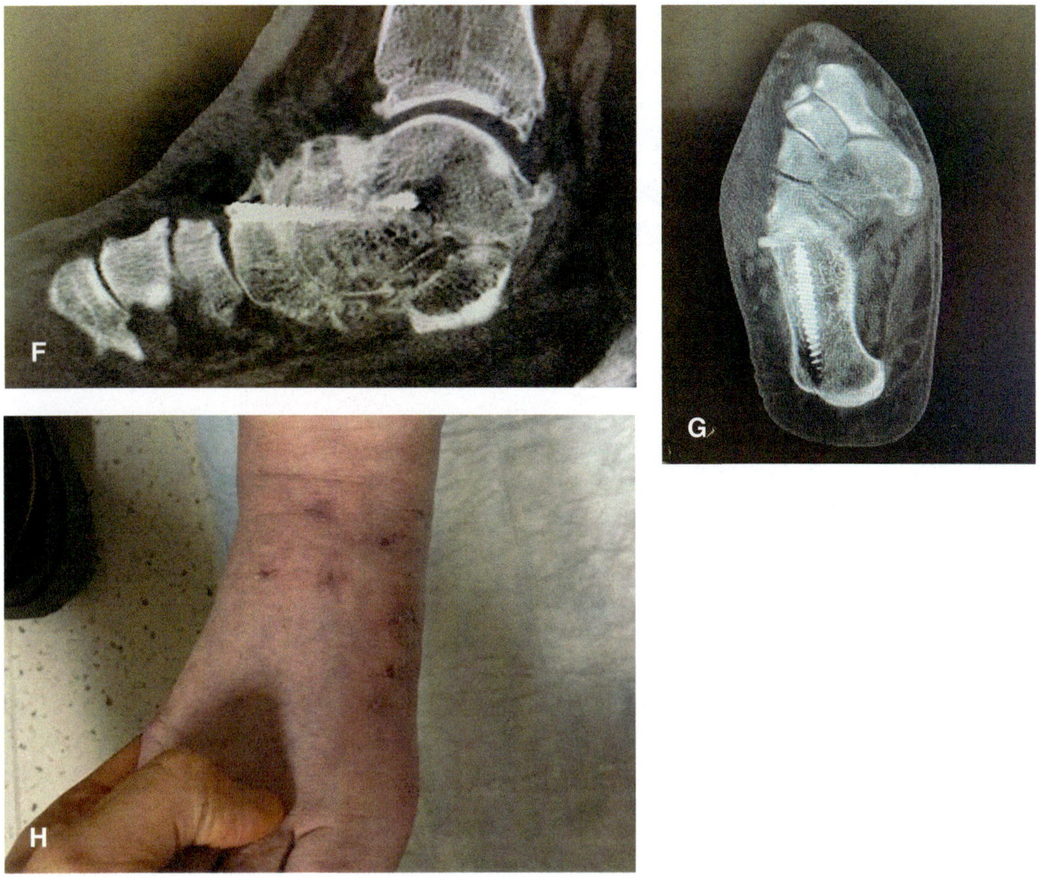

Figure 20.11 *(continued)*

21 Minimally Invasive Percutaneous Dorsal Cheilectomy With Hallux Metatarsophalangeal Joint Arthroscopy

Tyler Gonzalez

INTRODUCTION AND BACKGROUND

Similar to open cheilectomy, minimally invasive percutaneous dorsal cheilectomy (MIDC) is indicated for removal of the dorsal osteophyte of the metatarsal head and proximal phalanx to relieve pain and stiffness in patients with mild to moderate hallux rigidus.[1] The touted benefits of MIDC include less pain, less stiffness, improved cosmesis, and comparable functional outcomes to an open procedure.[2-5] Several studies have looked at MIDC showing improved functional outcomes and pain with quick return to work and normal shoe wear.[4-6] Early results of this new technique are encouraging with high patient satisfaction and low complication rates.[7,8]

INDICATIONS

- Mild to moderate hallux rigidus with pain at the extremes of range of motion (ROM), negative grind test, and no mid-arch of motion pain
- Presence of dorsal osteophyte causing impingement pain with dorsiflexion of the hallux metatarsophalangeal (MTP) joint or pain from shoe pressure directly on the osteophyte dorsally
- Failure of nonoperative interventions

CONTRAINDICATIONS

- Advanced articular surface osteoarthritis as shown clinically by a positive grind test
- Pain with mid-arch motion or plantar pain suggesting inferior sesamoid degeneration
- Night pain or pain that occurs at rest
- Absence of dorsal osteophyte
- Any sign of infection

PATIENT HISTORY AND PHYSICAL EXAMINATION

- A detailed history of present illness should be preformed.
- Patients with hallux rigidus usual present with pain over the dorsal osteophyte and pain with shoe wear.
- They may complain of pain going up stairs and hills, and pain with stepping up on their toes and with walking. They may express limited range of motion of the toe.
- Specific activities such as running, hiking, and dancing may be limited due to limited range of motion of the toe.
- Examination should include the following:
  - Standing physical examination.
  - Detailed neurovascular examination.
  - Examination of the hallux MTP joint should include range of motion in dorsiflexion and plantarflexion as well as evaluation of the presence of dorsal osteophyte should be recorded.
  - Pain at the extremes of motion or mid-arch should be recorded.
  - A grind test should be preformed.

IMAGING STUDIES

- Obtain standing, weight-bearing plain radiographs of the foot in anteroposterior (AP) and lateral views to evaluate severity of articular degeneration (Figure 21.1).
- Advanced imaging such as CT and MRI is usually not indicated for mild to moderate hallux rigidus. If there is a concern for osteochondral lesion or cystic changes with the metatarsal head, then an MRI should be done.

PREPARATION AND PATIENT POSITIONING

- This procedure is often performed in the outpatient setting.
- The patient is positioned supine, with the limb free to allow for dorsoplantar rotation and lateral fluoroscopy. The other leg is frog-legged out of the way of the surgeon, the operative limb, and the fluoroscopy machine (Figure 21.2).
- The heel hangs off the end of the table perpendicular to the mini C-arm, which is always positioned on the side of the surgeon's dominant hand (adjacent to the patient's right foot for a right-handed surgeon) regardless of which foot is being operated on.

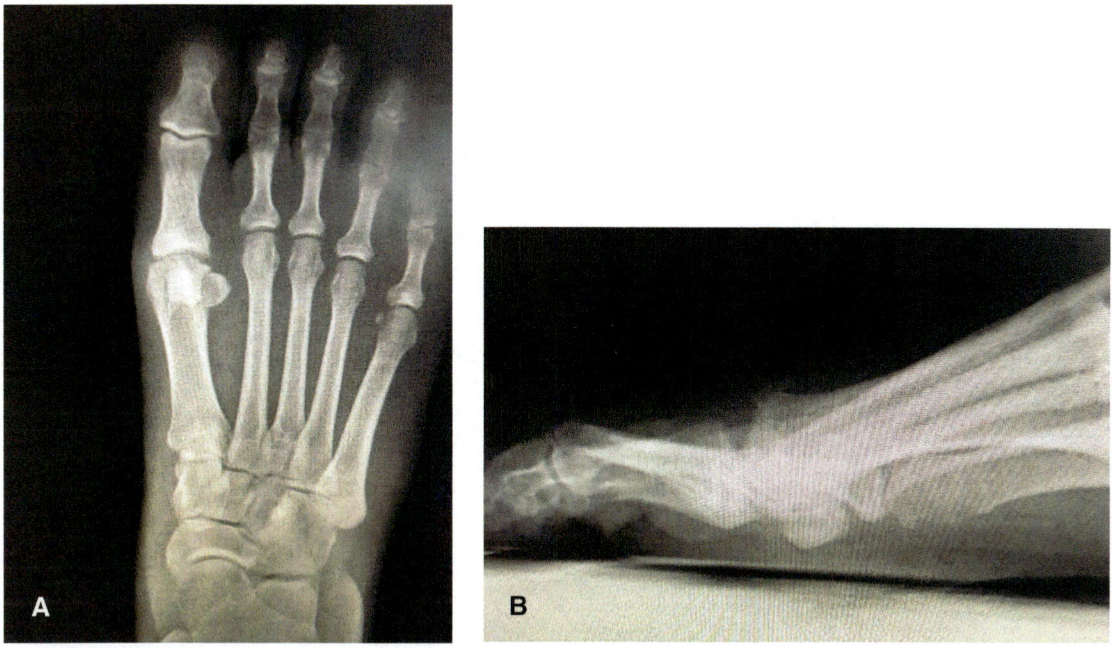

Figure 21.1 Weight-bearing **(A)** AP and **(B)** lateral view of the foot showing large dorsal osteophyte with slight joint space narrowing.

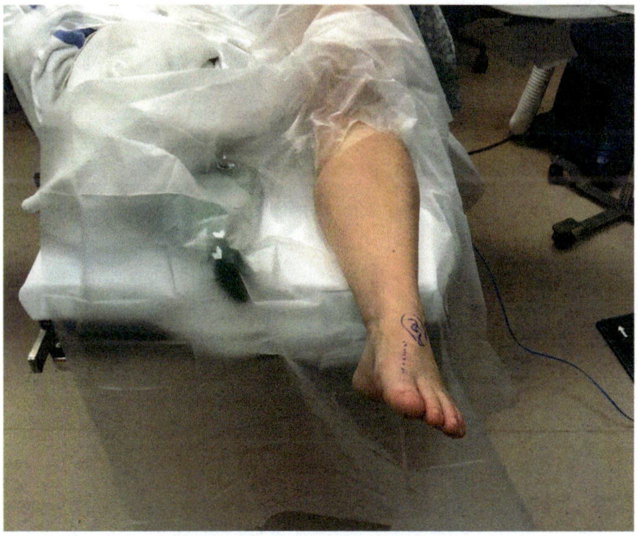

Figure 21.2 Position of patient for MIDC and metatarsophalangeal arthroscopy.

SURGICAL TECHNIQUE

1. Use of a tourniquet is discouraged as the restriction of blood flow may promote thermal injury and prevent the cooling of the surgical site.
2. A longitudinal incision only through skin measuring 4 mm is made over the dorsomedial aspect of the first metatarsal, approximately 2.5 cm from the hallux MTP joint. The incision should remain plantar to the dorsomedial cutaneous nerve. Caution should be taken to avoid damaging the dorsomedial cutaneous nerve during this procedure due to its proximity to the portal.
3. A blunt-tipped hemostat is utilized to mobilize the subcutaneous tissue, and then, a straight elevator is used to elevate the joint capsule off the dorsal osteophytes in order to create a working space between the bone and soft tissues.
4. A 3.1-mm wedge burr is employed via the portal, running at low speed but high torque (<6,000 rpm) to minimize heat generation as it engages the osteophyte. Fluoroscopic imaging is used here to check the resection angle of the cut (Figure 21.3).
5. It is recommended to use chilled saline and stopping every 10 to 20 seconds during the burring process to

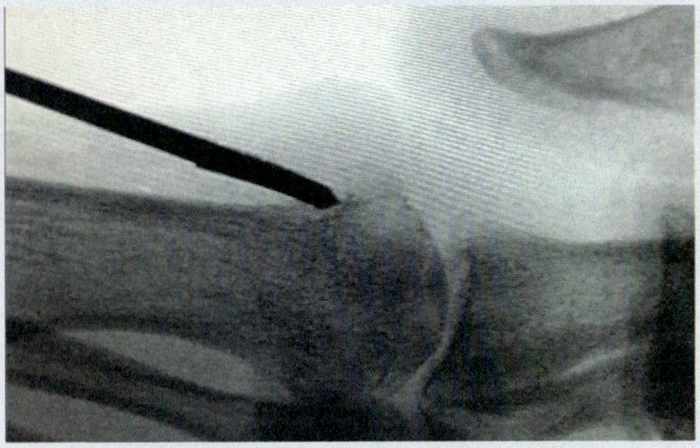

Figure 21.3 Resection level set with burr. Notice that the burr is NOT on top of the osteophyte but engaging it at its base.

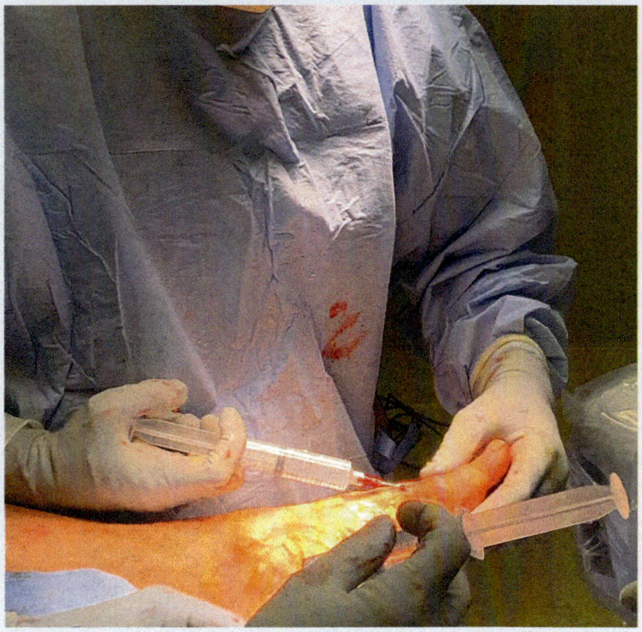

Figure 21.4 Irrigating out the wound after resection of osteophyte.

allow the unit to cool down to avoid thermal necrosis of the soft tissue and bone.

6. The surgeon should not approach the osteophyte dorsally as this endangers the extensor hallucis tendons. Rather, the burr should engage the osteophyte from the base as seen in Figure 21.3 and advance distally until the osteophyte is completely removed. Avoid plantarflexing the hallux during this process as tension on the dorsal soft tissues puts the extensor tendons and nerve at risk for damage or rupture from the burr.
7. As the osteophyte is pulverized, the author recommends removing the burr and checking the resection level. The bone debris is then expressed and flushed from the wound with insertion of a syringe using copious irrigation. The author recommends using an 18-gauge blunt tip needle or a large angiocatheter and 30-mL syringe to irrigate the working space (Figure 21.4).
8. After irrigation, a rasp should be used to remove residual bone fragments adherent to the capsule to minimize bone debris that can cause irritation postoperatively. This debris can usually be visualized fluoroscopically and should not be left in the joint. Regardless of fluoroscopy use during resection, AP, lateral, and oblique views should be obtained at the end of the case to ensure that no bone debris remains in the region of the resection. An opacity dorsal to the resection is indicative of likely remaining debris that requires further removal.
9. Burring should continue until fluoroscopic imaging confirms resection of the dorsal osteophytes; clinically, the surgeon can palpate the metatarsal head to make sure that there are no more palpable spurs.
10. While the amount of bone resected depends on the surgeon's preference, the surgeon should aim for roughly 30% resection and/or until 70° dorsiflexion is achieved (Figure 21.5A and B).
11. MTP arthroscopy may be employed at this point per surgeon's preference. Kerlix gauze attached to a noninvasive distractor device is used to distract the toe (Figure 21.6).

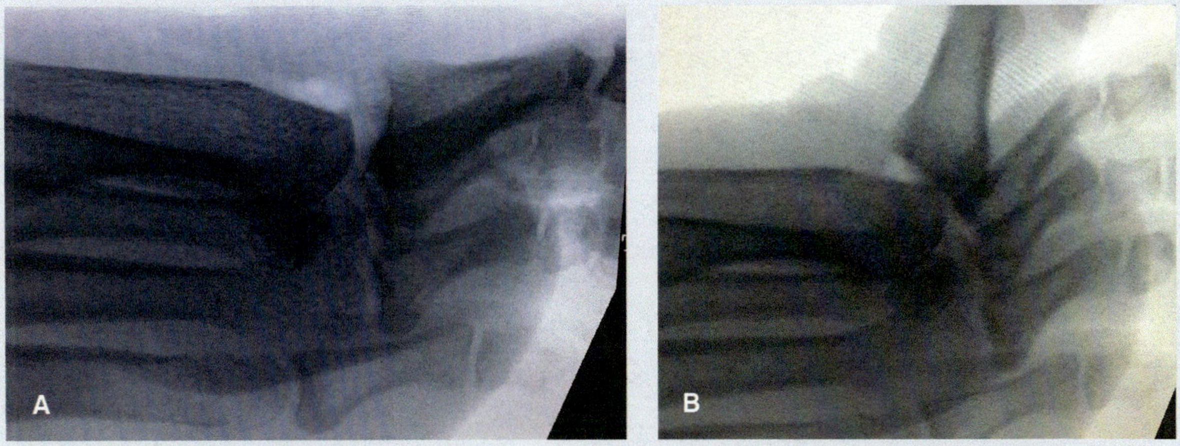

Figure 21.5 **A, B.** Final resection level and dorsiflexion view showing appropriately 30% head resection with 90° of dorsiflexion.

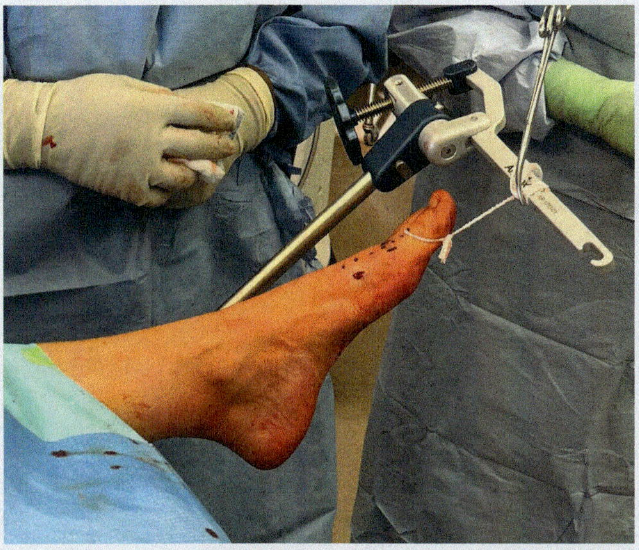

Figure 21.6 Noninvasive distraction set up for metatarsophalangeal arthroscopy.

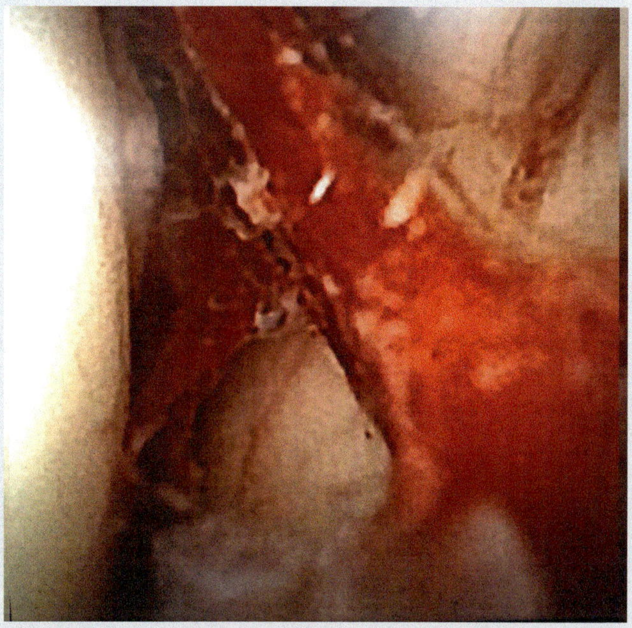

Figure 21.7 Metatarsophalangeal arthroscopy showing débride within the joint upon diagnostic arthroscopy.

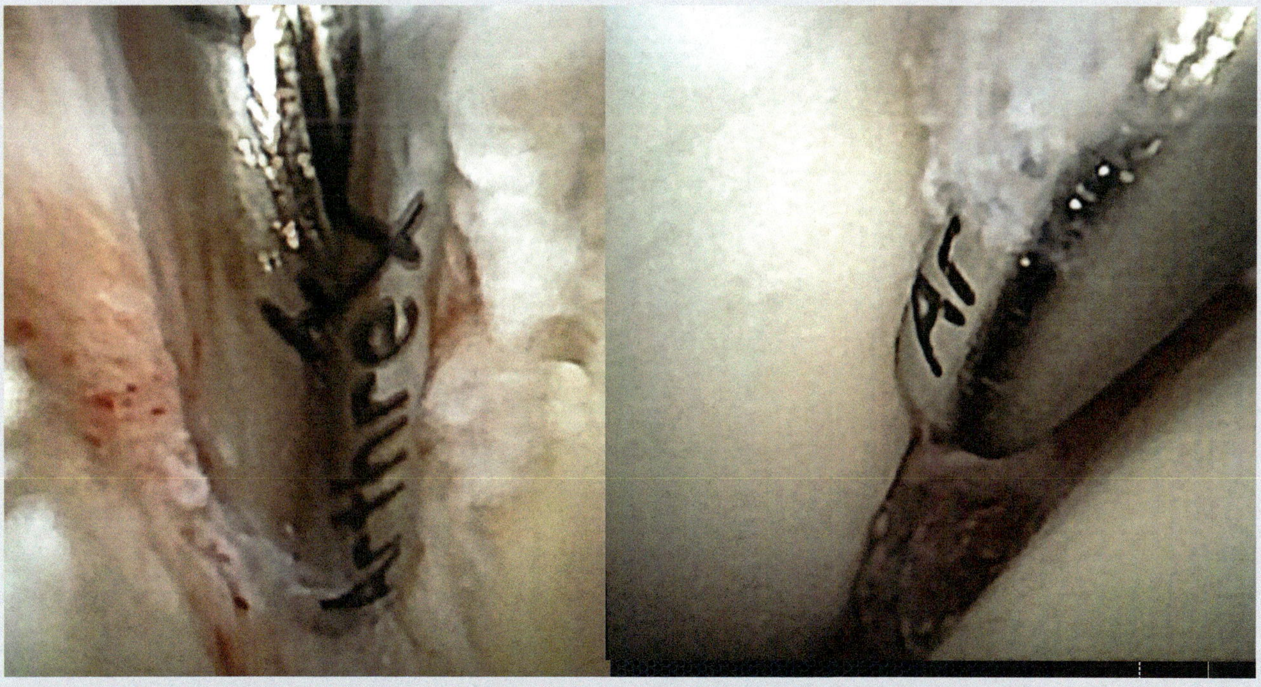

Figure 21.8 Débridement of the metatarsophalangeal joint with 2.0 shaver.

12. Standard medial and lateral portals are made, medial and lateral to the extensor hallucis longus, and a 2.7-mm arthroscope (size per surgeon's preference) is advanced into the joint.
13. Diagnostic arthroscopy ensures appropriate resection of the osteophytes and removal of debris was completed and assesses the joint to better understand the degree of cartilage damage (Figure 21.7A).
14. Any remaining bony debris and synovitis is then débrided with a 2.0 shaver (Figure 21.8). Loose bodies and osteochondral defect can also be addressed at this time.
15. At this point, the arthroscopy and shaver are removed.
16. The portals are closed with Steri-Strips or 4-0 nylon sutures based on the surgeon's preference and simple dry dressing bandages.

◆ POSTOPERATIVE CARE

- Patients immediately go into a stiff-soled shoe, and over-the-counter pain medications are recommended as needed for 1 to 3 days.
- Full weight bearing as tolerated is permitted, but the foot should be elevated for most of the first 72 hours.
- Simple ROM exercises of the hallux can begin on postoperative day 1.
- Patients may return to their own footwear on postoperative day 7. Physiotherapy may be initiated to restore normal gait and ROM.
- Patients will refrain from heavy activity, sports, or prolonged periods of weight bearing for the first 4 weeks and may return to full activity as tolerated afterward.

◆ COMPLICATIONS AND MANAGEMENT

- Dorsomedial cutaneous nerve injury
  - This is an iatrogenic complication that has been cited to occur in 3% of cases.
  - Teoh et al. showed damage to the nerve in 15% of cases in a cadaveric study, highlighting the importance of adequate pocket space for the burr and identifying the nerve prior to incision whenever possible to mitigate risk.[2]
- Bone debris within soft tissue
  - This is also an iatrogenic complication.
  - Meticulous irrigation and rasping along with fluoroscopic imaging should be used to make sure that there are no opacities within the soft tissue after burring is complete.
- Infection
  - This is extremely rare. Superficial infections may be treated with oral antibiotics, while deep infections may necessitate irrigation and débridement.
- Persistent pain and worsening arthritis
  - This may necessitate repeat cheilectomy, other joint reserving surgeries, or fusion.
  - Patients should be counseled preoperatively that this surgery only addresses pain related to dorsal osteophytes and will likely not improve pain related to the underlying arthritis within the joint.

◆ OUTCOMES

Teoh and colleagues demonstrated that at an average follow-up of 50 months, patients treated with MIDC achieved significant improvement in the Manchester-Oxford Foot Questionnaire and visual analog scale pain scores. The authors concluded that MIDC is a safe technique with minimal complications like open cheilectomy. They reported 7 cases of first MTP joint arthrodesis, 4 repeat cheilectomies, 2 wound infections, and 2 cases of permanent numbness out of a cohort of 98 feet.[2]

A case series comparing a cohort of 22 patients treated with MIDC with median 11-month follow-up to a matched cohort of 25 patients treated with open cheilectomy with median 17-month follow-up demonstrated that both groups had statistically significant improvement in Manchester-Oxford Foot Questionnaire.[3] The investigators reported 3 cases of first MTP joint arthrodesis in the open group versus none in the percutaneous cheilectomy group.[3]

Glenn et al. looked at 20 patients with MIDC and MTP arthroscopy with average follow-up of 1.5 years. They showed improved in visual analog scale scores from 7 to 0.75, statistically significant improvement in range of motion in dorsiflexion and plantarflexion, and back to normal shoe wear on average at 2.1 weeks. Additionally, they found that 100% of the patients had intra-articular pathology and concluded that some of the prior studies early revisions might have occurred due to inability to address the MTP pathology. Therefore, the authors recommend MTP arthroscopy with MIDC.[4]

Stevens et al. compared 133 MIDC to 38 open procedures. They reported a reoperation rate of 12.8% in the MIDC versus 2.6% open cohort. Additionally, they reported 1 complication in the open versus 15 in the MIDC cohort. They concluded that MIDC is a viable option; however, there appears to be a relative risk of requiring further procedures with MIDC. There were limitations of the study that the authors stated such as the higher number of reoperations in the MIDC cohort. This could be related to selection bias as there was no randomization and earlier in the study more MIDC were being done than open procedures. Additionally, no patient report outcomes were done. Therefore, no conclusion could be drawn regarding functional outcomes or pain compared between the two groups.[9]

In summary, early results of this technique are encouraging with patient satisfaction as well as return to normal function and footwear similar to open cheilectomy.[2-5]

Larger prospective comparative trials to identify a benefit over open cheilectomy need to be done to truly assess long-term functional outcomes, relative risk of complications, and reoperations.

References

1. Walter R, Perera A. Open, arthroscopic, and percutaneous cheilectomy for hallux rigidus. *Foot Ankle Clin*. 2015;20(3):421-431.
2. Teoh KH, Tan WT, Atiyah Z, Ahmad A, Tanaka H, Hariharan K. Clinical outcomes following minimally invasive dorsal cheilectomy for hallux rigidus. *Foot Ankle Int*. 2019;*40*(2):195-201.
3. Morgan S, Jones C, Palmer S. Minimally invasive cheilectomy: functional outcome and comparison with open cheilectomy. *Orthop Proc*. 2012;94(SUPP_XLIII):14-14.
4. Glenn RL, Gonzalez TA, Peterson AB, Kaplan J. Minimally invasive dorsal cheilectomy and hallux metatarsal phalangeal joint arthroscopy for the treatment of hallux rigidus. *Foot Ankle Orthop*. 2021;6(1):2473011421993103.
5. Dawe E, Ball T, Annamalai S, Davis J. Early results of minimally invasive cheilectomy for painful hallux rigidus. *Orthop Proc*. 2012;*94*(SUPP_XXII):33.
6. Loveday D, Guha A, Singh D. Arthritis great toe MTPJ. *Consensus of the Round Table. Aspects of Orthopaedic Foot and Ankle Surgery. Paris*; 2012:1-9.
7. Razik A, Sott A. Cheilectomy for hallux rigidus. *Foot Ankle Clin*. 2016;*21*(3):451-457.
8. Redfern D, Vernois J, Legré BP. Percutaneous surgery of the forefoot. *Clin Podiatr Med Surg*. 2015;*32*(3):291-332.
9. Stevens R, Bursnall M, Chadwick C, et al. Comparison of complication and reoperation rates for minimally invasive versus open cheilectomy of the first metatarsophalangeal joint. *Foot Ankle Int*. 2020;41(1):31-36.

22 Percutaneous Ankle Arthrodesis

Gerard F. Marciano and Ettore Vulcano

◆ INTRODUCTION

Ankle arthrodesis is indicated as a primary surgical treatment option for disabling end-stage ankle osteoarthritis. In a review of Medicare patients from 2005 to 2014, a total of 19,120 ankle fusions were performed.[1] Fusion rates for ankle arthrodesis have been reported between 80% to 100%, depending on technique and indication.[2-5] Complication rates ranging between 0% and 50% have been reported with any of the described techniques, including infection, wound dehiscence, nonunion, and painful hardware.[5,6]

Percutaneous fusion is an uncommonly employed technique consisting of joint preparation through two 3-mm portals, without the use of arthroscopy. As such, the literature on percutaneous fusion remains limited. In an early study by Lauge-Pedersen, percutaneous ankle fusion was performed in 10 patients with end-stage ankle rheumatoid arthritis. Ankle fusion was observed in all patients with a 100% patient satisfaction rate.[7] More recently, a comparison of minimally invasive percutaneous joint preparation versus open techniques in a cadaver model was reported in the literature. Zhao et al. compared the percentage of joint surface preparation in various foot/ankle joints in a cadaveric model using percutaneous and open techniques. No significant differences were noted except for the talonavicular and calcaneocuboid joints where the percutaneous method prepared more of the joint surface. Of interest, more of the tibiotalar joint surface was able to be prepared percutaneously but not to a statistically significant difference.[8]

◆ INDICATIONS AND CONTRAINDICATIONS

Any patient with a diagnosis of end-stage ankle arthritis, talus or tibia avascular necrosis, severe ankle deformity, complex pilon fractures, paralytic foot drop, or any other indication for ankle fusion is a potential candidate for the procedure.

Contraindications include active ankle infections and recent steroid injections (<3 months) in the affected area.

◆ PATIENT HISTORY AND PHYSICAL EXAMINATION

Patients typically complain of pain at the ankle joint, which most commonly affects the anterior aspect of the joint. Many patients will also complain of limited ankle range of motion. On clinical examination, patients will complain of tenderness to palpation at or around the ankle joint and can present with decreased range of motion. Individuals with certain deformities might also present with objective or subjective gross ankle instability.

◆ IMAGING STUDIES

Weight-bearing three-view foot and ankle radiographs are usually sufficient to diagnose and study the ankle. However, CT and MRI may be indicated in less clear situations such as deformities, avascular necrosis, fractures, Charcot's, and other complex etiologies.

◆ SURGICAL PREPARATION

Room Setup

The authors routinely place the patient supine with the surgical foot at the edge of the table. A bump under the ipsilateral hip ensures that the ankle is facing "straight up" or the sagittal plane of the ankle is directly perpendicular to the floor. The contralateral leg is frog-legged to avoid interference with the mini C-arm and/or the operator. Regardless of surgical site laterality, the power box and the scrub technician are always at the left side of the patient and the mini C-arm is always on the right side of the patient (Figure 22.1). The power box should be set at 6,000 rpm. The use of a tourniquet is highly discouraged as intraosseous bleeding may help cool down the burr during the procedure reducing the risk of heat necrosis.

Saline irrigation of the burr throughout the procedure is crucial to reduce the risk of thermal injury to the soft tissues. This may be achieved by automated irrigation systems or manual irrigation by the surgical assistant with the use of a bulb syringe. Automated irrigation systems can be provided by several manufacturers that distribute minimally invasive surgical instrumentation.

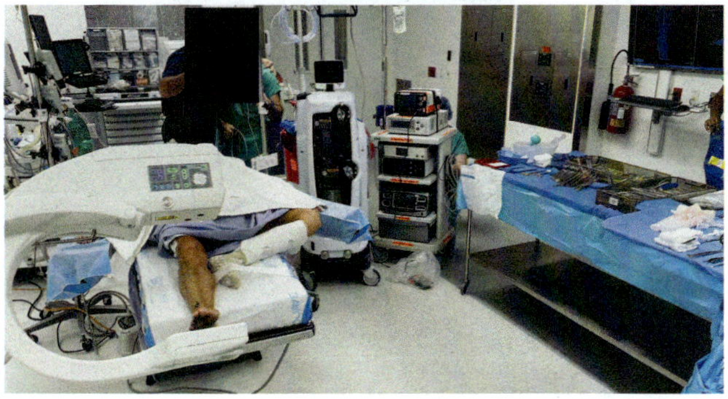

Figure 22.1 Room setup with fluoroscopy at the right side of the patient, regardless of operative side.

SURGICAL TECHNIQUE

The surgeon will stand at the end of the bed and may move to the side of the patient as needed. The first step is to perform a percutaneous Achilles tenotomy in patients with a fixed equinus contracture. Next, two portals (anteromedial and anterolateral, equivalent to those made for standard ankle arthroscopy) are established at the ankle. The entry point can be determined under fluoroscopic guidance, if necessary (Figure 22.2). The 3-mm skin incisions are made superficially and then the subcutaneous tissues are bluntly dissected with a mosquito clamp until the joint capsule is violated. Use an elevator to palpate the joint and familiarize with the anatomy (Figure 22.3).

Next, a 3 × 30 mm cutting burr is advanced in either of the two portals and activated inside the joint. The author's preference is to start débriding the tibia from the posterior to the anterior aspect of the joint, first addressing the medial half of the surface through the anteromedial portal and then the lateral half of the plafond through the anterolateral portal (Figure 22.4). Anteroposterior and lateral fluoroscopy should be used repeatedly to confirm position of the burr throughout the case. If desired, the cutting burr can be exchanged for a 3-mm wedge burr to continue débriding the joint, especially in patients with harder bone. Once the tibial side has been addressed, the same steps are performed at the level of the talus. To help débride, the posterior aspect of the talus the ankle can be plantarflexed as needed (Figure 22.5). Lastly, the medial gutter is débrided of all cartilage (Figure 22.6).

Next, a small curette (regular or arthroscopic) is inserted into the joint to palpate for any areas of remaining cartilage and be removed with the same instrument if needed. To irrigate the joint, a 50-mL syringe with an 18-gauge blunt needle is used to vigorously rinse the ankle. A bone rasp that is often available with most minimally invasive sets in the market, or a pituitary rongeur, is also recommended to remove debris from the joint.

The final step of joint preparation is the drilling of the joint with the use of a 2-mm wire advanced through the portals. As with the joint débridement, the senior author's preference is to

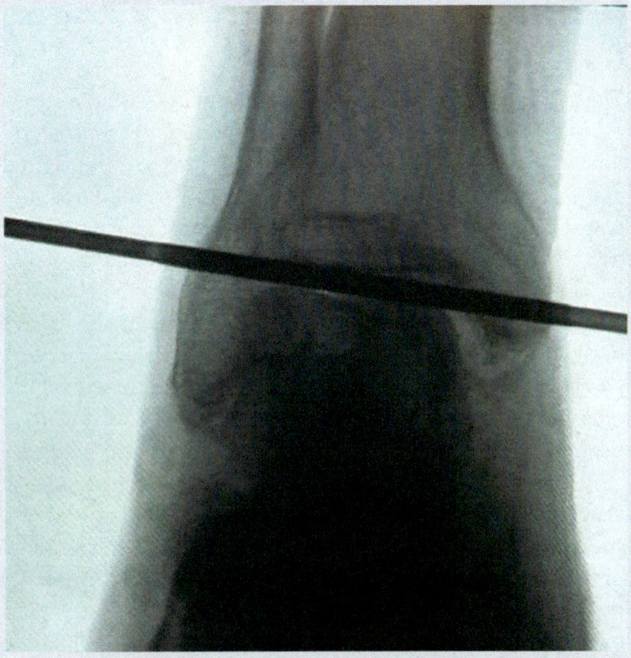

Figure 22.2 Identify the ankle joint under fluoroscopy.

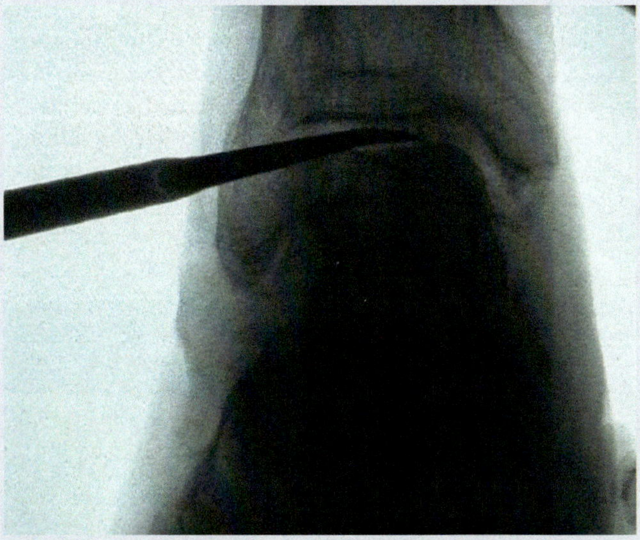

Figure 22.3 Once the anteromedial and anterolateral portals are established, palpate the joint with a freer to familiarize with the anatomy.

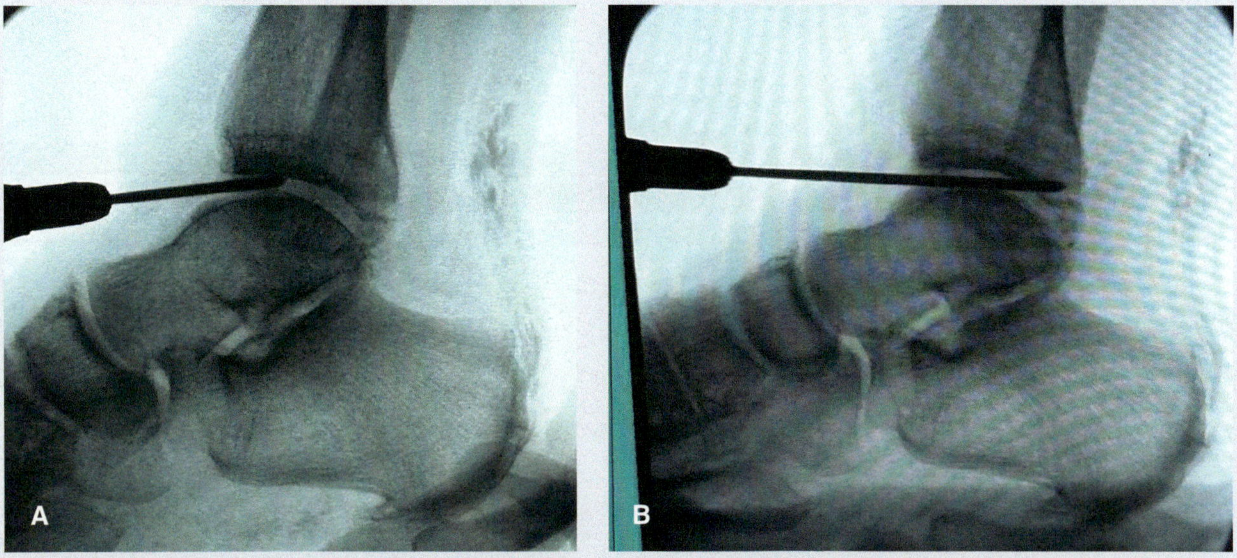

Figure 22.4 The images demonstrate débridement of the posterior aspect of the tibia plafond **(A)** and the anterior tibia plafond **(B)**.

move from posterior to anterior, first medially and then laterally. Bone graft or bone graft substitute can be inserted as needed into the joint with the use of a mosquito clamp. Due to the size of the portals, multiple passages will be necessary to advance the graft.

Once the ankle is ready for stabilization, all portals are closed with the surgeon's preferred suture. The joint is aligned in neutral dorsiflexion, mild valgus (<5°), and 5° of external rotation and stabilized with the guidewires for the screws of choice. The senior author's preferred configuration is to have two 7-mm headless compression screws from medial to lateral and one headless compression screw (5 or 7 mm) from lateral to medial (Figure 22.7). Upon fluoroscopic confirmation of the wire position, the skin is incised, the wires are measured and overdrilled, and the screws sequentially advanced.

Lastly, all wounds are closed with sutures, and a well-padded splint is applied to the surgical leg (Figure 22.8).

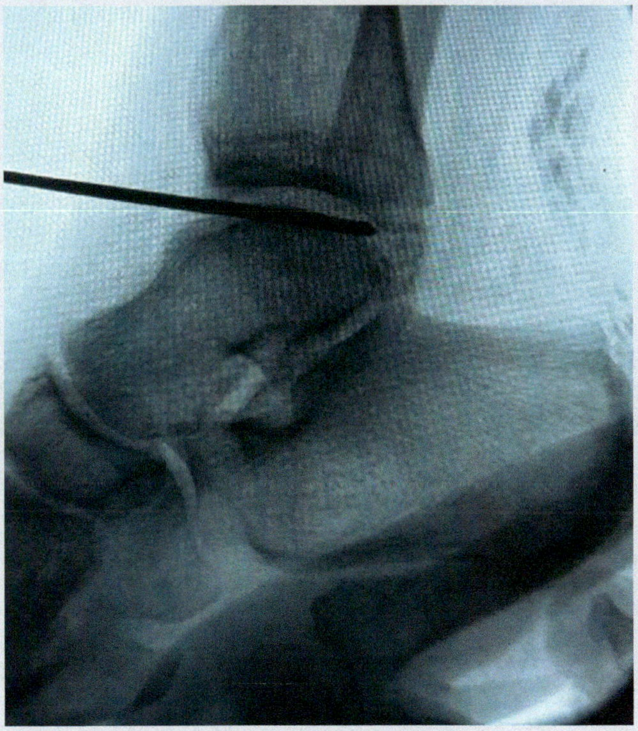

Figure 22.5 The image demonstrates débridement of the posterior aspect of the tibia plafond.

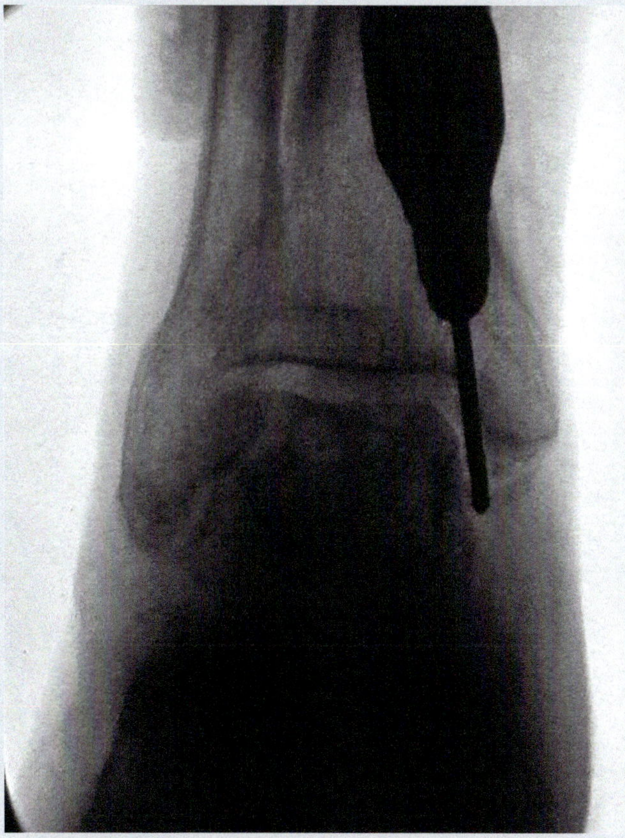

Figure 22.6 The image demonstrates débridement of the medial gutter through the anteromedial portal.

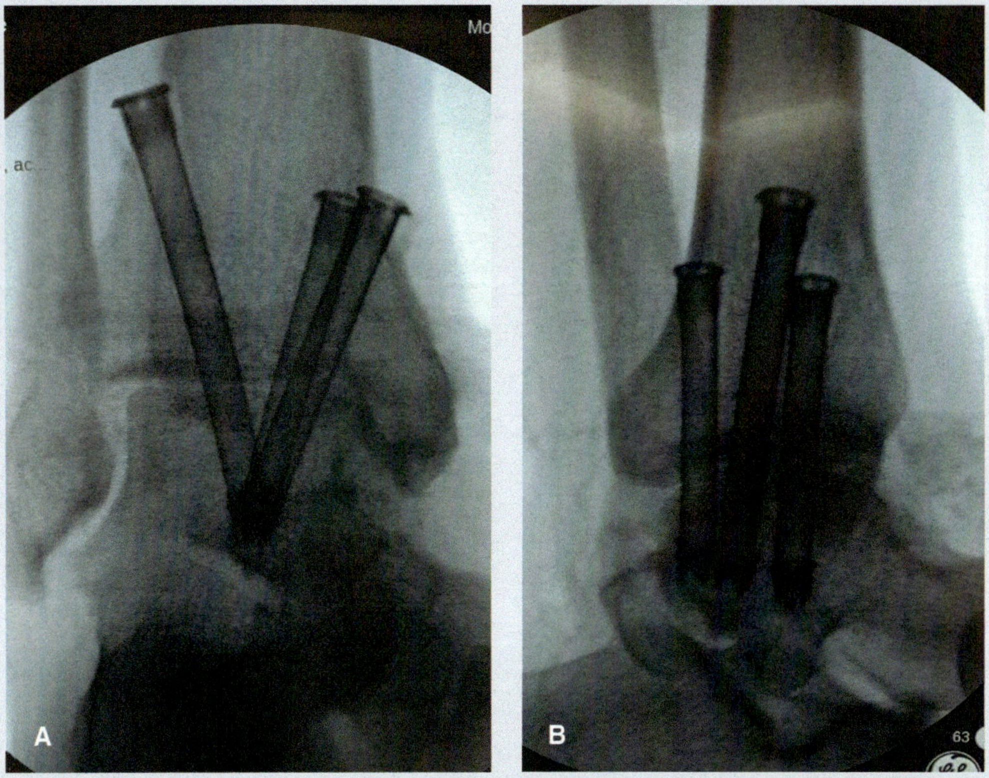

Figure 22.7 The images demonstrate final fluoroscopy of the ankle fusion in the anteroposterior **(A)** and lateral **(B)** views.

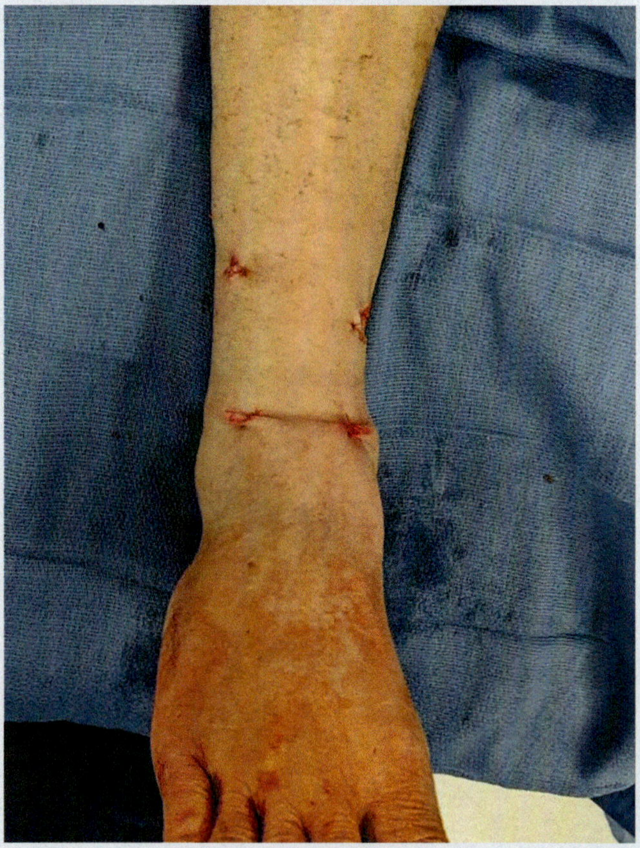

Figure 22.8 The image demonstrates closure of all incisions.

PEARLS AND PITFALLS

- Do not keep the burr activated for more than 8 to 10 seconds. This may lead to thermal injury to the tissues. Stop the power, allow a few seconds to cool down without removing the burr from its position, and resume the procedure.
- While débriding the joint, exert sufficient pressure to remove the cartilage but not excessive to cause over-resection of the bone. Until good tactile feedback is developed by the surgeon, frequent use of fluoroscopy is helpful in preventing such complications.
- Remember to use a rotational hand movement while making the osteotomy. Imagine the hinge of the burr to be at the skin incision. Ignoring this will cause a widening of the skin incision.

POSTOPERATIVE MANAGEMENT

Patients are kept non–weight bearing for 6 weeks. Deep vein thrombosis chemoprophylaxis consists of aspirin 81 mg daily for low-risk patients or rivaroxaban 10 mg daily for high-risk patients. At 2 weeks postoperatively, the splint is removed and exchanged for a controlled ankle motion boot. Three-view weight-bearing radiographs of the ankle are obtained to confirm alignment at this time. Additionally, patients are allowed to bathe the surgical foot and can wear socks at 2 weeks. Six weeks postoperatively, new radiographs are obtained, and patients are allowed to start weight bearing as tolerated in the surgical boot.

Three months postoperatively, patients are allowed comfortable shoes, and a CT scan is obtained to confirm bone healing. At this time, it is recommended to remind the patient that postoperative swelling will resolve around 4 months postoperatively.

OUTCOMES

There are minimal published studies on percutaneous ankle arthrodesis. However, in a soon to be published study by the authors utilizing the included technique, the results obtained were excellent. In the retrospective study of 27 adult patients, fusion was achieved in 26/27 (96.3%) patients at 3 months. There were only four patients (14.7%) with complications that were all easily treated. These included symptomatic hardware, superficial wound dehiscence, transient superficial peroneal neuritis, and one nonunion in a diabetic patient converted to a tibiotalocalcaneal nail.[9] Overall, the rate of fusion reported is similar to the literature for more invasive techniques.[2-5] Similarly, the reported complication rate of 15% is either consistent with or lower than previously reported complication rates of other techniques.[5] With further study, the authors suspect the minimally invasive percutaneous method will continue to show high rate of fusion with low rate of easily treated complications.

References

1. Tucker WA, Barnds BL, Morris BL, et al. Nationwide analysis of total ankle replacement and ankle arthrodesis in Medicare patients: trends, complications, and cost. *Foot Ankle Spec.* 2022;15(3):201-208.
2. Chalayon O, Wang B, Blankenhorn B, et al. Factors affecting the outcomes of uncomplicated primary open ankle arthrodesis. *Foot Ankle Int.* 2015;36(10):1170-1179.
3. Zvijac JE, Lemak L, Schurhoff MR, Hechtman KS, Uribe JW. Analysis of arthroscopically assisted ankle arthrodesis. *Arthroscopy.* 2002;18(1):70-75.
4. Ogilvie-Harris DJ, Lieberman I, Fitsialos D. Arthroscopically assisted arthrodesis for osteoarthrotic ankles. *J Bone Joint Surg Am.* 1993;75(8):1167-1174.
5. Nihal A, Gellman RE, Embil JM, Trepman E. Ankle arthrodesis. *Foot Ankle Surg.* 2008;14(1):1-10.
6. Hirose C, Coughlin MJ, Stevens F. Ankle arthritis. In: Coughlin MJ, Saltzman CL, Anderson R, eds. *Mann's Surgery of the Foot and Ankle.* 9th ed. Saunders; 2014:867-1007.
7. Lauge-Pedersen H. Percutaneous arthrodesis. *Acta Orthop Scand Suppl.* 2003;74(307):I. 1-30.
8. Zhao JZ, Kaiser PB, DeGruccio C, Farina EM, Miller CP. Quality of MIS vs open joint preparations of the foot and ankle. *Foot Ankle Int.* 2022;43(7):948-956.
9. Marciano G, Vulcano E. Minimally invasive percutaneous ankle fusion outcomes and technique. *Int Orthop.* 2021;45(1):217-223.

Index

Note: Page numbers followed by *f* and *t* indicates figure and table respectively.